COLOR ATLAS AND SYNOPSIS OF ADULT CONGENITAL HEART DISEASE

NOTICE

COLOR ATLAS AND SYNOPSIS OF ADULT CONGENITAL HEART DISEASE

EDITORS

Curt J. Daniels, MD

Director, Columbus Ohio Adult Congenital Heart (COACH) Disease Program

Director, Pulmonary Hypertension Program

Professor of Internal Medicine and Pediatrics

The Heart Center, Nationwide Children's Hospital

The Ohio State University Wexner Medical Center

Columbus, Ohio

Ali N. Zaidi, MD

Director, Montefiore Adult Congenital Heart Disease Program (MAtCH)

Montefiore Heart and Vascular Care Institute

The Children's Hospital at Montefiore

Assistant Professor of Internal Medicine and Pediatrics

Albert Einstein College of Medicine

Bronx, New York

SERIES EDITOR

William T. Abraham, MD, FACP, FACC, FAHA, FESC

Professor of Medicine, Physiology, and Cell Biology

Chair of Excellence in Cardiovascular Medicine

Director, Division of Cardiovascular Medicine

Deputy Director, Davis Heart and Lung Research Institute

The Ohio State University

Columbus, Ohio

New York   Chicago   San Francisco   Athens   London   Madrid   Mexico City
Milan   New Delhi   Singapore   Sydney   Toronto

Color Atlas and Synopsis of Adult Congenital Heart Disease

Copyright © 2015 by McGraw-Hill Education. All rights reserved. Printed in China. Except as permitted under the United States Copyright Act of 1976, no part of this publication may be reproduced or distributed in any form or by any means, or stored in a data base or retrieval system, without the prior written permission of the publisher.

1 2 3 4 5 6 7 8 9 0   CTP/CTP   19 18 17 16 15

ISBN 978-0-07-174943-5
MHID 0-07-174943-8

This book was set in Perpetua by Cenveo® Publisher Services.
The editors were Karen G. Edmonson and Robert Pancotti.
The production supervisor was Richard Ruzycka.
Project management was provided by Sonam Arora, Cenveo Publisher Services.
The cover designer was Thomas DePierro.
China Translation & Printing Services Ltd. was the printer and binder.

Library of Congress Cataloging-in-Publication Data

Color atlas and synopsis of adult congenital heart disease/editors,
    Curt J. Daniels, Ali N. Zaidi.
        p. ; cm.
    Includes bibliographical references.
    ISBN 978-0-07-174943-5 (alk. paper)—
    ISBN 0-07-174943-8 (alk. paper)
    I. Daniels, Curt J., editor.   II. Zaidi, Ali N., editor.
    [DNLM: 1. Heart Defects, Congenital—Atlases.   WG 17]
    RC687
    616.1′2043—dc23
                                2014042106

McGraw-Hill Education books are available at special quantity discounts to use as premiums and sales promotions or for use in corporate training programs. To contact a representative, please visit the Contact Us pages at www.mhprofessional.com.

DEDICATION

To my wonderful family Nicole, Zac, Makenzie, and Alayna for always supporting me through all of my training and work. For understanding my efforts in trying to balance being a caring husband, a dad who is always there, and also an academic physician on a mission to change how we deliver ACHD care in the United States.

To my mentors Hugh Allen MD, Tim Feltes MD, William Abraham MD, and John Cheatham MD for their tremendous support of ACHD and in building an ACHD program by giving me the tools to develop a high-quality program and provide the care our patients deserve.

To our ACHD nurses Jenne Hickey, Steve Crumb, Tracey Sisk, Kathy Junge, Renee Schnug, and Deb Mitchell for your unrelenting commitment to patient care each and every day—without the fanfare, but for all the right reasons.

Finally to Ali Zaidi MD, colleague and friend, for all of your hard work, organization and dedication to the field of ACHD and to this color atlas for ACHD.

As you read through the chapters and pages in this atlas, my hope is that you gain a greater appreciation for the complexity of ACHD and the ACHD patient. Each picture is a patient and each patient deserves our best. The outcomes today are not what we expect for this population. In order to truly change the outcome for ACHD patients, WE MUST:

(1) train more specialists in ACHD, (2) develop high-quality ACHD programs, and (3) advocate and vehemently pursue multi-center federal funding of ACHD-specific research. Patients, professionals, and elected officials, all have the power and the ability to change the outcome for the next generation of CHD patients reaching adulthood.

Curt J. Daniels, MD

To Ami and Aboo....for their selfless dedication, affection and guidance.
To the Aans....for with you two lies the future—I love you guys.
To TFF, HDA, JPC, SCC and Curt.....for teaching me the nuances of CHD.
To DV....for letting the *Force* be with me.
To all my patients......for being the best teachers a student could ever ask for.
And to Saki, without whom nothing would have come together.......for being my rock, I love you more and more every day!

Ali N. Zaidi, MD

CONTENTS

Jamil Aboulhosn, MD, FACC, FSCAI

Director, Ahmanson/UCLA Adult Congenital Heart Disease Center
Associate Professor of Medicine
Departments of Medicine and Pediatrics
David Geffen School of Medicine
Los Angeles, California

Anish Amin, MD

Adult Electrophysiology Fellow
The Ohio State University Wexner Medical Center
Columbus, Ohio

Craig Broberg, MD

Associate Professor
Director, Adult Congenital Heart Program
Knight Cardiovascular Institute
Oregon Health and Science University
Portland, Oregon

Scott Cohen, MD

Wisconsin Adult Congenital Heart Disease Program (WAtCH)
Assistant Professor of Medicine and Pediatrics
Medical College of Wisconsin
Milwaukee, Wisconsin

Stephen C. Cook, MD

Associate Professor of Pediatrics and Internal Medicine
Director, Adult Congenital Heart Disease Center
Heart Institute, Children's Hospital of Pittsburgh
UPMC Heart and Vascular Institute
Pittsburgh, Pennsylvania

Marc G. Cribbs, MD, MS

Director, Adult Congenital Heart Disease
Assistant Professor of Medicine
University of Alabama
Birmingham, Alabama

Curt J. Daniels, MD

Director, Columbus Ohio Adult Congenital Heart Disease Program
(COACH)
Director, Pulmonary Hypertension Program
Professor of Internal Medicine and Pediatrics
The Heart Center, Nationwide Children's Hospital
The Ohio State University Wexner Medical Center
Columbus, Ohio

Michael G. Earing, MD

Director, Wisconsin Adult Congenital Heart Disease Program
(WAtCH)
Associate Professor of Medicine and Pediatrics
Medical College of Wisconsin
Milwaukee, Wisconsin

Jennifer Huang, MD

Pediatric Cardiology Fellow
Doernbecher Children's Hospital
Oregon Health and Science University
Portland, Oregon

John Lynn Jefferies, MD, MPH, FACC, FAHA

Director, Cardiomyopathy and Advanced Heart Failure
Associate Professor, Adult Cardiovascular Diseases and Pediatric
    Cardiology
Division of Human Genetics
The Heart Institute
Cincinnati Children's Hospital Medical Center
Cincinnati, Ohio

Steven Kalbfleisch, MD

Professor of Medicine
The Ohio State University Wexner Medical Center
Columbus, Ohio

W. Aaron Kay, MD

Director, Adult Congenital Heart Disease Program
Indiana University
Indianapolis, Indiana

Naomi J. Kertesz, MD

Associate Professor of Pediatrics
Director of Pediatric Electrophysiology
The Nationwide Children's Hospital
The Ohio State University
Columbus, Ohio

Amber Khanna, MD

Assistant Professor of Medicine
Division of Cardiology
Adult Congenital Heart Disease Program
University of Colorado School of Medicine
Aurora, Colorado

Eric V. Krieger, MD

Assistant Professor of Medicine
Seattle Adult Congenital Heart Service
University of Washington Medical Center & Seattle Children's
    Hospital
University of Washington School of Medicine
Seattle, Washington

Mary Hunt Martin, MD

Assistant Professor of Pediatrics and Internal Medicine
University of Utah
Salt Lake City, Utah

Megan Barnhart McGreevy, MD

Heart Institute
Children's Hospital of Pittsburgh
Pittsburgh, Pennsylvania

Alexander R. Opotowsky, MD

Boston Adult Congenital Heart and Pulmonary Hypertension Service
Boston Children's Hospital
Brigham and Women's Hospital
Boston, Massachusetts

Sara L. Partington, MD

Philadelphia Adult Congenital Heart Center
Assistant Professor of Clinical Medicine
Perelman School of Medicine, University of Pennsylvania
Philadelphia, Pennsylvania

Sharon Roble, MD

Columbus Ohio Adult Congenital Heart Disease Program (COACH)
Assistant Professor of Internal Medicine
Division of Cardiovascular Medicine
The Heart Center, Nationwide Children's Hospital
The Ohio State University
Columbus, Ohio

Karen K. Stout, MD

Associate Professor of Medicine
Director, Seattle Adult Congenital Heart Service
University of Washington Medical Center &
    Seattle Children's Hospital
University of Washington School of Medicine
Seattle, Washington

Jeffrey A. Towbin, MD, FACC, FAHA

Executive Co-Director and Chief, Pediatric Cardiology
The Heart Institute
Cincinnati Children's Hospital
Cincinnati, Ohio

Anne Marie Valente, MD, FACC

Boston Adult Congenital Heart Program (BACH)
Department of Cardiology
Boston Children's Hospital
Outpatient Director, Boston Adult Congenital Heart Service
Assistant Professor of Internal Medicine; Assistant Professor of
    Pediatrics
Harvard Medical School
Boston, Massachusetts

Gary D. Webb, MD, FACC, FAHA

Director, Cincinnati Adolescent and Adult Congenital Heart Disease
    Program
The Heart Institute
Cincinnati Children's Hospital Medical Center
Cincinnati, Ohio

Angela T. Yetman, MD

Director, Vascular Medicine
Professor of Pediatrics
University of Nebraska
Children's Hospital & Medical Center
Omaha, Nebraska

Ali N. Zaidi, MD

Director, Montefiore Adult Congenital Heart Disease Program
    (MAtCH)
Montefiore Heart and Vascular Care Institute
The Children's Hospital at Montefiore
Assistant Professor of Internal Medicine and Pediatrics
Albert Einstein College of Medicine
Bronx, New York

Congenital heart disease (CHD) remains the most common birth defect and leading cause of birth defect–related infant mortality. Nearly 40,000 infants in the United States are born each year with CHDs. With increasing medical treatment options, survival is improving with more than 90% of these patients living into adulthood, resulting in a growing population of adults with CHD (ACHD). There are currently more than 1.3 million adults with CHD and this prevalence is expected to increase 5% annually. These patients frequently develop complications characteristic of the defect or its treatment. Consequently, adult cardiologists participating in the care of these patients need a working knowledge of the more common defects. Fewer than 10% of ACHD in the United States are receiving recommended specialized care for their CHD.

Occasionally, some patients with congenital heart defects such as atrial septal defect, Ebstein's anomaly, or physiologically corrected transposition of the great arteries present for the first time in adulthood, which often creates diagnostic and therapeutic dilemmas that may be difficult to manage later in life. Adults with moderate or complex CHD are at higher risk of long-term complications, morbidity, and early mortality. More often patients previously treated in pediatric cardiology centers have transitioned to Adult Congenital Heart Disease centers for ongoing care. Some of the more important defects in this category are tetralogy of Fallot, transposition of the great arteries,

functionally single ventricle defects, and coarctation of the aorta. There is a higher than expected burden of sudden cardiac death in CHD patients once reaching adulthood—with many cases occurring 20 years or more after initial surgical repair. CHD represents a medical challenge that spans the life of a patient from birth through adolescence and into adulthood, including pregnant women with CHD. This includes an increasing number of women with CHD who are in their childbearing years. Between 1998 and 2007, the number of annual deliveries in women with CHD rose by 35% as compared with a 21% increase in women with no CHD.

Through this field guide, we provide an overview of selected defects commonly seen in an adult congenital cardiology practice using clinical cases, imaging studies, and pathology specimens to provide a brief overview of the anatomy, physiology, clinical presentation, common complications, treatment options, and long-term outcomes for adults with congenital heart disease. This Atlas is meant for the general audience including internists, pediatricians, general practitioners, nurse practitioners, physician assistants, and general cardiologists. We would like to offer our heartfelt gratitude to all the authors who contributed in the preparation of this Color Atlas.

Curt J. Daniels, MD, and Ali N. Zaidi, MD

1 INTRODUCTION

Curt J. Daniels, MD
Ali N. Zaidi, MD

A GROWING POPULATION

Congenital heart disease (CHD) is the most common birth defect with an incidence ranging from 4 to 50/1000 live births, a range that is dependent on definitions and global variation.[1] With improved medical, surgical, and intensive care, over the past several decades, the survival to adulthood has exponentially improved. It is now expected that greater than 90% of children born with CHD will survive to adulthood (Figure 1-1). Consequently, in the United States, there are now greater than 1 million adults with congenital heart disease (ACHD), with a 5% increase or 20,000 new patients reaching adulthood each year (Figure 1-2). In fact, it is estimated that for the first time in history, there has been a shift in the CHD population (Figures 1-3A, 1-3B, and 1-3C) with more adults living with CHD than children (Figure 1-4)[2].

With the rise in the ACHD population, there has been a similar surge in clinics caring for this unique and complex population (Figure 1-5), as well as fellowship programs to train cardiologists in the field of ACHD. In the United States and around the world, there is a focused and directed effort to create comprehensive ACHD

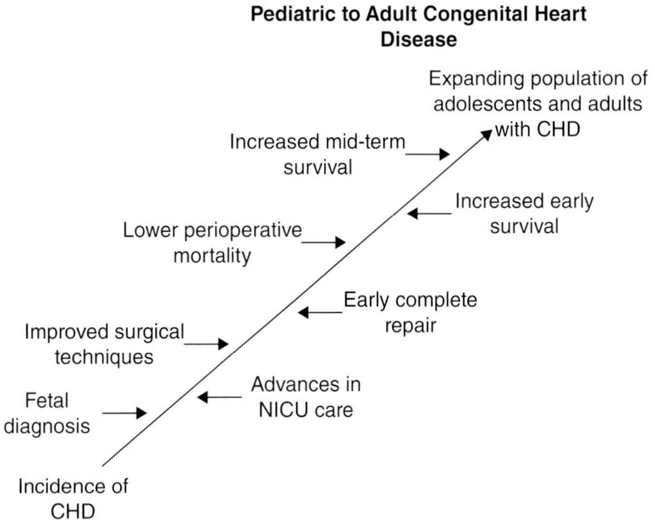

Pediatric to Adult Congenital Heart Disease
Expanding population of adolescents and adults with CHD
Increased mid-term survival
Increased early survival
Lower perioperative mortality
Early complete repair
Improved surgical techniques
Advances in NICU care
Fetal diagnosis
Incidence of CHD

FIGURE 1-1 Factors leading to improved congenital heart disease (CHD) care and expanding population of adolescent and adults with CHD.

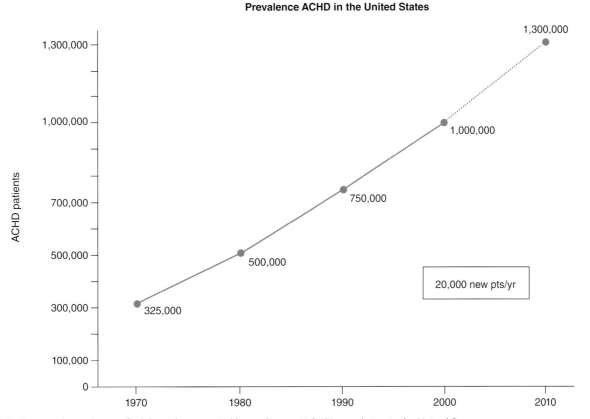

Prevalence ACHD in the United States
ACHD patients
1,300,000
1,000,000
700,000
500,000
300,000
100,000
0
1970
1980
1990
2000
2010
325,000
500,000
750,000
1,000,000
1,300,000
20,000 new pts/yr

FIGURE 1-2 Estimated prevalence of adults with congenital heart disease (ACHD) population in the United States.

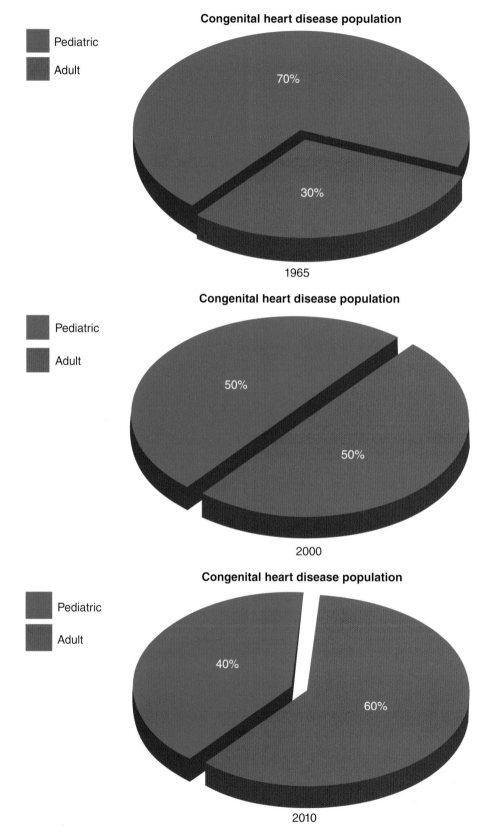

FIGURE 1-3 Shifting congenital heart disease (CHD) population over time from 1965 to 2000, and 2010. There are now more adults than children with CHD.

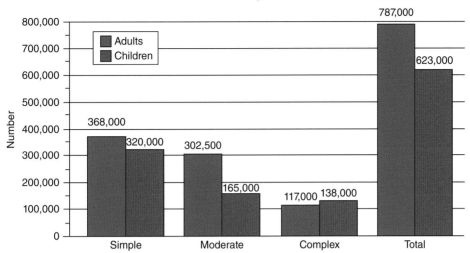

FIGURE 1-4 Adult versus pediatric congenital heart disease (CHD) population in the United States for simple, moderate, and complex forms of CHD.[2] *(Reproduced with permission from Williams RG, Pearson GD, Barst RJ, et al. The report of the National Heart, Lung, and Blood Institute working group on research in adult congenital heart disease. J Am Coll Cardiol 2006;47:701-707.)*

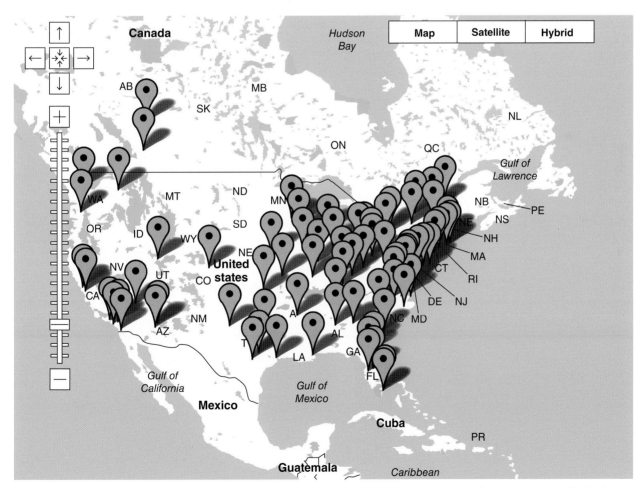

FIGURE 1-5 Adult congenital heart disease (ACHD) programs in North America. *(From Adult Congenital Heart Association [ACHA] www.achaheart.org)*

centers and establish training guidelines for cardiologists. This process was well outlined in 2000 at the American College of Cardiology 32nd Bethesda Conference and published in 2001.[3] There are now established training guidelines, to become an ACHD specialist. Cardiologists have to spend two extra years training in ACHD after finishing either their general pediatric or adult cardiology fellowships.

After several years of deliberation, the first sub-specialty board exam for Adult Congenital Heart Disease will be administered in the United States in 2015 by the American Board of Internal Medicine (ABIM) and the American Board of Medical Specialties (ABMS).

LONG-TERM OUTCOMES FOR ACHD

As epidemiologic data sets clearly define the rise and continual growth of the ACHD population, at the same time, outcome data reported a more dismal outlook for the same CHD patients reaching adulthood describing early mortality and substantial morbidity.

The explanation for the outcome data is rooted in the natural history of unrepaired and repaired congenital heart defects. It is well established that many patients who have undergone total corrective surgery for mild forms of CHD with no risk factors or postoperative complications will have few, if any, hemodynamic residua (eg, atrial septal defect, ventricular septal defect, patent ductus arteriosus, mild pulmonary stenosis).

However, patients with more complex lesions, or complications of less complex lesions, such as residual shunts, valvular disease, ventricular dysfunction, and arrhythmias require more frequent evaluation, medical treatment, and consideration for further surgical or catheter-based interventions. This population of moderate or complex CHD, despite adequate childhood repair dominates the majority of long-term complications, with substantial morbidity and early mortality.

In 1998, a study from Oregon Health Systems reported a higher than expected burden of sudden cardiac death in CHD patients once reaching adulthood.[4] In fact, many cases occurred 20 years or more after initial surgical repair, confirming the ideology that CHD patients are repaired but not cured. The highest risk patients in the study were those with tetralogy of Fallot, aortic stenosis, d-transposition of the great arteries, and coarctation of the aorta (Figure 1-6). A group from Belgium showed that the survival benefits for pediatric CHD patients gained over time, attributed in part to improved technology, were lost once patients reached 18 years of age.[5]

In a large Dutch registry of ACHD patients, 77% of the long-term mortality was attributed to a cardiovascular etiology with 45% due to heart failure and arrhythmia combined (Figure 1-7). In this study of almost 7000 patients, the mean age of death was 48.8 years. When compared to the general Dutch population there was a much higher than expected mortality rate especially in the young adult population.[6]

Increasing morbidity has also plagued the ACHD population with several studies demonstrating, that when compared to the general population at the same age, ACHD patients have higher hospitalization rates, need for ICU care and emergency room visits. In a Quebec ACHD population study, hospitalization rates were 2 to 3 times higher than expected for those with moderate and severe forms of CHD (Figure 1-8).[7] In the Netherlands, across all age spectrums, hospitalization rates for ACHD patients were significantly higher than expected in the general population[8] (Figure 1-9).

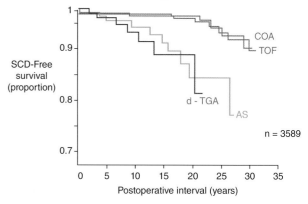

FIGURE 1-6 Actuarial probability of sudden cardiac death (SCD)-free survival after surgical treatment. AS, aortic stenosis; COA, coarctation of the aorta; d-TGA, d-transposition of the great arteries; TOF, tetralogy of Fallot.[4]

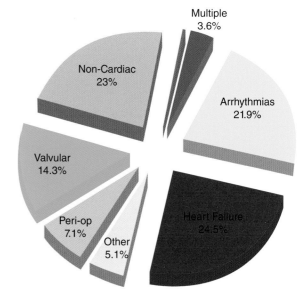

FIGURE 1-7 Causes of ACHD mortality.[4] (*Data from the Dutch ACHD Registry.*)

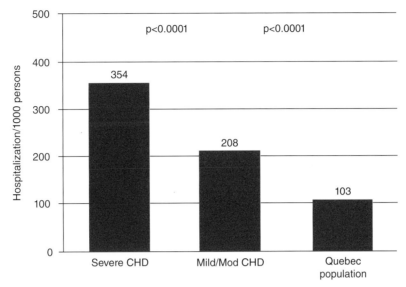

FIGURE 1-8 One-year hospitalization rate of patients with severe and other cardiac lesions compared with the adult population of Quebec.[8] *(Reprinted from The American Journal of Cardiology, Vol 99, Mackie AS, Pilote L, Ionescu-Ittu R, Rahme E, Marelli AJ. Health care resource utilization in adults with congenital heart disease, pages 839-843. Copyright 2007, with permission from Elsevier.)*

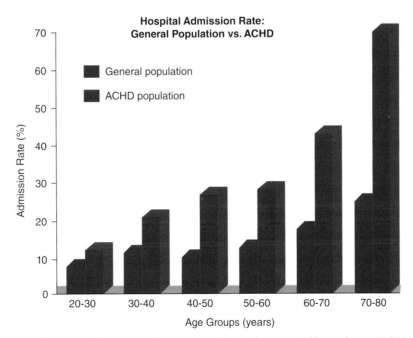

FIGURE 1-9 Hospital admission rate for general Dutch population versus adults with congenital heart disease (ACHD) population.[8] *(Reproduced from Heart, Verheugt CL, Uiterwaal CSPM, van der Velde ET, Meijboom FJ, Pieper PG, et al. Vol 96, pages 872-878, Copyright 2010 with permission from BMJ Publishing Group Ltd.)*

COMPLEXITY OF ACHD

The ACHD population remains one of the most complex cohorts of patients that health care providers will care for during their career. Their underlying cardiac complexity and growing noncardiac or nonmedical issues contribute to the complexity of these patients.[9]

General internal medicine, family practice, or adult cardiovascular training programs do not require a formal understanding of CHD and therefore cardiologists evaluating patients frequently do not have an adequate knowledge base of CHD anatomy, physiology, surgical repairs, adult long-term complications, and indications for further intervention. Interpretation of diagnostic studies is also unique in this population and therefore understanding the significance of findings on echocardiograms and cardiac magnetic resonance imaging (MRI), for example, becomes less accurate leading to the possibility of misdiagnosis and delayed treatment. Defined data sets have demonstrated that many patients diagnosed with CHD as infants or children, eventually are lost in transition going from pediatric to adult CHD care.

In a Quebec population, patients born with CHD were followed to determine whether they maintained specialized CHD care throughout childhood and into young adulthood. At the age interval of 18 to 22 years, only 40% were still in CHD care[10] (Figure 1-10). The lost to care issue plays a significant role leading to the poor outcome data for ACHD patients.

Finally, being a young adult population carries other important complex issues that must be addressed as below:

- Psychosocial needs
- Economic/job security
- Health insurance
- Pregnancy
- Family planning

Pregnancy for women must be appropriately addressed to determine whether they are safe to be become pregnant with their CHD. If the CHD patient becomes pregnant, then ACHD cardiologists and the

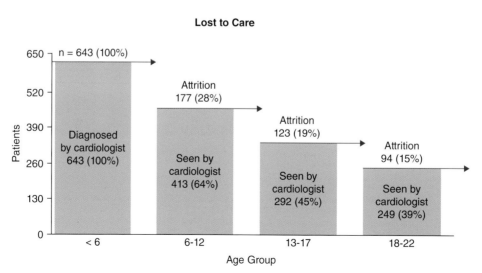

FIGURE 1-10 Loss of follow-up from age 6 to 22 years among a study cohort diagnosed with congenital heart disease (CHD). Only 39% were still being seen by CHD specialists at age 18 to 22.[10] *(Reproduced from Circulation, Vol 120, Mackie AS, Ionescu-Ittu R, Therrien J, Pilote L, Abrahamowicz M, Marelli AJ, Children and adults with congenital heart disease lost to follow up: who and when?, pages 302-309.)*

appropriate consultants must consider treatment options during pregnancy, mode of delivery, risk of transmission of CHD to offspring, and postdelivery care.

CHANGING THE OVERALL OUTCOME

Despite this well-documented but poorer than expected outcome, a concerted effort is underway to improve the care for ACHD patients. Organizations such as Adult Congenital Heart Association (ACHA), the American College of Cardiology (ACC), the American Heart Association (AHA) are sponsoring and participating in several ongoing national initiatives, to improve the quality of care and the outcome for ACHD patients. Some of these initiatives include the following:

- Improved training requirements for cardiologists caring for ACHD patients. There is now a mandatory two year dedicated ACHD sub-speciality fellowship, followed by a national board examination for ACHD starting in 2015.
- Establishing criteria for ACHD programs with a multidisciplinary team approach including ACHD trained cardiologists, midlevel practitioners, and registered nurses with dedicated ACHD site visits to be performed at each center which will begin in 2015.
- Legislation enacted (The Congenital Heart Futures Act) to provide more accurate prevalence and surveillance data
- Published guidelines to care for ACHD patients through the ACC and AHA[1,9]
- Develop multicenter research trials

Over the following chapters, we outline in a lesion-specific format, the long-term adult complications of CHD and discuss the current state-of-the-art therapeutic options for this growing, complex and highly unique population for the internist, general practitioner, pediatrician, and general cardiologist.

REFERENCES

1. Hoffman JIE, Kaplan S. The incidence of congenital heart disease. *J Am Coll Cardiol*. 2002;39:1890-1900.

2. Williams RG, Pearson GD, Barst RJ, et al. The report of the national heart, lung, and blood institute working group on research in adult congenital heart disease. *J Am Coll Cardiol*. 2006;47:701-707.

3. Webb GD, Williams RG. 32nd Bethesda conference: care of the adult with congenital heart disease. *J Am Coll Cardiol*. 2001;37:1166.

4. Silka MJ, Hardy BG, Menashe VD, Morris CD. A population-based prospective evaluation of the risk of sudden cardiac death after operation for common congenital heart defects. *J Am Coll Cardiol*. 1998;32:245-251.

5. Moons P, Bovijn L, Budts W, Belman A, Gewillig M. Temporal trends in survival to adulthood among patients born with congenital heart disease from 1970 to 1992 in Belgium. *Circulation*. 2010;122:2264-2272.

6. Verheugt CL, Uiterwaal C, Van der Velde ET, et al. Mortality in adult congenital heart disease. *Eur Heart J*. 2010;31:1220-1229.

7. Mackie AS. Health care resource utilization in adults with congenital heart disease. *Am J Cardiol*. 2007;99:839-843.

8. Verheugt CL, Uiterwaal CS, van der Velde ET, et al. The emerging burden of hospital admissions of adults with congenital heart disease. *Heart*. 2010;96:872-878.

9. Warnes C, Williams RG, Bashore TM, et al. ACC/AHA 2008 guidelines for the management of adults with congenital heart disease. *Circulation*. 2008;118:2395-2451.

10. Mackie AS, Ionescu-Ittu R, Therrien J, Pilote L, Abrahamowicz M, Marelli A. Children and adults with congenital heart disease lost to follow-up: who and when. *Circulation*. 2008;120:302-309.

2 THE ADULT WITH INTRACARDIAC SHUNT LESIONS: ASD, VSD, AND AVSD

Megan Barnhart McGreevy, MD
Stephen C. Cook, MD

Atrial Septal Defects

PATIENT STORY

A 35-year-old woman presented to the Adult Congenital Heart Disease Clinic 1 month after successful caesarean section (C-section) of her second child. A C-section was performed only as a result of fetal distress. She reported that compared to her prior pregnancy, symptoms of increasing shortness of breath in the third trimester that persisted postpartum. At the time of her initial outpatient clinic visit she experienced dyspnea with routine activities.

Her physical examination revealed the following vital signs: blood pressure (BP) 111/72 mm Hg, heart rate (HR) 74 bpm with 98% oxygen saturations in room air. Chest examination demonstrated no evidence of a right ventricular (RV) lift or heave. Cardiac examination demonstrated a regular rate and rhythm with a normal S1 and a fixed, split S2. The P2 component of the second heart sound was not accentuated. There was a soft II/VI systolic ejection murmur best appreciated at the left, upper sternal border. No diastolic murmurs, rubs, or gallops were heard. Extremities were warm and well perfused without clubbing, cyanosis, or edema.

A 12-lead electrocardiography (ECG) demonstrated a normal sinus rhythm, normal axis, and incomplete right bundle branch pattern (Figure 2-1). A transthoracic echocardiogram (TTE) demonstrated right atrial and ventricular enlargement (Figures 2-2 and 2-3) as a consequence of a large atrial septal defect, secundum type.

CASE EXPLANATION

- Patients with an atrial septal defect (ASD) often have fixed splitting of the second heart sound. However, its absence does not exclude an ASD. The absence of a loud P2 component of the second heart sound minimizes the possibility of pulmonary hypertension. The systolic ejection murmur is consistent with increased pulmonary blood flow.

- The incomplete right bundle branch block pattern on 12-lead ECG suggests right ventricular volume overload.

- Findings of right atrial and ventricular enlargement on echocardiogram should prompt an evaluation for possible ASD.

EPIDEMIOLOGY

- ASDs are common and can present at any age. Interatrial communications are the third most common type of congenital heart defect and the type most likely to be diagnosed in adulthood.

- Female gender constitutes 65% to 75% of patients with secundum ASDs.[1]

ANATOMY

- There are 3 major types of interatrial communications: ostium secundum, ostium primum, and sinus venosus defects.[1] The secundum defect is a true defect of the atrial septum and it involves the region of the fossa ovalis. The ostium primum defect is within a spectrum of defects known as atrioventricular (AV) septal defects. Finally, the sinus venosus defect is located at the junction of the right atrium and superior vena cava and often associated with partial anomalous pulmonary venous return, most often of the right sided pulmonary veins.

- Uncommon types of ASD include the coronary sinus defect and the inferior vena cava form of ASD.

- Down syndrome is associated primarily with AV septal defects, but secundum defects occur with increased frequency.[1] Ostium primum defects have been associated with both DiGeorge and Ellis-van Creveld syndromes.

- ASDs are the most common cardiac manifestation of Holt-Oram syndrome, which has been caused by mutation of *TBX5*.[2]

ETIOLOGY AND PATHOPHYSIOLOGY

- Failure of normal development of the septum secundum between the left and right atrial chambers will result in a secundum-type ASD that permits blood to flow in either direction (left to right or right to left).[3]

- Flow across an interatrial communication is determined in part by the size of the defect and in part by the relative ventricular compliances. Small defects (usually less than 8-10 mm) can be restrictive and limit both blood flow and pressure transmission.

- Flow across a large, unrestrictive defect is dependent on the difference in compliance between the right and left ventricle, rather than the pressure difference between the atria. Since the RV compliance is usually higher than LV, shunt flow is from left to right across the defect. The shunt causes volume loading of the right heart, resulting in both right atrial and right ventricular enlargement.

- Increased pulmonary blood flow over time can damage the pulmonary vascular endothelium leading to an increase in pulmonary vascular resistance called pulmonary vascular obstructive disease.

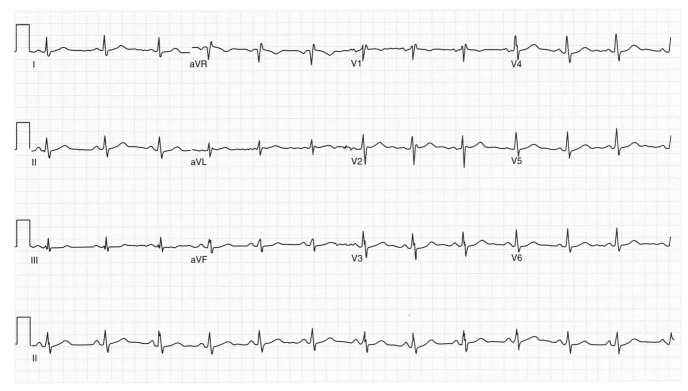

FIGURE 2-1 A 12-lead electrocardiogram demonstrates a normal sinus rhythm with an incomplete right bundle branch block.

DIAGNOSTIC TESTING

Clinical Presentation/History

- The history and clinical examination are pivotal to determine the presence of key clinical features associated in the adolescent or young adult with unoperated ASD.

- Clinical features to identify include shortness of breath or palpitations due to atrial arrhythmias as the presenting symptoms, cardiac enlargement on chest x-ray (CXR), or a heart murmur is detected.

- The clinical examination should document evaluation of the right ventricular impulse if present, the presence of a wide and fixed split second heart sound, commonly associated in ASD physiology, a pulmonary systolic ejection murmur at the left upper sternal border, and the presence of an accentuated pulmonary component of the second heart sound. This last physical examination finding is of great importance as this may represent increased pulmonary arterial pressure in the unoperated adult with ASD physiology.

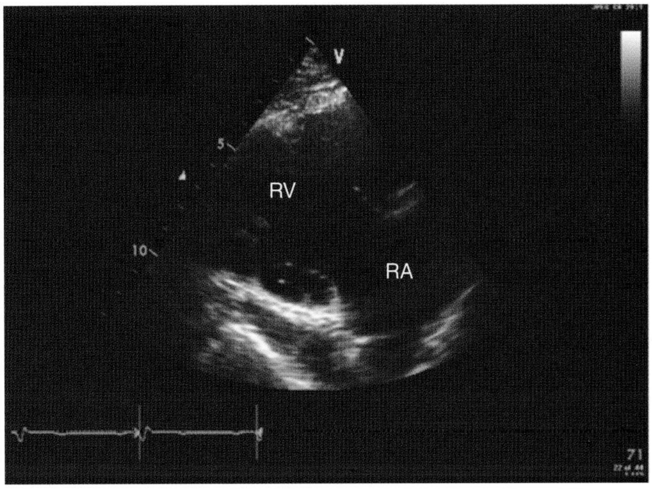

ECG

- A 12-lead ECG when obtained may show right-axis deviation and incomplete right bundle branch block pattern (rSr′ or rsR′).[4] A complete bundle branch block is not uncommon with increasing age.

- The presence of an abnormal P-wave axis may suggest the finding of a sinus venosus ASD. Left-axis deviation (moderate to extreme) may suggest a primum ASD.

FIGURE 2-2 Right ventricular inflow view demonstrating moderate right atrial and ventricular enlargement on outpatient 2-dimensional transthoracic imaging. RA, right atrium; RV, right ventricle.

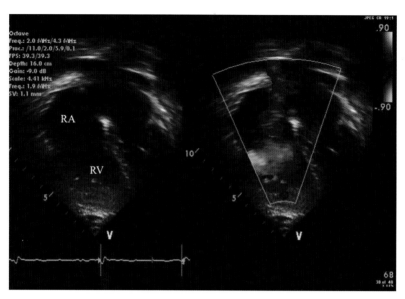

FIGURE 2-3 Apical 4-chamber view on a transthoracic echocardiogram with right atrial and ventricular chamber enlargement (left) and left-to-right shunt with color Doppler interrogation suggestive of secundum-type defect (right). RA, right atrium; RV, right ventricle.

Echocardiography

- A transthoracic echocardiogram often confirms the diagnosis of ASD through a combination of both color Doppler interrogation and a wide variety of views that include subcostal, parasternal, and apical 4-chamber views.

- Ostium secundum defects are best visualized in the midportion of the atrial septum from the subcostal 4-chamber view. Typically, these defects are bordered on all sides by atrial septal tissue. They are differentiated from the sinus venosus defect as this defect is located in the most posterior and superior location of the atrial septum and no tissue is visualized between the defect and the posterior right atrial wall. Often with sinus venosus–type defect, one or more pulmonary veins often drain anomalously to the right atrium.

- Atrial septal defects are often difficult to diagnose using the apical 4-chamber view alone. This is because the atrial septum is parallel to the ultrasound beam, and as a result, artifactual dropout is frequently noted in the region of the atrial septum. Therefore, in patients with poor acoustic windows (eg, obese, pregnant patient) where subcostal windows cannot be obtained, the atrial septum can be visualized from the parasternal window by sliding the transducer to a "low parasternal 4-chamber view" to image the atrial septum nearly perpendicular to the sound beam (Figure 2-4A).

- Echocardiography is often the noninvasive imaging modality of choice to assess the atrial septum in the assessment of the adult patient with suspected ASD. However, complementary imaging with cardiac magnetic resonance has become increasingly utilized in the adult congenital patient population to provide information to clarify the nature of the defect, nature of the shunt (Qp:Qs), biventricular size and function, and associated defects, particularly anomalous pulmonary venous abnormalities[5] (Figure 2-4B).

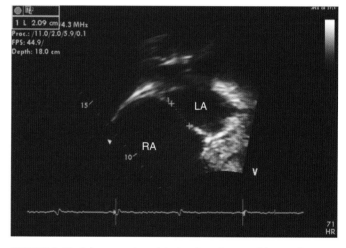

FIGURE 2-4A A low parasternal 4-chamber view provides an alternative imaging method to assess the atrial septum. The atrial septal defect measures 2.09 cm from this view. LA, left atrium; RA, right atrium.

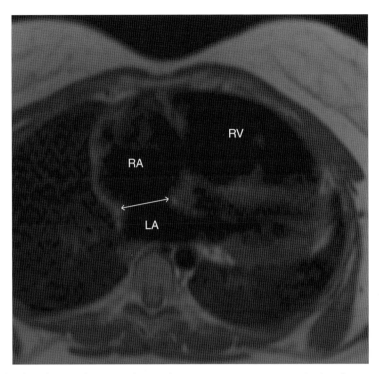

FIGURE 2-4B An oblique dark blood axial image from a cardiovascular magnetic resonance examination demonstrates an atrial septal defect (arrows), mild right atrial (RA), and right ventricular enlargement (RV).

Cardiac Catheterization

- Cardiac catheterization is no longer utilized to make a diagnosis or evaluate the anatomy of the ASD.

- Cardiac catheterizations may be performed to determine patient suitability for transcatheter closure of the ASD (see later).

MANAGEMENT

- Patients with a significant ASD, such as the case outlined above with signs of right heart dilation, should be offered elective closure soon after the diagnosis of ASD is established, irrespective of age.

- Potential benefits of ASD closure include improved exercise capacity and functional class. Closure of ASD prevents both the development of right heart failure and pulmonary arterial hypertension. Although the risk of these complications is relatively small, it is inversely related to the age of patient at time of ASD closure.

- Indications for ASD closure include the following[1]:
  - Right atrial and ventricular enlargement identified by noninvasive imaging studies (transthoracic echocardiography, cardiac magnetic resonance, computed tomography angiography)
  - ASD greater than 10 mm
  - No evidence of advanced pulmonary hypertension
  - Qp:Qs greater than 1.5:1 measured by transthoracic echocardiography, cardiac magnetic resonance or cardiac catheterization

- However, several important caveats should be kept in mind as to why an ASD should **not** be closed include the following:
  - Conservative management of the small ASD (<10 mm) without evidence of right heart enlargement on noninvasive imaging studies.

○ Advanced pulmonary arterial hypertension that requires the ASD as a physiologic "pop-off." Such patients often demonstrate cyanosis at rest and increasing cyanosis during peak exercise.

○ Similarly, the ASD that serves as a pop-off in the presence of severe left ventricular (LV) systolic dysfunction.

○ ASD that is identified during pregnancy should be followed and when appropriate, therapy may be deferred approximately 6 months postpartum.

• All secundum ASDs should be considered for transcatheter closure with currently available devices.

• Defects up to 40 mm in diameter can be considered for device closure with multiple different closure devices including the Amplatzer Septal Occluder (ASO; AGA Medical Corp., Golden Valley, Minnesota, USA) device guided by transesophageal or intracardiac echocardiography[6] (Figures 2-5 and 2-6).

• These imaging techniques are often performed simultaneously to evaluate those patients with inadequate septal rims that may not permit stable device deployment, defects in close proximity to the atrioventricular valves, the coronary sinus, or those with defects in close proximity to the vena cava. Patients with anatomy unsuitable for transcatheter intervention should be considered for surgical repair.

• Otherwise, device closure is considered a safe and effective procedure with reported complications such as cardiac perforation or device embolization occurring in fewer than 1% of patients.[7]

FOLLOW-UP

• Currently, there is no consensus available for appropriate follow-up of the adult late after ASD device closure. Although device-related complications are rare (device migration, erosion, or other complications), this patient population should be evaluated periodically.

• The American College of Cardiology/American Heart Association 2008 Guidelines for the Management of Adults with Congenital Heart Disease recommends evaluation 3 months to 1 year after device closure and periodically thereafter.[8]

LONG-TERM COMPLICATIONS

• Atrial arrhythmias (atrial flutter or fibrillation) are very common in older adults with large ASDs. In a surgical series reported by Roos-Hesselink et al., demonstrated that pre- and postoperative risk of atrial flutter and fibrillation correlated closely with patient's age above 40 years.[9] Patients who undergo repair of an atrial communication prior to 25 years of age appear to have a normal lifespan and low risk for pulmonary hypertension and arrhythmias.

• One may speculate that increased utilization of device closure at a younger age may reduce the atrial arrhythmia burden in this patient population.

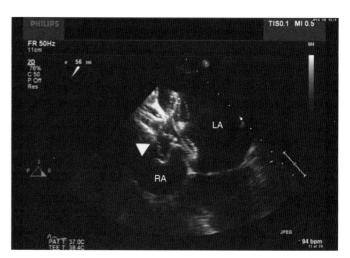

FIGURE 2-5 Transesophageal echocardiogram demonstrating the placement of a 32-mm Amplatzer Septal Occluder (arrowhead) device prior to deployment within the atrial septum. LA, left atrium; RA, right atrium.

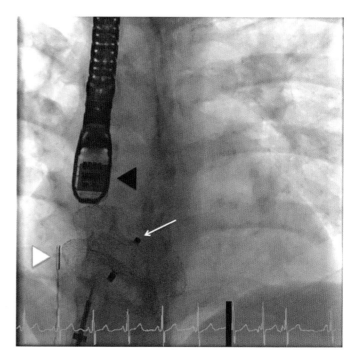

FIGURE 2-6 Both transesophageal (black arrowhead) and intracardiac echocardiographic (white arrowhead) imaging was performed to assess the atrial septum during transcatheter closure of an atrial septal defect. A 32-mm Amplatzer Septal Occluder device (white arrow) was deployed.

Ventricular Septal Defect

PATIENT STORY

A 24-year-old man with a history of a small, perimembranous ventricular septal defect (VSD) presents to the Adult Congenital Heart Disease Clinic for initial evaluation and consultation. He reports normal exercise tolerance and no evidence of functional decline since his last outpatient visit with his pediatric cardiologist several years ago. He denies symptoms of palpitations or syncope.

Physical examination revealed the following vital signs: BP 118/70 mm Hg, HR 62 bpm with oxygen saturations of 100% on room air. He is a well-appearing, well-built young adult man. Chest examination shows a normal active precordium. On auscultation there is a normal S1 and physiologic split S2 with a harsh, grade III/VI S1 coincident or holosystolic murmur best heard at the left sternal border in the fourth intercostal space. No diastolic murmurs, rubs, or gallops are appreciated. Normal pulses are noted throughout all extremities. No clubbing, cyanosis, or edema was appreciated and his extremities were warm and well perfused.

A 12-lead ECG demonstrates sinus bradycardia with sinus arrhythmia and an incomplete right bundle branch block pattern (Figure 2-7). A TTE demonstrated a small, perimembranous VSD with partial closure by tricuspid valve tissue. The defect measured 2 to 3 mm in diameter (Figure 2-8). There was evidence of a left-to-right shunt by color Doppler interrogation (Figure 2-9). The peak gradient (99 mm Hg) confirmed the restrictive physiology of the defect as well as normal right ventricular pressures (Figure 2-10).

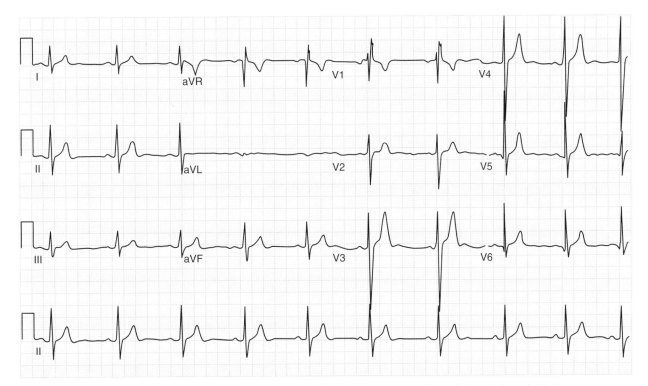

FIGURE 2-7 A 12-lead electrocardiogram demonstrates a normal sinus rhythm with an incomplete right bundle branch block.

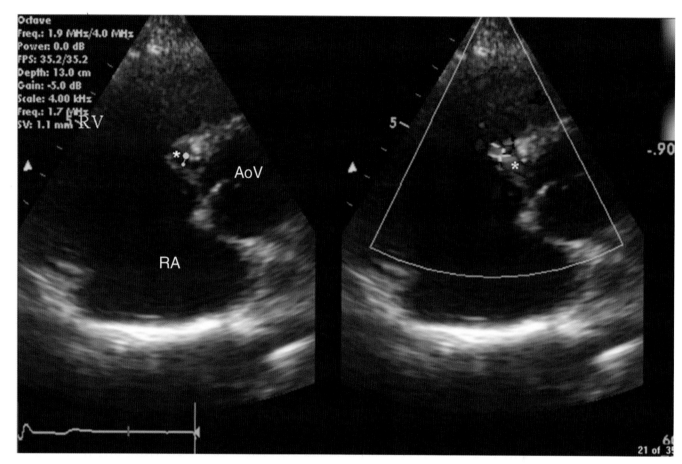

FIGURE 2-8 Parasternal short-axis view from a transthoracic echocardiogram view demonstrating a perimembranous ventricular septal defect (*). With color Doppler (right), the left-to-right shunt is also visualized. AoV, aortic valve; RA, right atrium; RV, right ventricle.

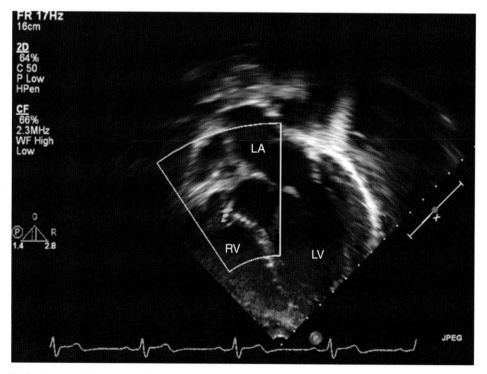

FIGURE 2-9 An apical 5-chamber view from a transthoracic echocardiogram showing a perimembranous VSD with left-to-right shunt with color Doppler. LA, left atrium; LV, left ventricle; RV, right ventricle.

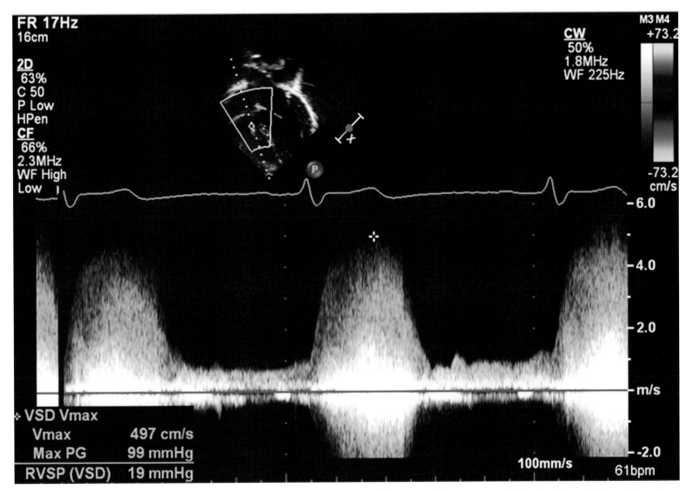

FIGURE 2-10 Continuous wave Doppler interrogation of the ventricular septal defect (VSD) shows restrictive VSD physiology with a peak gradient of approximately 99 mm Hg estimated by the modified Bernoulli equation.

CASE EXPLANATION

- A harsh, holosystolic murmur is consistent with a diagnosis of a restrictive VSD. Most adults with small VSDs remain asymptomatic as they have restrictive, or limited, blood flow across the defect without increased pulmonary blood flow.

- The findings of an incomplete right bundle branch block on an ECG can be interpreted as a variant of "normal" in the adolescent. Alternatively, this may suggest evidence of right ventricular volume overload. Other ECG findings with VSD include LV enlargement in patients with a large VSD.

- The TTE demonstrated normal left ventricular size and systolic function. A small VSD with left-to-right shunt was identified at the perimembranous portion of the ventricular septum with partial closure by the tricuspid valve. Color Doppler was helpful in improving the sensitivity of identifying this small defect. The Doppler gradient across the ventricular septum confirmed normal right ventricular systolic pressure and restrictive VSD physiology.

EPIDEMIOLOGY

- VSDs make up 20% to 30% of all congenital heart defects historically, however, estimates now show VSDs occur in up to 50 per 1000 births.[10]

- The majority of smaller defects will close spontaneously during childhood.
- VSDs are the most common lesion in many chromosomal syndromes, including trisomy 13, trisomy 18, trisomy 21, and other relatively rare syndromes. However, in more than 95% of patients with VSDs, the defects are not associated with a chromosomal abnormality.
- A VSD that causes congestive heart failure, left-sided volume overload (left atrial or left ventricular enlargement), or pulmonary blood flow (Qp) to be twice as much as systemic blood flow (Qs) will be surgically closed during childhood.
- A new diagnosis of VSD is uncommon in adults.

ANATOMY

- Although there are many different classification systems for VSDs, it is simplest to describe their anatomic location as seen from the right ventricle.
- Perimembranous defects are the most common (70%) and are often located in the upper region of the ventricular septum beneath the septal leaflet of the tricuspid valve.
- Muscular VSDs (20%) are located between the left and right ventricles in any portion of the muscular septum.
- Inlet VSDs (5%) are located in the posterior portion of the septum behind the tricuspid valve.
- Lastly, outlet VSDs (5%) are found between the left and right ventricular outflow tracts.[11]

ETIOLOGY AND PATHOPHYSIOLOGY

- The etiology of VSD remains unknown, but a combination of genetic as well as other factors has been suggested. Failure of the normal development and fusion of the membranous, conotruncal, or muscular regions of the ventricular septum can lead to a variety of ventricular septal defects.
- A VSD allows shunting between the ventricles. With normal systemic and pulmonary vascular resistances, the resultant shunt is left-to-right. Small, "restrictive" defects provide an inherent resistance to flow. Surgery is often recommended for moderate- and larger-sized VSDs within the first year of life to prevent the irreversible vascular damage to the lungs if left unrepaired.
- Larger defects, left untreated, may develop into Eisenmenger syndrome. At this stage, patients present with cyanosis, right-to-left shunt, and signs of pulmonary vascular disease.

DIAGNOSIS

Clinical Presentation/History

- Although it is uncommon to make a new diagnosis of VSD in an adolescent or adult patient, the history and physical examination are essential to the diagnosis. A small, restrictive VSD is unlikely to cause symptoms. Here, the physical examination likely shows a normally active precordium and normal first and second heart sounds.
- The characteristic murmur associated with a small, restrictive VSD (Qp:Qs <1.5:1) is an S1 coincident or holosystolic murmur.

- A medium-pitched holosystolic murmur, with mid-diastolic rumble, suggestive of increased flow across the mitral valve, may be appreciated in the younger child with moderate-to-large VSD prior to surgical repair.
- In adult patients with large defects left uncorrected, the amount of left-to-right shunting may decrease and present later with signs of pulmonary vascular disease. Clinical symptoms may include shortness of breath and increasing fatigue with routine activities.
- The chest examination may demonstrate a prominent right ventricular heave. The characteristic VSD murmur may be absent with a pronounced P2 component of the second heart sound consistent with features of pulmonary hypertension. It is important to evaluate extremities for both clubbing and cyanosis.

ECG

- A 12-lead ECG may be normal with small VSDs. With larger VSDs there may be signs of left atrial and left ventricular enlargement. With disease progression, right-axis deviation, right atrial and ventricular hypertrophy occur.

Radiography

- A chest radiograph is typically normal in small VSDs, but may show cardiomegaly and increased pulmonary vascularity in larger defects (Figure 2-11).
- In the unoperated adult with Eisenmenger syndrome, chest radiography demonstrates decreased pulmonary vascularity with pruning of pulmonary vasculature, right heart enlargement, and dilation of the main pulmonary artery.

Echocardiography

- TTE is the most common noninvasive imaging modality to routinely diagnose and evaluate patients with VSD.[12] This single modality provides pertinent information regarding the VSD that includes size and location, surrounding anatomic relations, assessment of right ventricular pressure, and left ventricular size and systolic function.
- Although in most individuals with VSDs, adequate diagnostic information can be obtained from clinical examination and echocardiography, cardiac magnetic resonance imaging might be of use, particularly in patients with poor echocardiographic images.[13]

Cardiac Catheterization

- Cardiac catheterization is not typically performed for the routine diagnosis or management of VSD. This procedure is reserved to calculate pulmonary vascular resistance for those suspected of pulmonary vascular disease. Very rarely patients may be assessed for transcatheter closure of a muscular VSD (Figure 2-12).[14]

MANAGEMENT

- The majority of adult patients with VSD will have undergone intervention earlier in life. Some adult patients with small and even moderate defects that have not been closed should be monitored during late-onset complications that would warrant closure.

- Indications for late VSD closure include the following[8]:
  - Qp:Qs>2:1
  - Prolapse of the aortic valve leading to aortic valve insufficiency
  - Infective endocarditis
- Patients with Eisenmenger syndrome require medical management and close follow-up evaluation with specialists in adult congenital heart disease and pulmonary hypertension. Advances in vasodilator therapy have provided significant benefit with demonstrated improvements in functional capacity.[15]

FOLLOW-UP

- The American College of Cardiology/American Heart Association 2008 Guidelines for the Management of Adults with Congenital Heart Disease recommends routine follow-up every 3 to 5 years for small, uncomplicated VSDs.[8]
- Annual follow-up is recommended for patients with evidence of aortic regurgitation, left ventricular dilation, or pulmonary arterial hypertension.

LONG-TERM COMPLICATIONS

- In the unoperated patient, long-term complications include aortic valve leaflet prolapse with or without resultant aortic insufficiency. The debate continues regarding surgical closure of the VSD that causes aortic valve prolapse with stable, trivial aortic insufficiency.
- In patients with progressive or severe aortic insufficiency, VSD closure is warranted. Another potential complication is infective endocarditis. In a review of the natural history of VSDs by Corone et al., 3.7% developed infective endocarditis and 6.3% developed aortic insufficiency.[16]
- Surgical closure of a VSD (Qp:Qs >2) in the adult has low surgical mortality. In a surgical series by Mongeon et al. for adults undergoing VSD closure, there were no early deaths.[17] Indications for reoperation in this cohort included aortic regurgitation, left ventricular enlargement, and pulmonary hypertension.

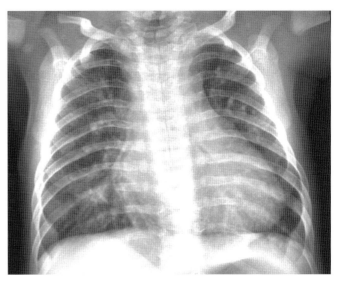

FIGURE 2-11 Chest radiograph demonstrating cardiomegaly and increased pulmonary vascularity obtained in an infant with a moderate-to-large ventricular septal defect (VSD).

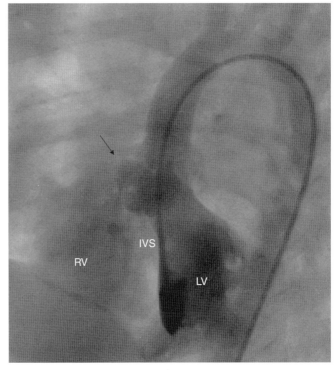

FIGURE 2-12 Left ventriculogram in the left anterior oblique projection demonstrates a perimembranous VSD (arrow). IVS, interventricular septum; LV, left ventricle; RV, right ventricle.

Atrioventricular Septal Defects

PATIENT STORY

A 27-year-old woman who has a history of a complete atrioventricular septal defect (AVSD) repaired at 1 year of age presents for her annual visit with the Adult Congenital Heart Disease Clinic. Most recently, she underwent reoperation for resection of a subaortic membrane 6 months ago that was discovered at the time of her initial consultation. Compared to her initial outpatient visit, she now reports both increased energy level and exercise tolerance. She works full time and is able to perform her activities of daily living that also include caring for her 7-year-old son without fatigue.

Physical examination revealed a BP of 125/73 mm Hg, HR of 86 bpm, and oxygen saturation of 97% on room air. Chest examination showed a well-healed midline sternotomy scar. There was no lift or heave noted on palpation. On auscultation there was a normal S1 and physiologically split S2. There was a II/VI systolic ejection murmur appreciated along the right upper sternal border and a soft, early II/IV diastolic murmur along the left sternal border. Extremities were warm and well perfused without clubbing, cyanosis, or edema.

A 12-lead ECG (Figure 2-13) demonstrated a normal sinus rhythm, normal axis, and first-degree heart block. A TTE demonstrated trivial right-sided AV valve insufficiency, mild left-sided AV valve insufficiency, and mild left-sided AV valve stenosis. There was no evidence of residual left ventricular outflow obstruction (Figures 2-14 through 2-16) or residual intracardiac shunt. Biventricular volumes and function were normal.

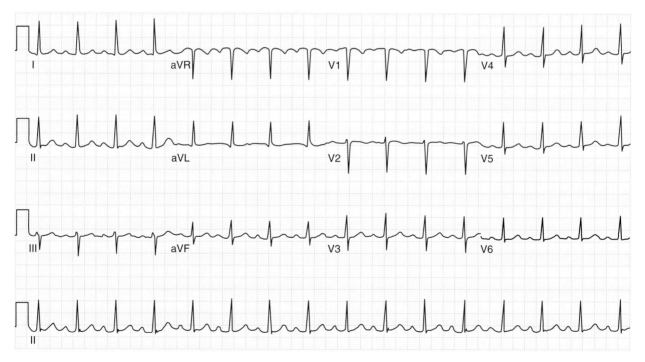

FIGURE 2-13 A 12-lead electrocardiogram shows prolonged PR interval.

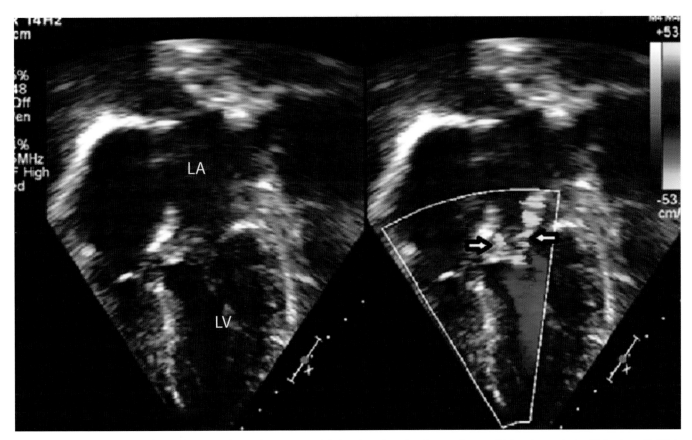

FIGURE 2-14 A 2-dimensional transthoracic echocardiogram apical 4-chamber view showing an abnormal left atrioventricular (AV) valve with 2 jets of left AV regurgitation (arrows). LA, left atrium; LV, left ventricle.

CASE EXPLANATION

- Patients born with a complete form of AVSD will undergo surgical repair within the first year of life. Because there is a common AV valve, there is no true tricuspid or mitral valve. The surgical repair consists of dividing the valve into right and left AV valves and closing both the primum atrial and ventricular septal defects.

- Because the AV valves are surgically created, patients are often left with some degree of insufficiency and less commonly stenosis. Atrioventricular valve insufficiency can often be appreciated as a holosystolic murmur. The systolic ejection murmur is likely secondary to residual left ventricular outflow tract obstruction after subaortic membrane resection.

- A subaortic membrane can be present prior to initial surgical repair, but occurs more commonly late after initial surgical intervention.[18]

- About 25% of patients with a complete AVSD will have PR prolongation prior to surgery. The PR prolongation is secondary to intra-atrial conduction delay.

EPIDEMIOLOGY

- Also commonly called endocardial cushion defects or AV canal defects.

- Atrioventricular septal defects account for 2% to 9% of congenital heart disease in various series. It also accounts for 5% of all congenital heart disease or 0.19 per 1000 live births.[19]

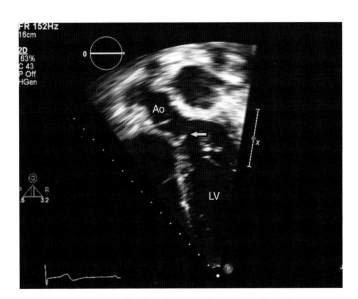

FIGURE 2-15 An apical 5-chamber view showing a subaortic membrane (arrow) located just below the aortic valve. Ao, aorta; LV, left ventricle.

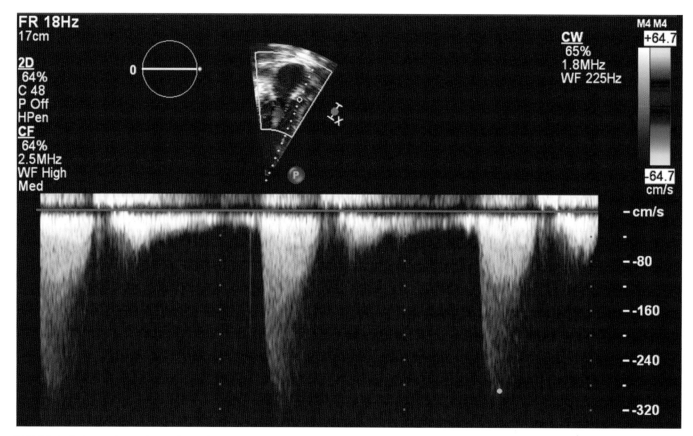

FIGURE 2-16 Spectral Doppler performed to estimate the peak gradient in the presence of a subaortic membrane. Using the modified Bernoulli equation a peak gradient of approximately 34 mm Hg was estimated.

- The male-to-female distribution of atrioventricular septal defect is approximately equal.
- Most commonly associated with trisomy 21. About 45% of patients with Down syndrome have congenital heart disease and about 45% of them have an AVSD.[20]
- AVSDs are also associated with patients who have a heterotaxy syndrome.[21]

ANATOMY

- The following classifications are used to describe the various forms of AVSD:
  - A partial (incomplete) defect is defined by a primum atrial septal defect, 2 discrete AV valves with contiguous right and left AV valve annuli, and varying degrees of left AV valve malformation leading to regurgitation.
  - A transitional (intermediate) AVSD is similar to the partial defect with the exception that there is an inlet VSD (Figure 2-17).
  - A complete AVSD has a primum ASD that extends to an inlet ventricular septal defect. There is a common AV valve bridging both the right and left sides of the heart. In complete atrioventricular septal defect, a single atrioventricular valve annulus, a common atrioventricular valve, and a defect of the inlet ventricular septum are observed. The deficiency of the atrioventricular septum also results in the presence of a large primum atrial septal defect. The common AV valve consists of at least 4 leaflets.

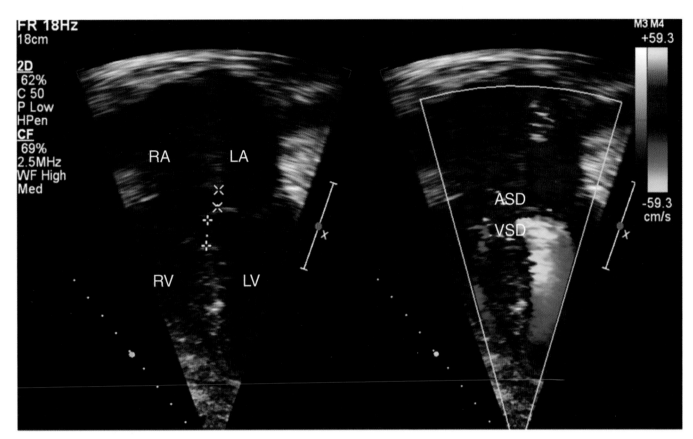

FIGURE 2-17 Apical 4-chamber view on transthoracic echocardiogram showing a transitional type atrioventricular septal defect (AVSD). With color Doppler (right) showing left-to-right shunt at both the level of the atrium and ventricular septal defects. ASD, atrial septal defect; LA, left atrium; LV, left ventricle; RA, right atrium; RV, right ventricle; VSD, ventricular septal defect.

These include the anterior and posterior bridging leaflets and 2 lateral leaflets. The anterior leaflet may be further subdivided to produce a total of 5 leaflets.

- Balanced versus unbalanced AVSD

  ○ With a balanced defect the valve opens equally into 2 appropriately sized ventricles.

  ○ In the unbalanced defect the AV inlet is preferential to one of the ventricles, called right or left ventricular dominance.

  ○ This accounts for about 10% of all AVSDs.[22]

ETIOLOGY AND PATHOPHYSIOLOGY

- The etiology of an AVSD is thought to be a lack of fusion of the endocardial cushions. The endocardial cushions are involved in the development of the mitral and tricuspid valves and their support apparatus during embryogenesis.

- In all types of atrioventricular septal defects, the initial physiology is that of a large left-to-right shunt. In patients with partial defects, this occurs through the ostium primum atrial septal defect. When a complete endocardial cushion defect is present, a large ventricular septal defect as well as valvular insufficiency may develop, resulting in volume overload of both the left and right ventricles associated with heart failure in early life.

- Pulmonary overcirculation and congestive heart failure symptoms are common in the first several months of life as pulmonary vascular resistance continues to fall throughout infancy.

- In contrast, the adult with an uncorrected complete AVSD, the pulmonary vasculature is subjected to both increased blood flow and systemic pressure and eventually develops irreversible pulmonary vascular disease (Eisenmenger syndrome).

DIAGNOSIS

Clinical Presentation/History

- A complete AVSD will present in the first few months of life with tachypnea and failure to thrive secondary to increased pulmonary blood flow. A partial or transitional AVSD is usually detected in childhood. However, some may present later in the adolescent or young adult. The key historical details would include shortness of breath, exercise intolerance, or atrial arrhythmia.
- Physical examination may show a normal S1, a fixed split S2, and a systolic ejection murmur over the left upper sternal border with radiation to lung fields caused by increased flow across the pulmonary valve.
- A loud holosystolic murmur heard along the left sternal border and at the cardiac apex suggests the presence of left-sided AV valve regurgitation. A low-pitched mid-diastolic murmur may also be appreciated if there is increased flow from significant left AV valve regurgitation or large left-to-right shunt. In the presence of increased pulmonary arterial pressures, the P2 component of S2 becomes increasingly accentuated.

ECG

- A 12-lead ECG in an unrepaired partial AVSD may show left-axis deviation while a superior or northwest axis deviation is common in complete AVSD.
- A prolonged PR interval preoperatively is thought to be secondary to intra-atrial conduction delay. An RSR' pattern can be seen when right volume overload is present. Left ventricular hypertrophy may also be seen.

Chest Radiography

- Chest radiography may show cardiomegaly with enlargement of the right atrium and ventricle. There is often increased pulmonary vascularity in patients with a complete AVSD.
- The main pulmonary artery usually is prominent with increased pulmonary vascular markings. After pulmonary hypertension develops, a reduction in pulmonary vascular markings is observed.

Echocardiography

- For all 3 types of AVSDs transthoracic echocardiography remains the noninvasive imaging modality of choice. It provides the detailed anatomy assessment required to differentiate between partial, transitional, and complete AVSDs.
- This technique should demonstrate the diagnosis of AVSD, the morphology of the AV valves, associated valvular abnormalities, level and direction of shunt, ventricular function, presence of left or right ventricular outflow tract obstruction, estimate of pulmonary pressures, and exclusion of other associated anomalies.

- Echocardiography can often show the lack of displacement of the left and right AV valves which is a characteristic finding in this condition.

Cardiac Catheterization

- Cardiac catheterization is not routinely performed for the evaluation of AVSD. In the adolescent or adult with an unoperated defect, cardiac catheterization is performed to assess pulmonary vascular resistance.
- If other lesions are suspected or if operative planning cannot be performed adequately after noninvasive testing, then catheterization should be undertaken.
- Left ventricular angiography in the frontal plane shows an elongated left ventricular outflow tract, called a "gooseneck deformity," which is characteristically seen in patients with unrepaired defects.
- It should involve quantitation of the shunts and valvular insufficiency and calculation of pulmonary vascular resistance.

MANAGEMENT

- A review of the Pediatric Heart Network data of primary surgical repair for AVSD performed prior to 1 year of age demonstrated both low mortality (3%) and a 20-year survival of about 95%.[23,24] The most common residual lesion postoperatively is left AV valve regurgitation. This finding is present in about 25% of patients as soon as 6 months postoperatively.
- Many of these patients may require reoperation. The current recommendations for reoperation include the following[8]:
  - Left AV vale repair/replacement for regurgitation or stenosis causing symptoms, arrhythmias, LV dilation, or LV dysfunction.
  - Left ventricular outflow tract obstruction (subaortic stenosis) with a mean gradient of more than 50 mm Hg or peak greater than 70 mm Hg. In the setting of mitral regurgitation, surgical intervention should be considered with a gradient greater than 50 mm Hg.
  - Residual ASD or VSD that meets criteria for closure.
- Patients with unrepaired defects in adulthood should undergo evaluation for pulmonary vascular obstructive disease. If pulmonary vascular resistance is acceptable, the patient should undergo complete repair of the defect. If pulmonary vascular disease is severe (Eisenmenger syndrome) the patient should have close follow-up with specialists in adult congenital heart disease and pulmonary hypertension.
- Advances in pulmonary vasodilator therapy have provided significant benefit with demonstrated improvements in functional capacity.

FOLLOW-UP

- The American College of Cardiology/American Heart Association 2008 Guidelines for the Management of Adults with Congenital Heart Disease recommends all patients with an AVSD should follow routinely with an Adult Congenital Heart Disease specialist.[8] Most often patients undergo annual evaluation.
- However, this guideline can be tailored appropriately in the presence of residual sequelae such as AV valve regurgitation, subaortic obstruction, arrhythmias, and decreased ventricular function that

develop after surgical repair or the presence of pulmonary hypertension that warrants closer surveillance.

- Routine evaluation should include a focused TTE that includes AV valve function, left ventricular outflow tract, and ventricular function. Routine ECG and intermittent Holter monitor evaluation should be considered to evaluate for AV block (~2%) as there is an increased risk of injury during surgical repair to the posteriorly displaced AV node.

LONG-TERM COMPLICATIONS

- In both the repaired and unrepaired patient, atrial arrhythmias can be common. In a study by Garson et al. of 380 pediatric patients, mean age 10.3 years, with atrial arrhythmias, 5% of these patients had an AVSD. Of these patients, 80% had a previous surgical repair.[25]

- As atrial arrhythmias may contribute to a significant source of morbidity and mortality in this growing adult congenital population, the patient with AVSD (repaired or unrepaired) who presents with an atrial arrhythmia warrants a detailed evaluation of hemodynamics, specifically AV valve regurgitation, functional assessment, and any residual defects. (ASD/VSD).

REFERENCES

1. Webb G, Gatzoulis MA. Atrial septal defects in the adult: recent progress and overview. *Circulation*. 2006;114:1645-1653.

2. Basson CT, Huang T, Lin RC, et al. Different TBX5 interactions in heart and limb defined by Holt-Oram syndrome mutations. *Proc Natl Acad Sci USA*. 1999;96:2919-2924.

3. Krasuski RA. When and how to fix a 'hole in the heart': approach to ASD and PFO. *Cleve Clin J Med*. 2007;74:137-147.

4. Khairy AP, Marelli AJ. Clinical use of echocardiography in adults with congenital heart disease. *Circulation*. 2007;116:2734-2746.

5. Kilner PJ. Imaging congenital heart disease in adults. *Br J Radiol*. 2011;84:S258-S268.

6. Fu Y, Cao Q, Hijazi Z. Device closure of large atrial septal defects: technical considerations. *J Cardiovasc Med*. 2007;8:30-33.

7. Landzberg MJ, Khairy P. Indications for the closure of patent foramen ovale. *Heart*. 2004;90:219-224.

8. Warnes CA, Williams RG, Bashore TM, et al. ACC/AHA 2008 guidelines for the management of adults with congenital heart disease: a report of the American College of Cardiology/ American Heart Association task force on practice guidelines (Writing committee to develop guidelines on the management of adults with congenital heart disease) developed in collaboration with the American Society of Echocardiography, Heart Rhythm Society, International Society for Adult Congenital Heart Disease, Society for Cardiovascular Angiography and Interventions, and Society of Thoracic Surgeons. *J Am Coll Cardiol*. 2008;52:e1-e121.

9. Roos-Hesselink JW, Meijboom FJ, Spitaels SE, et al. Excellent survival and low incidence of arrhythmias, stroke and heart failure long-term after surgical ASD closure at young age: a prospective follow-up study of 21-33 years. *Eur Heart J*. 2003;24:190-197.

10. Roguin N, Du ZD, Barack M, et al. High prevalence of muscular ventricular septal defects in neonates. *J Am Coll Cardiol*. 1995;26:1545-1548.

11. McDaniel NL. Ventricular and atrial septal defects. *Pediatr Rev*. 2001;22:265-269.

12. Minette MS, Sahn D. Ventricular septal defect. *Circulation*. 2006;114:2190-2197.

13. Kilner PJ, Geva T, Kaemmerer H, et al. Recommendations for magnetic resonance imaging in adults with congenital heart disease from the respective working groups of the European Society of Cardiology. *Eur Heart J*. 2010;31:794-805.

14. Butera G, Carminati M, Chessa M, et al. Transcatheter closure of perimembranous ventricular septal defects: early and long-term results. *J Am Coll Cardiol*. 2007;50:1189-1195.

15. Galie N, Beghetti M, Gatzoulis M, et al. Bosentan therapy in patients with Eisenmenger syndrome. *Circulation*. 2006;114:48-54.

16. Corone P, Doyon F, Gaudeau S, et al. Natural history of ventricular septal defect: a study involving 790 cases. *Circulation*. 1977;55:908-915.

17. Mongeon FP, Burkhart HM, Ammash NM, et al. Indications and outcomes of surgical closure of ventricular septal defect in adults. *J Am Coll Cardiol Cardiovasc Interv*. 2010;3:290-297.

18. Kalfa D, Ghez O, Kreitmann B, Metra D. Secondary subaortic stenosis in heart defects without any initial subaortic obstruction: a multifactorial post-operative event. *Eur J Cardiothorac Surg*. 2007;32:582-587.

19. Fyler DC, Buckley LP, Hellenbrand WE, et al. Endocardial cushion defect. Report of the New England Regional Infant Cardiac Program. *J Pediatr*. 1980;65:441-444.

20. Freeman SB, Bean LH, Allen EG, et al. Ethnicity, sex and the incidence of congenital heart defects: a report from the National Down Syndrome Project. *Genet Med*. 2008;10:173-180.

21. Qureshi AU, Kazmi U, Kazmi T, Sadiq M. Congenital heart defects associated with left atrial isomerism. *J Coll Physicians Surg Pak*. 2012;22:549-552.

22. Cohen MS, Spray TL. Surgical management of unbalanced atrioventricular canal defect. *Semin Thorac Cardiovasc Surg Pediatric Card Surg Annu*. 2005;8:135-144.

23. Atz AM, Hawkins JA, Lu M, et al. Surgical management of complete atrioventricular septal defects: associations with surgical technique, age and trisomy 21. *J Thorac Cardiovasc Surg*. 2010;141:1371-1379.

24. McGrath LB, Gonzalezo-Lavin L. Actuarial survival, freedom from reoperation, and other events after repair of atrioventricular septal defects. *J Thorac Cardiovasc Surg*. 1987;94:582.

25. Garson A, Bink-Boelkens M, Hesslei PS, et al. Atrial flutter in the young: collaborative study of 380 cases. *J Am Coll of Cardiol*. 1985;6:871-878.

3 THE ADULT WITH COARCTATION OF THE AORTA

Eric V. Krieger, MD
Karen K. Stout, MD

PATIENT STORY

A 23-year-old man was seen for difficult-to-control hypertension. On initial presentation he had a blood pressure (BP) of 160/90 mm Hg. Despite initiation of multiple antihypertensive medications including hydrochlorothiazide and lisinopril, the patient remained hypertensive with systolic BP of greater than 140 mm Hg. The patient was asymptomatic but reported a lifelong murmur. Physical examination revealed a right upper extremity BP of 146/82 mm Hg. Cardiovascular examination was significant for a grade II/VI systolic ejection murmur and a posterior systolic murmur in the left infrascapular region. Lower extremity pulses were diminished. A transthoracic echocardiogram demonstrated a bicuspid aortic valve, mild aortic dilation, and flow acceleration across the aortic isthmus.

CASE EXPLANATION

- This patient has coarctation of the aorta (CoA) and its most common manifestation is systemic arterial hypertension.
- Patients with CoA often present in infancy with congestive heart failure.[1] However, those who escape diagnosis in childhood most commonly present with difficult-to-control hypertension later in life.
- This patient also had a bicuspid aortic valve (BAV) which is present in approximately 50% to 60% of patients with CoA.
- Aortic dilation along with a BAV can also be seen in such patients.

EPIDEMIOLOGY

- The incidence of CoA is approximately 0.3 per 1000 live births[2,3] and accounts for approximately 5% to 8% of congenital heart disease making it the eighth most common congenital heart defect.[4,5]
- CoA, like other forms of left-sided heart obstruction, is more common in males than females.[4]
- While CoA can be isolated, it often coexists with other forms of heart disease: Of patients with simple CoA, 42% have a patent ductus arteriosus. Approximately 50% to 60% of patients with CoA have bicommissural aortic valve (BAV). Approximately 10% have an intracranial aneurysm.[6,7]
- CoA often coexists with other forms of left heart obstruction including mitral stenosis, subaortic stenosis, and aortic stenosis. In addition, CoA is associated with atrial septal defects, ventricular septal defects, and complex congenital heart disease (eg, hypoplastic left heart syndrome, atrioventricular canal defect, transposition of the great arteries).[3]
- Women with Turner syndrome (gonadal dysgenesis with 45,X karyotype) have an increased risk (12%-35%) of CoA.[8-10]

ETIOLOGY

- The etiology of CoA is multifactorial and incompletely understood.
- There is a compelling evidence for a genetic contribution to CoA.[11-14] CoA is more common in the children of women with CoA.[15] The genetics is not simple, however, while *NOTCH1* mutations have been described in patients with CoA, this mutation is absent in most patients.[16] Linkage analysis has identified multiple candidate genes[17] although progress has been hindered by the relative rarity of the disorder and phenotypic variability. As CoA often coexists with other forms of left heart obstruction, as described above, some have speculated whether CoA, BAV, and other forms of left-sided obstruction are different phenotypic manifestations of the same disease process.[18]
- Seasonal variability is present with peak incidence in spring and fall suggesting a possible role of infection or other unidentified environmental factors.[19]
- Environmental risk factors may play a role in the pathogenesis, including organic solvents, although this has not been confirmed.[20]
- Traditionally, the etiology of CoA was thought to be due to either incomplete regression of ductal tissue causing aortic constriction or reduced aortic growth in response to inadequate anterograde flow.[21] CoA is now known to be part of a diffuse arteriopathy with abnormalities throughout the pre-coarctation arterial tree.[6]

ANATOMY

- Most commonly CoA is a discrete fibrotic posterior ridge or shelf which narrows the aorta at the insertion of the ductus arteriosus—called juxtaductal (Figure 3-1).
- Anatomic variations exist including discrete CoA, long-segment CoA, hypoplastic aortic arch in association with CoA.
- Histologic changes to the arterial tree include cystic medial necrosis, elastic tissue fragmentation, smooth muscle hypertrophy, and loss of elastic fibers. These changes are found throughout the arterial tree and are not merely a response to pressure load.[22-24]
- Often vascular function is abnormal, with impaired endothelium-dependent and endothelium-independent vasoreactivity with abnormal vasodilation in response to flow and exogenous nitric oxide.[25,26]

PATHOPHYSIOLOGY

- CoA causes upper extremity hypertension which can result in hypertension and left ventricular hypertrophy.
- Hypertension affects 25% to 75% of patients with repaired CoA.[27-35] Age at repair is an important determinant of late hypertension.

- In several studies, those who are repaired during infancy have a less than 5% chance of developing hypertension by early adulthood while those operated on after the age of 1 had a 25% to 33% chance of developing hypertension early in life.[28,29,36]

- Late hypertension is strongly associated with residual or recurrent aortic arch obstruction.[30] Therefore, in patients with repaired CoA who present with hypertension, residual obstruction must be excluded.[37]

- Nonetheless, some patients with early repair and no residual arch obstruction still develop hypertension due to vascular dysfunction (discussed later). For example, in a study of 119 children repaired in early infancy, 19% of patients with no residual arch obstruction had an ambulatory blood pressure greater than the 95th percentile.[30]

- Patients with CoA have diffuse arterial disease manifested by increased vascular stiffness, decreased arterial elasticity, and impaired endothelial function.[6,26,36,38-46] The mechanisms underlying hypertension in these patients is complex. Reduced vascular compliance and accelerated pulse wave velocity contribute to augmentation of systolic blood pressure via reflected waves which fall in systole.[42,47] Additionally, stiff proximal conduit arteries fail to dampen pulsatile flow thereby raising vascular impedance and ventricular afterload.[48]

- When the left ventricle is coupled to abnormal vasculature, remodeling occurs.[48,49] Increased pressure results in left ventricular hypertrophy in order to normalize wall strain.[50] Ventricular systolic stiffness increases and, in combination with the increased arterial elastance, contributes to hypertension both at rest and with adrenergic stimulation.[39]

- Hypertension can lead to cardiovascular events as early as the third and fourth decade. Patients with repaired CoA are at increased risk for premature myocardial infarction, cerebrovascular accidents, dissection, left ventricular systolic dysfunction, and endocarditis.[28,51] However, with increased recognition of late hypertension and treatment of modifiable risk factors[37] the incidence of premature cardiovascular disease in this population may be improving.[52,53]

- The prevalence of hypertension also depends on how blood pressure is measured and the age of the population is studied. In one study, ambulatory blood pressure measurement diagnosed hypertension in 54% of patients with repaired CoA while resting BP detected hypertension in only 21%.[38]

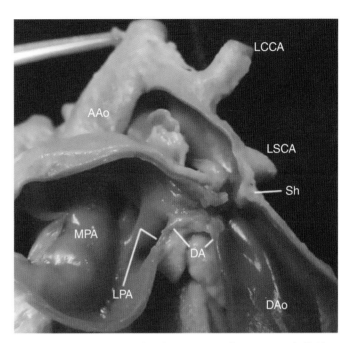

FIGURE 3-1 Discrete juxtaductal coarctation. The posterior shelf (Sh) is seen just distal to the left subclavian artery (LSCA). The ductus arteriosus (DA) is opposite the posterior shelf. Note the fleshy, corrugated appearance of the ductus tissue, completely different from either the main pulmonary artery (MPA) or the descending aorta (DAo). The distal arch (*) is mildly narrow. AAo, ascending aorta; LCCA, left common carotid artery; LPA, left pulmonary artery. (*Reproduced with permission from Stephen P. Sanders, MD, Professor of Pediatrics [Cardiology], Harvard Medical School; Director, Cardiac Registry, Departments of Cardiology, Pathology, and Cardiac Surgery, Children's Hospital Boston, Boston, Massachusetts.*)

DIAGNOSIS

- The diagnosis of CoA depends on appropriate clinical suspicion. Not all patients with hypertension require imaging of the aorta to exclude CoA as the physical examination can diagnose a hemodynamically significant CoA in most patients.

Physical Examination

- Measurement of the blood pressure in the arm and leg with the patient in a supine position should be performed. Normally the lower extremity blood pressure is 10% to 20% higher than the upper extremity blood pressure due to wave amplification.[54] If leg blood pressure is substantially lower (10 mm Hg) than arm BP then CoA or other forms of peripheral arterial disease should be suspected. A gradient of greater than 35 mm Hg has a very high specificity for CoA.[55] Collateral vessels which bridge the region of CoA are common so blood pressure gradient may not be very high even in patients with hemodynamically important CoA.

- Simultaneous palpitation of right radial and femoral arteries should also be performed if CoA is suspected. If femoral pulse is weak or delayed in relation to the radial pulse then CoA should be suspected and imaging should be performed.

- A systolic or continuous murmur over the back may be present in patients with CoA.

- As more than 5% of patients with bicommissural aortic valve have CoA, all patients with bicommissural aortic valve should be evaluated for CoA. A careful physical examination may be adequate to exclude CoA but echocardiography or cross-sectional imaging of the thoracic aorta with magnetic resonance (MR) or computed tomography (CT) angiography is reasonable.[37]

Echocardiography

- Transthoracic echocardiography (TTE) is widely available but has significant limitations in the evaluation of CoA. Suprasternal acoustic windows are often difficult in the adult and the distance between the transducer and the aortic isthmus make echocardiographic imaging challenging. Nonetheless, the directed goals of the TTE are listed in Table 3-1 should be to evaluate the aortic

Table 3-I Echocardiogram of Native Coarctation

Goal	Window	Challenges	Solutions
Arch anatomy and relationship of coarctation to brachiocephalic vessels	Suprasternal notch, left subclavicular window	Long distance from transducer	Neck extension, low-frequency transducer, left subclavicular window, harmonic imaging
Gradients across the coarctation site	Suprasternal notch, right and left subclavicular window	Overestimation of gradients due to issues with modified Bernoulli equation, underestimation due to poor angle of intercept	Adjust for proximal velocity using: $\Delta P = 4(v_2^2 - v_1^2)$
Flow profile in abdominal aorta	Subcostal short axis		
Aneurysmal disease in ascending aorta (in case of bicommissural aortic valve) or distal to the coarctation site.	High right parasternal, suprasternal notch	Poor acoustic windows, distance from transducer	Low-frequency transducer, harmonic imaging. Cross-sectional imaging with MR or CT angiography may be needed

CT, computed tomography; ΔP, pressure gradient; MR, magnetic resonance; v_1 = velocity proximal to coarctation obtained from pulse-wave Doppler; v_2, maximum velocity through coarctation, obtained via continuous-wave Doppler.

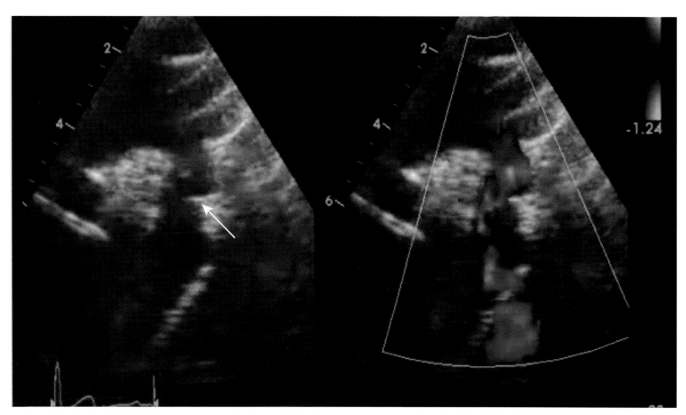

FIGURE 3-2 Suprasternal notch view on 2D transthoracic echocardiogram with color compare demonstrating coarctation by 2D (left) and color Doppler (right). Arrow notes point of coarctation.

isthmus, hemodynamic significance of the gradient across the CoA, and aortic aneurysms (either proximal or distal to the CoA). The left subclavian artery should be identified from long-axis views and the proximal descending thoracic aorta should be imaged to evaluate for narrowing and poststenotic dilation (Figure 3-2). Use of a low-frequency imaging probe and harmonic imaging can improve 2D imaging of the aortic isthmus.

- Spectral Doppler across the CoA is valuable but has potential pitfalls. From the suprasternal window continuous Doppler can be used to estimate gradient across CoA. As in all applications of spectral Doppler, the beam must be aligned with the direction of flow.

- Qualitative assessment of the continuous-wave Doppler signal across the CoA provides valuable information about the degree of obstruction: high maximum velocity across the isthmus with prolonged diastolic deceleration phase (Figure 3-3). Caution must be used in analyzing this pattern as alterations in arterial compliance, common in patients with CoA, can alter the appearance such that stiffer conduit arteries accelerate the pressure decay and potentially mask a hemodynamically significant CoA.[56]

- The modified Bernoulli equation (pressure gradient $= 4v^2$) often overestimates the pressure gradient measured at the time of cardiac catheterization.[57,58] The accuracy of continuous-wave Doppler estimation of gradients across the isthmus can be improved by expanding the modified Bernoulli equation to include the proximal velocity measured by pulse-wave Doppler (v_1) such that pressure gradient $= 4(v_2^2 - v_1^2)$.[58,59] The presence of significant collateral arteries bridging the CoA can cause spectral Doppler to underestimate the severity of obstruction.[60] Very severe obstruction,

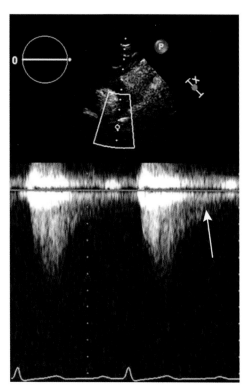

FIGURE 3-3 Continuous-wave Doppler signal from the aortic arch with long diastolic "tail" (arrows) and increased systolic velocity.

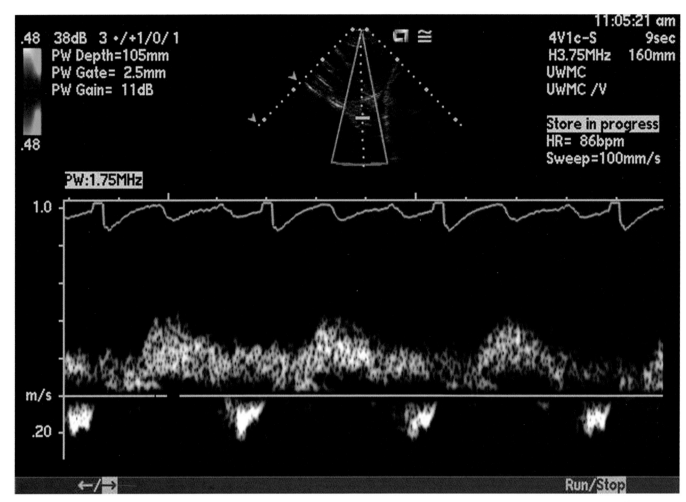

FIGURE 3-4 Abdominal Doppler signal with decreased and delayed systolic velocity and continuous antegrade diastolic flow or "runoff."

stiff arteries, long, torturous, or eccentric gradients can also lead to misleading Doppler estimation of gradient.[56,57,61,62]

- Abdominal aortic flow pattern provides important information on severity of obstruction. When a pulse-wave Doppler sample is placed in the abdominal aorta in patients without aortic obstruction, there is a rapid systolic upstroke, a short deceleration time, a brief early diastolic flow reversal, and little anterograde flow throughout diastole (Figure 3-4).[63-65] Loss of early diastolic flow reversal is highly sensitive for the detection of upstream stenosis. Blunted systolic velocity, continuous anterograde flow, and increased diastolic flow velocity in the abdominal aorta are important indicators of aortic obstruction. A greater than 50-ms delay between the R-wave and the peak velocity in the abdominal aorta is also associated with significant CoA.[63] Prolonged deceleration time also indicated significant upstream obstruction.[6]

Magnetic Resonance Imaging

- Magnetic resonance (MR) imaging has emerged as a comprehensive method to evaluate CoA. MR provides anatomic data, is not limited by acoustic windows, and does not expose the patient to ionizing radiation which is an important concern in young patients who will need to undergo serial examinations.

- Black blood double-inversion recovery spin echo imaging in the long-axis images provides static images with excellent anatomic definition of the CoA (Figure 3-5). Black blood images are less susceptible to artifact from implanted metallic devices than other MR techniques.

- Balanced steady-state free precession (bright blood cine) images also provide good anatomic detail and can show turbulence across the region of CoA. These cine images are also used to evaluate for the hemodynamic consequence of chronic pressure overload such as alterations in left ventricular size, mass, and systolic function.[35]

- Phase-contrast MR provides information about the quantity, direction, and velocity of blood flow. As is true in Doppler echocardiography, high-velocity flow across the CoA is likely indicative of a significant obstruction but precise measurement of gradients is difficult. A high-velocity encoding (VENC) setting may be required. The degree of collateral circulation can be quantified using phase-contrast MR techniques. A sample can be obtained just proximal to the CoA to determine the volume per beat. A second sample is obtained at the diaphragm. In patients without collateral vessels the flow at the diaphragm should be slightly lower than the flow proximal to the CoA due to blood sent to the intercostal and bronchial arteries. However, in patients with significant collaterals the flow at the diaphragm will be higher than the flow proximal to the CoA.[66-68] Analysis of the pattern of phase-contrast MR in the descending thoracic aorta at the level of the diaphragm provides information similar to that obtained by pulse-wave Doppler in the abdominal aorta. A long rate-corrected diastolic deceleration time is associated with hemodynamically significant CoA[69,70] (Figure 3-6).

- Gadolinium-enhanced MR angiography provides useful information regarding CoA anatomy, proximity to brachiocephalic vessels, aneurysmal disease, and collaterals (Figures 3-7A and 3-7B). Multiplanar reconstructions should be used to evaluate lumen diameter (Figure 3-8). Maximum-intensity projections (MIP) and 3-dimensional, volume rendered reconstructions provide an anatomic roadmap for surgical or transcatheter therapy (Figure 3-9).

- Four-dimensional (4D) phase contrast is an emerging technique which can combine anatomic information with flow mapping to quantify collateral flow and visualize blood flow in 3 dimensions throughout the cardiac cycle.[71]

- Approximately 10% of patients with CoA have cerebral aneurysms.[7,72] The natural history and clinical significance of these aneurysms are unknown. Magnetic resonance angiography to search for intracranial aneurysms is appropriate.[37] The optimal age for screening and frequency of reevaluation is unknown.

MANAGEMENT: MEDICAL, TRANSCATHETER, AND SURGICAL

- A hemodynamically significant CoA requires intervention in order to alleviate upper extremity hypertension and reduce long-term cerebrovascular and cardiovascular risk. A significant CoA is defined as a greater than or equal to 20-mm Hg systolic gradient at catheterization or a CoA associated with collaterals.[37] Cardiac catheterization is not usually necessarily required to establish significance; classic physical examination findings as described earlier (arm-leg blood pressure gradient, posterior murmur, and

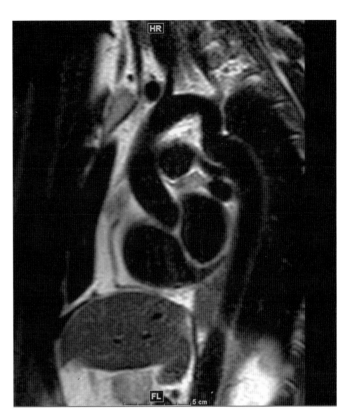

FIGURE 3-5 T$_2$-weighted black blood oblique sagittal image demonstrating coarctation.

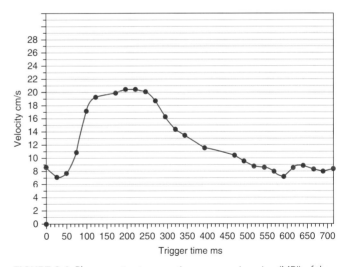

FIGURE 3-6 Phase-contrast magnetic resonance imaging (MRI) of the post-coarctation aorta demonstrating blunted upstroke and prolonged deceleration time.

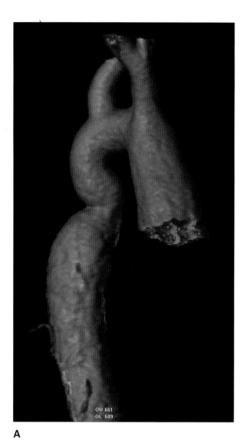

A

FIGURE 3-7A Three-dimensional gadolinium-enhanced contrast magnetic resonance angiogram (MRA) showing a native coarctation of the aorta.

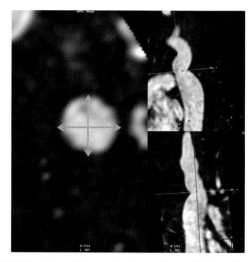

FIGURE 3-8 Double-oblique technique using multiplanar formatting for measuring minimal luminal diameter of a coarctation of the aorta.

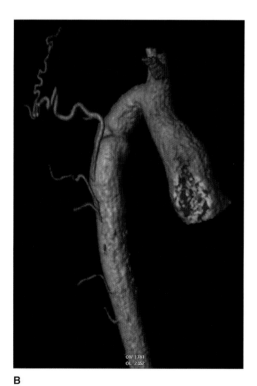

B

FIGURE 3-7B Three-dimensional (3D) gadolinium-enhanced contrast magnetic resonance angiogram showing a native coarctation of the aorta with significant collaterals supplying the descending thoracic aorta.

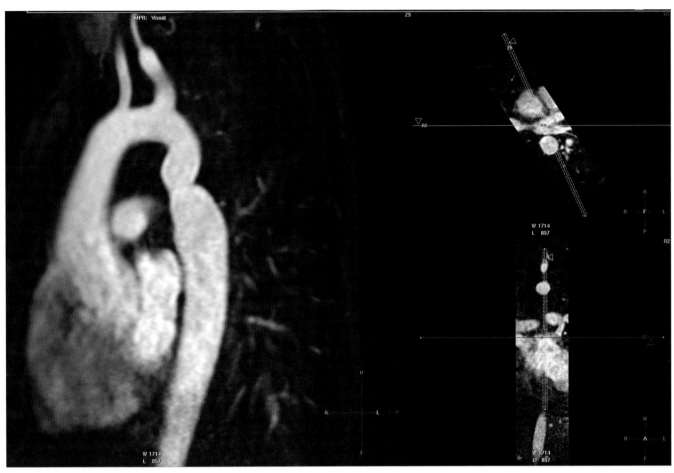

FIGURE 3-9 Maximum-intensity projection (MIP) from a contrast-enhanced magnetic resonance angiogram (MRA) demonstrating coarctation of the aorta.

radio-femoral pulse delay) accompanied by corroborative findings on imaging are usually adequate to establish the significance of a CoA.

- Both transcatheter and surgical approaches are available to treat native CoA in the adult. No trials have effectively compared surgery to transcatheter therapy in adults.[73]

- Surgery has a long track record of efficacy, long follow-up, low operative mortality, and the risk of spinal injury appears to be low in the modern era,[74-77] although publication bias may limit the number of poor outcomes reported. Patients with robust collaterals are at higher risk for operative bleeding.

- Transcatheter therapy with balloon angioplasty has been available for more than 30 years. Balloon angioplasty is effective with excellent relief of obstruction but has been limited by residual stenosis, late restenosis, aneurysm formation, or occasional dissection.[78,79] Balloon expandable stents provide support to the arterial wall and appose torn intima to the media. They also allow for redilation with reduced risk in the case of residual or recurrent stenosis.[80] For this reason angioplasty with stent implantation is emerging as the preferred method for treatment of discrete native CoA of the aorta in older children and adults.[81-88] Patients with long-segment CoA or complex arch anatomy are often less suitable for transcatheter therapy. Choice of transcatheter or surgical intervention of a native CoA should be determined in consultation with a team adult congenital cardiologists, surgeons, and interventional cardiologists with advanced training/experience in adult congenital heart disease.[37]

- Acute and midterm results of CoA stenting are excellent (Figure 3-10). The most robust data come from The Congenital Cardiovascular Interventional Study Consortium who reported on results from 565 bare metal stent implantations.[81,85] Mean luminal diameter increased by 180% and in 98% of cases the gradient across the CoA was reduced to less than 20 mm Hg. However, complications were present: There were 2 procedural deaths, 4 strokes, and at 1 year of follow-up 9% developed aneurysms (which were mostly small) and 3% had dissection or intimal tear. Risk factors for sub-optimal outcome included angioplasty prior to stent deployment or the use of an oversized balloon.

- Covered stents have been developed in an effort to increase procedural safety and reduce complications of aortic wall injury. Covered stents can reduce bleeding after intimal tear and can be used to exclude aneurysm, often obviating the need for surgery in patients with concomitant aneurysmal disease.[80] Covered Cheatham platinum (CP) stents have approval in Europe and are under active investigation in the United States.[89]

- Many patients have a reduction in upper extremity hypertension after intervention for CoA. In some studies more than half of treated patients became normotensive after surgery.[76,77] However, patients who were older at the time of intervention are considerably less likely to become normotensive than those who were treated at a younger age.[77] It is important to remember that patients with CoA have inherent vascular abnormalities with increased arterial stiffness which does not resolve after relief of isthmus obstruction. For that reason many patients have persistent hypertension at rest and with exercise even after a technically successful intervention.[90] Nonetheless many patients have a greater than 20-mm Hg reduction in their blood pressure even 3 years after their intervention and require fewer antihypertensive medications.[80,91-93]

- Residual hypertension should be aggressively treated medically once re-coarctation has been excluded. Large-scale trials are not available in this population to mandate one class of therapy over another although beta-blockers and ACE-inhibitors have been used successfully.[37,94]

LONG-TERM FOLLOW-UP AND COMPLICATIONS

- Suggested follow-up for patients with CoA is shown in Table 3-2. Patients with repaired CoA remain at lifelong risk for hypertension and premature cardiovascular complications. Therefore, lifelong follow-up is needed and should be done in consultation with an adult congenital heart disease specialist.[37]

- Hypertension should be aggressively sought out. Minimum screening should include annual 4-extremity blood pressure measurements with the patient lying flat. Left arm blood pressure may be misleadingly low if the left subclavian artery was sacrificed during repair. If upper extremity hypertension is discovered then re-coarctation must be excluded as hypertension is the most common presenting sign of re-coarctation.

- More sensitive screening techniques to detect occult hypertension are available and include exercise testing to evaluate for exercise-induced hypertension and ambulatory blood pressure monitoring.

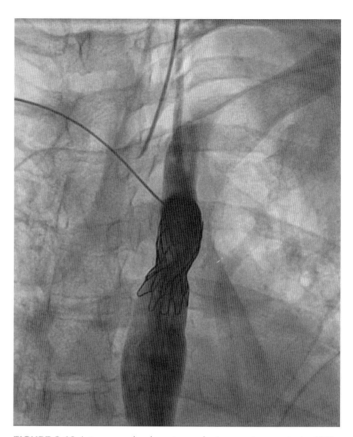

FIGURE 3-10 Intraprocedural angiography in an anteroposterior (AP) view demonstrating stent placement in a severe native coarctation of the aorta.

Table 3-2 Suggested Follow-Up for Patients With Coarctation

	Initial	Annual	Every 3-5 years	Situational
History and directed physical examination	X	X		
Arm and leg blood pressure measurements	X	X		
Echocardiogram	X		X	
MR or CT angiography of aorta	X		X	
Exercise testing				X
Brain MR angiography	X			

CT, computed tomography; MR, magnetic resonance.
(Adapted from ACC/AHA guidelines for the management of adults with congenital heart disease.)

Exercise-induced hypertension is common in patients with repaired CoA[27,31,33,43,95-99] and may be prognostically important: many patients with normal resting blood pressure and exercise-induced hypertension develop resting hypertension in follow-up.[34] Additionally, patients with exercise-induced hypertension are more likely to have adverse ventricular remodeling than those with normal exercise blood pressure.[35] Exercise testing, therefore, identifies patients who may be at increased risk of developing hypertension or ventricular hypertrophy.[100,101] It may be particularly useful in patients who are normotensive at rest. However, whether treating exercise-induced hypertension in patients with repaired CoA changes outcomes has not been established.

- Premature atherosclerotic disease was common in patients with repaired CoA prior to widespread recognition and treatment of hypertension and dyslipidemia in this population.[28,51,102] While early atherosclerotic death appears to be less common in the modern era (when CoA is treated much earlier and risk factors are aggressively modified), contemporary studies do still demonstrate subclinical disease in patients with repaired CoA of the aorta.[103-105] Therefore, aggressive treatment of modifiable cardiovascular risk factors is warranted in patients with CoA.[37]

- Re-coarctation of a previously repaired CoA is common, particularly in the case of neonatal CoA repair.[100,106] Therefore, annual surveillance should be performed to exclude re-coarctation. Directed physical examination with arm-leg blood pressure gradients, listening for a posterior murmur, and checking for radio-femoral pulse delay is the first step. If re-coarctation is suspected, imaging with echocardiography, CT or MR angiography should be performed (Figure 3-11). If the patient has a stented CoA, MR angiography is a poor choice to evaluate for re-coarctation due to limitations from susceptibility artifact. Re-coarctation should be treated if there are symptoms, hypertension, a high gradient or collateral vessels.[37] Transcatheter therapy with angioplasty, and increasingly stenting, are first-line therapy for re-coarctation of the aorta.[84,91]

- Aortic aneurysms or pseudoaneurysms can occur either at the site of repair or in the mid-ascending aorta[6,107] (Figures 3-12A and 3-12B). After surgery, Dacron patch repair is associated with aneurysm formation and rupture and should be treated aggressively.[108-110] Due to intimal injury aneurysm formation can also occur at the margins of the stent.[81,84,85,87,89] Because CoA site aneurysms cannot be detected by physical examination and are difficult to see by echocardiography, surveillance with CT or MR angiography should be considered approximately every 3 to 5 years. Covered stents can often be used to exclude the aneurysm from the circulation as long as there is an adequate landing zone.[80,89] Ascending aortic aneurysm is often found in patients with CoA and bicuspid aortic valve.[107]

- In women with a well-repaired CoA and normal resting blood pressure, pregnancy and delivery are usually possible. Women with CoA who become pregnant should be cared for at a referral center with expertise in perinatology and adult congenital heart disease. The vast majority of women with CoA can have a vaginal delivery.[111] Cesarean delivery should be reserved for special circumstances or fetal indications.[37] Women with CoA are at an approximately 3-fold increased risk for hypertensive complications of pregnancy.[15,111-113] Maternal hypertension can predispose to

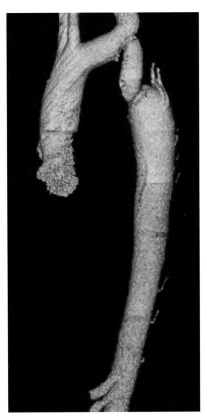

FIGURE 3-11 Three-dimensional (3D) reconstruction of computed tomography (CT) aortogram demonstrating long-segment, complex obstruction due to interposition graft placed in childhood.

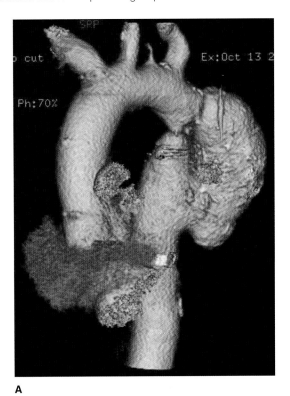

A

FIGURE 3-12A Three-dimensional (3D) reconstruction of aneurysm at prior repair site. The repair bypassed the narrowed segment with a tube graft, and the long-standing pseudoaneurysm is at the distal anastomosis of the graft.

low birth weight or premature delivery.[114,115] Rates of preeclampsia and eclampsia do not seem to be increased in CoA.[112] During pregnancy heart rate, stroke volume, and cardiac output increase placing additional hemodynamic stress on the arterial system. Aortic dissection and rupture have been described in women with repaired and unrepaired CoA[116,117] and women with CoA and Turner syndrome who have undergone in vitro fertilization are at very high risk of acute aortic syndromes.[118,119]

CONCLUSION

- CoA is a lifelong disease with a guarded prognosis.

- These patients need to be followed and screened with cardiology clinic visits, BP evaluation, directed imaging with echo, cardiac MRI, or CT when needed to screen for long-term complications.

- Patients with repaired CoA remain at lifelong risk for recurrent obstruction or re-coarctation, development of aneurysms or pseudoaneurysms, hypertension, and premature cardiovascular complications.

- Therefore, lifelong follow-up is imperative and should be done in consultation with an adult congenital heart disease specialist.

- Women with a well-repaired CoA and normal resting blood pressures may undergo pregnancy and delivery but should be cared for at a referral center with expertise in perinatology and adult congenital heart disease.

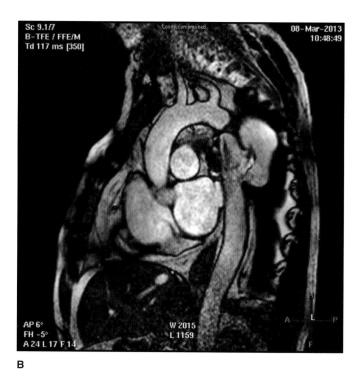

B

FIGURE 3-12B Sagittal image from magnetic resonance imaging (MRI) demonstrating the same pseudoaneurysm.

REFERENCES

1. Shinebourne EA, Tam AS, Elseed AM, Paneth M, Lennox SC, Cleland WP. Coarctation of the aorta in infancy and childhood. *Br Heart J*. 1976;38:375-380.

2. Gatzoulis MA, Webb GD, Daubeney PEF. *Diagnosis and Management of Adult Congenital Heart Disease*. 2nd ed. Philadelphia, PA: Elsevier/Churchill Livingstone; 2011.

3. Keane JF, Lock JE, Fyler DC, Nadas AS. *Nadas Pediatric Cardiology*. 2nd ed. Philadelphia, PA: Saunders; 2006.

4. Talner CN. Report of the New England Regional Infant Cardiac Program, by Donald C. Fyler, MD, Pediatrics, 1980;65(suppl):375-461. *Pediatrics*. 1998;102:258-259.

5. Botto LD, Correa A, Erickson JD. Racial and temporal variations in the prevalence of heart defects. *Pediatrics*. 2001;107:E32.

6. Krieger EV, Stout K. The adult with repaired coarctation of the aorta. *Heart*. 2010;96:1676-1681.

7. Cook SC, Hickey J, Maul TM, et al. Assessment of the cerebral circulation in adults with coarctation of the aorta. *Congenit Heart Dis*. 2013;8:289-295.

8. Ho VB, Bakalov VK, Cooley M, et al. Major vascular anomalies in Turner syndrome: prevalence and magnetic resonance angiographic features. *Circulation*. 2004;110:1694-1700.

9. Lopez L, Arheart KL, Colan SD, et al. Turner syndrome is an independent risk factor for aortic dilation in the young. *Pediatrics*. 2008;121:e1622-e1627.

10. Prandstraller D, Mazzanti L, Picchio FM, et al. Turner's syndrome: cardiologic profile according to the different

chromosomal patterns and long-term clinical follow-up of 136 nonpreselected patients. *Pediatr Cardiol*. 1999;20:108-112.

11. Loffredo CA, Chokkalingam A, Sill AM, et al. Prevalence of congenital cardiovascular malformations among relatives of infants with hypoplastic left heart, coarctation of the aorta, and d-transposition of the great arteries. *Am J Med Genet A*. 2004;124A:225-230.

12. McBride KL, Pignatelli R, Lewin M, et al. Inheritance analysis of congenital left ventricular outflow tract obstruction malformations: segregation, multiplex relative risk, and heritability. *Am J Med Genet A*. 2005;134A:180-186.

13. Lewin MB, McBride KL, Pignatelli R, et al. Echocardiographic evaluation of asymptomatic parental and sibling cardiovascular anomalies associated with congenital left ventricular outflow tract lesions. *Pediatrics*. 2004;114:691-696.

14. Bruneau BG. The developmental genetics of congenital heart disease. *Nature*. 2008;451:943-948.

15. Beauchesne LM, Connolly HM, Ammash NM, Warnes CA. Coarctation of the aorta: outcome of pregnancy. *J Am Coll Cardiol*. 2001;38:1728-1733.

16. McBride KL, Riley MF, Zender GA, et al. NOTCH1 mutations in individuals with left ventricular outflow tract malformations reduce ligand-induced signaling. *Hum Mol Genet*. 2008;17:2886-2893.

17. McBride KL, Zender GA, Fitzgerald-Butt SM, et al. Linkage analysis of left ventricular outflow tract malformations (aortic valve stenosis, coarctation of the aorta, and hypoplastic left heart syndrome). *Eur J Hum Genet*. 2009;17:811-819.

18. Warnes CA. Bicuspid aortic valve and coarctation: two villains part of a diffuse problem. *Heart*. 2003;89:965-966.

19. Miettinen OS, Reiner ML, Nadas AS. Seasonal incidence of coarctation of the aorta. *Br Heart J*. 1970;32:103-107.

20. Loffredo CA. Epidemiology of cardiovascular malformations: prevalence and risk factors. *Am J Med Genet*. 2000;97:319-325.

21. Rudolph AM, Heymann MA, Spitznas U. Hemodynamic considerations in the development of narrowing of the aorta. *Am J Cardiol*. 1972;30:514-525.

22. Jimenez M, Daret D, Choussat A, Bonnet J. Immunohistological and ultrastructural analysis of the intimal thickening in coarctation of human aorta. *Cardiovasc Res*. 1999;41:737-745.

23. Niwa K, Perloff JK, Bhuta SM, et al. Structural abnormalities of great arterial walls in congenital heart disease: light and electron microscopic analyses. *Circulation*. 2001;103:393-400.

24. Isner JM, Donaldson RF, Fulton D, Bhan I, Payne DD, Cleveland RJ. Cystic medial necrosis in coarctation of the aorta: a potential factor contributing to adverse consequences observed after percutaneous balloon angioplasty of coarctation sites. *Circulation*. 1987;75:689-695.

25. Brili S, Tousoulis D, Antoniades C, et al. Evidence of vascular dysfunction in young patients with successfully repaired coarctation of aorta. *Atherosclerosis*. 2005;182:97-103.

26. Brili S, Tousoulis D, Antoniades C, et al. Effects of ramipril on endothelial function and the expression of proinflammatory cytokines and adhesion molecules in young normotensive subjects with successfully repaired coarctation of aorta: a randomized cross-over study. *J Am Coll Cardiol*. 2008;51:742-749.

27. Earley A, Joseph MC, Shinebourne EA, de Swiet M. Blood pressure and effect of exercise in children before and after surgical correction of coarctation of aorta. *Br Heart J*. 1980;44:411-415.

28. Cohen M, Fuster V, Steele PM, Driscoll D, McGoon DC. Coarctation of the aorta. Long-term follow-up and prediction of outcome after surgical correction. *Circulation*. 1989;80:840-845.

29. Seirafi PA, Warner KG, Geggel RL, Payne DD, Cleveland RJ. Repair of coarctation of the aorta during infancy minimizes the risk of late hypertension. *Ann Thorac Surg*. 1998;66:1378-1382.

30. O'Sullivan JJ, Derrick G, Darnell R. Prevalence of hypertension in children after early repair of coarctation of the aorta: a cohort study using casual and 24 hour blood pressure measurement. *Heart*. 2002;88:163-166.

31. Hager A, Kanz S, Kaemmerer H, Hess J. Exercise capacity and exercise hypertension after surgical repair of isolated aortic coarctation. *Am J Cardiol*. 2008;101:1777-1780.

32. Hager A, Kanz S, Kaemmerer H, Schreiber C, Hess J. Coarctation long-term assessment (COALA): significance of arterial hypertension in a cohort of 404 patients up to 27 years after surgical repair of isolated coarctation of the aorta, even in the absence of restenosis and prosthetic material. *J Thorac Cardiovasc Surg*. 2007;134:738-745.

33. Toro-Salazar OH, Steinberger J, Thomas W, Rocchini AP, Carpenter B, Moller JH. Long-term follow-up of patients after coarctation of the aorta repair. *Am J Cardiol*. 2002;89:541-547.

34. Luijendijk P, Bouma BJ, Vriend JW, Vliegen HW, Groenink M, Mulder BJ. Usefulness of exercise-induced hypertension as predictor of chronic hypertension in adults after operative therapy for aortic isthmic coarctation in childhood. *Am J Cardiol*. 2011;108:435-439.

35. Krieger EV, Clair M, Opotowsky AR, et al. Correlation of exercise response in repaired coarctation of the aorta to left ventricular mass and geometry. *Am J Cardiol*. 2013;111:406-411.

36. Heger M, Willfort A, Neunteufl T, et al. Vascular dysfunction after coarctation repair is related to the age at surgery. *Int J Cardiol*. 2005;99:295-299.

37. Warnes CA, Williams RG, Bashore TM, et al. ACC/AHA 2008 Guidelines for the Management of Adults with Congenital Heart Disease: a report of the American College of Cardiology/American Heart Association Task Force on Practice Guidelines (writing committee to develop guidelines on the management of adults with congenital heart disease). *Circulation*. 2008;118:e714-e833.

38. de Divitiis M, Pilla C, Kattenhorn M, et al. Ambulatory blood pressure, left ventricular mass, and conduit artery function late after successful repair of coarctation of the aorta. *J Am Coll Cardiol*. 2003;41:2259-2265.

39. Senzaki H, Iwamoto Y, Ishido H, et al. Ventricular-vascular stiffening in patients with repaired coarctation of aorta: integrated pathophysiology of hypertension. *Circulation*. 2008;118:S191-S198.

40. Ou P, Celermajer DS, Jolivet O, et al. Increased central aortic stiffness and left ventricular mass in normotensive young subjects after successful coarctation repair. *Am Heart J*. 2008;155:187-193.

41. Celermajer DS, Greaves K. Survivors of coarctation repair: fixed but not cured. *Heart*. 2002;88:113-114.

42. de Divitiis M, Pilla C, Kattenhorn M, et al. Vascular dysfunction after repair of coarctation of the aorta: impact of early surgery. *Circulation*. 2001;104:I165-I170.

43. Guenthard J, Wyler F. Exercise-induced hypertension in the arms due to impaired arterial reactivity after successful coarctation resection. *Am J Cardiol*. 1995;75:814-817.

44. Gardiner HM, Celermajer DS, Sorensen KE, et al. Arterial reactivity is significantly impaired in normotensive young adults after successful repair of aortic coarctation in childhood. *Circulation*. 1994;89:1745-1750.

45. Gidding SS, Rocchini AP, Moorehead C, Schork MA, Rosenthal A. Increased forearm vascular reactivity in patients with hypertension after repair of coarctation. *Circulation*. 1985;71:495-499.

46. Sehested J, Baandrup U, Mikkelsen E. Different reactivity and structure of the prestenotic and poststenotic aorta in human coarctation. Implications for baroreceptor function. *Circulation*. 1982;65:1060-1065.

47. O'Rourke M. Mechanical principles in arterial disease. *Hypertension*. 1995;26:2-9.

48. Chirinos JA, Segers P. Noninvasive evaluation of left ventricular afterload: part 1: pressure and flow measurements and basic principles of wave conduction and reflection. *Hypertension*. 2010;56:555-562.

49. Chirinos JA, Segers P. Noninvasive evaluation of left ventricular afterload: part 2: arterial pressure-flow and pressure-volume relations in humans. *Hypertension*. 2010;56:563-570.

50. Grossman W, Jones D, McLaurin LP. Wall stress and patterns of hypertrophy in the human left ventricle. *J Clin Invest*. 1975;56:56-64.

51. Campbell M. Natural history of coarctation of the aorta. *Br Heart J*. 1970;32:633-640.

52. Cook SC, Ferketich AK, Raman SV. Myocardial ischemia in asymptomatic adults with repaired aortic coarctation. *Int J Cardiol*. 2009;133:95-101.

53. Verheugt CL, Uiterwaal C, van der Velde ET, et al. Mortality in adult congenital heart disease. *Eur Heart J*. 2010;31:1220-1229.

54. Park MK, Guntheroth WG. Direct blood pressure measurements in brachial and femoral arteries in children. *Circulation*. 1970;41:231-237.

55. Engvall J, Sonnhag C, Nylander E, Stenport G, Karlsson E, Wranne B. Arm-ankle systolic blood pressure difference at rest and after exercise in the assessment of aortic coarctation. *Br Heart J*. 1995;73:270-276.

56. Tacy TA, Baba K, Cape EG. Effect of aortic compliance on Doppler diastolic flow pattern in coarctation of the aorta. *J Am Soc Echocardiogr*. 1999;12:636-642.

57. Yoganathan AP, Valdes-Cruz LM, Schmidt-Dohna J, et al. Continuous-wave Doppler velocities and gradients across fixed tunnel obstructions: studies in vitro and in vivo. *Circulation*. 1987;76:657-666.

58. Marx GR, Allen HD. Accuracy and pitfalls of Doppler evaluation of the pressure gradient in aortic coarctation. *J Am Coll Cardiol*. 1986;7:1379-1385.

59. Lewin MB, Stout K. *Echocardiography in Congenital Heart Disease: Adult and Pediatric*. Philadelphia, PA: Elsevier/Saunders; 2012.

60. Houston AB, Simpson IA, Pollock JC, Jamieson MP, Doig WB, Coleman EN. Doppler ultrasound in the assessment of severity of coarctation of the aorta and interruption of the aortic arch. *Br Heart J*. 1987;57:38-43.

61. Stevenson JG, Kawabori I. Noninvasive determination of pressure gradients in children: two methods employing pulsed Doppler echocardiography. *J Am Coll Cardiol*. 1984;3:179-192.

62. Teirstein PS, Yock PG, Popp RL. The accuracy of Doppler ultrasound measurement of pressure gradients across irregular, dual, and tunnellike obstructions to blood flow. *Circulation*. 1985;72:577-584.

63. Silvilairat S, Cetta F, Biliciler-Denktas G, et al. Abdominal aortic pulsed wave Doppler patterns reliably reflect clinical severity in patients with coarctation of the aorta. *Congenit Heart Dis*. 2008;3:422-430.

64. Tan JL, Babu-Narayan SV, Henein MY, Mullen M, Li W. Doppler echocardiographic profile and indexes in the evaluation of aortic coarctation in patients before and after stenting. *J Am Coll Cardiol*. 2005;46:1045-1053.

65. Sanders SP, MacPherson D, Yeager SB. Temporal flow velocity profile in the descending aorta in coarctation. *J Am Coll Cardiol*. 1986;7:603-609.

66. Hom JJ, Ordovas K, Reddy GP. Velocity-encoded cine MR imaging in aortic coarctation: functional assessment of hemodynamic events. *Radiographics*. 2008;28:407-416.

67. Julsrud PR, Breen JF, Felmlee JP, Warnes CA, Connolly HM, Schaff HV. Coarctation of the aorta: collateral flow assessment with phase-contrast MR angiography. *Am J Roentgenol*. 1997;169:1735-1742.

68. Araoz PA, Reddy GP, Tarnoff H, Roge CL, Higgins CB. MR findings of collateral circulation are more accurate measures of hemodynamic significance than arm-leg blood pressure gradient after repair of coarctation of the aorta. *J Magn Reson Imaging*. 2003;17:177-183.

69. Nielsen JC, Powell AJ, Gauvreau K, Marcus EN, Prakash A, Geva T. Magnetic resonance imaging predictors of coarctation severity. *Circulation*. 2005;111:622-628.

70. Muzzarelli S, Meadows AK, Ordovas KG, et al. Prediction of hemodynamic severity of coarctation by magnetic resonance imaging. *Am J Cardiol*. 2011;108:1335-1340.

71. Hope MD, Meadows AK, Hope TA, et al. Clinical evaluation of aortic coarctation with 4D flow MR imaging. *J Magn Reson Imaging*. 2010;31:711-718.

72. Connolly HM, Huston J, 3rd, Brown RD, Jr., Warnes CA, Ammash NM, Tajik AJ. Intracranial aneurysms in patients with coarctation of the aorta: a prospective magnetic resonance angiographic study of 100 patients. *Mayo Clin Proc*. 2003;78:1491-1499.

73. Padua LM, Garcia LC, Rubira CJ, de Oliveira Carvalho PE. Stent placement versus surgery for coarctation of the thoracic aorta. *Cochrane Database Syst Rev*. 2012;5:CD008204.

74. Rokkas CK, Murphy SF, Kouchoukos NT. Aortic coarctation in the adult: management of complications and coexisting arterial abnormalities with hypothermic cardiopulmonary bypass and circulatory arrest. *J Thorac Cardiovasc Surg*. 2002;124:155-161.

75. Bauer M, Alexi-Meskishvili VV, Bauer U, Alfaouri D, Lange PE, Hetzer R. Benefits of surgical repair of coarctation of the aorta in patients older than 50 years. *Ann Thorac Surg*. 2001;72:2060-2064.

76. Carr JA. The results of catheter-based therapy compared with surgical repair of adult aortic coarctation. *J Am Coll Cardiol*. 2006;47:1101-1107.

77. Ozkokeli M, Gunduz H, Sensoz Y, et al. Blood pressure changes after aortic coarctation surgery performed in adulthood. *J Card Surg*. 2005;20:319-321.

78. Fawzy ME, Fathala A, Osman A, et al. Twenty-two years of follow-up results of balloon angioplasty for discreet native coarctation of the aorta in adolescents and adults. *Am Heart J*. 2008;156:910-917.

79. Kenny D, Hijazi ZM. Coarctation of the aorta: from fetal life to adulthood. *Cardiol J*. 2011;18:487-495.

80. Tzifa A, Ewert P, Brzezinska-Rajszys G, et al. Covered Cheatham-platinum stents for aortic coarctation: early and intermediate-term results. *J Am Coll Cardiol*. 2006;47:1457-1463.

81. Forbes TJ, Kim DW, Du W, et al. Comparison of surgical, stent, and balloon angioplasty treatment of native coarctation of the aorta: an observational study by the CCISC (Congenital Cardiovascular Interventional Study Consortium). *J Am Coll Cardiol*. 2011;58:2664-2674.

82. Bruckheimer E, Birk E, Santiago R, Dagan T, Esteves C, Pedra CA. Coarctation of the aorta treated with the Advanta V12 large diameter stent: acute results. *Catheter Cardiovasc Interv*. 2010;75:402-406.

83. Chessa M, Carrozza M, Butera G, et al. Results and mid-long-term follow-up of stent implantation for native and recurrent coarctation of the aorta. *Eur Heart J*. 2005;26:2728-2732.

84. Forbes TJ, Garekar S, Amin Z, et al. Procedural results and acute complications in stenting native and recurrent coarctation of the aorta in patients over 4 years of age: a multi-institutional study. *Catheter Cardiovasc Interv*. 2007;70:276-285.

85. Forbes TJ, Moore P, Pedra CA, et al. Intermediate follow-up following intravascular stenting for treatment of coarctation of the aorta. *Catheter Cardiovasc Interv*. 2007;70:569-577.

86. Mahadevan VS, Vondermuhll IF, Mullen MJ. Endovascular aortic coarctation stenting in adolescents and adults: angiographic and hemodynamic outcomes. *Catheter Cardiovasc Interv*. 2006;67:268-275.

87. Qureshi AM, McElhinney DB, Lock JE, Landzberg MJ, Lang P, Marshall AC. Acute and intermediate outcomes, and evaluation of injury to the aortic wall, as based on 15 years experience of implanting stents to treat aortic coarctation. *Cardiol Young*. 2007;17:307-318.

88. Johnston TA, Grifka RG, Jones TK. Endovascular stents for treatment of coarctation of the aorta: acute results and follow-up experience. *Catheter Cardiovasc Interv*. 2004;62:499-505.

89. Ringel RE, Gauvreau K, Moses H, Jenkins KJ. Coarctation of the Aorta Stent Trial (COAST): study design and rationale. *Am Heart J*. 2012;164:7-13.

90. Morgan GJ, Lee KJ, Chaturvedi R, Bradley TJ, Mertens L, Benson L. Systemic blood pressure after stent management for arch coarctation implications for clinical care. *JACC Cardiovasc Interv*. 2013;6:192-201.

91. Bentham JR, English K, Ballard G, Thomson JD. Effect of interventional stent treatment of native and recurrent coarctation of aorta on blood pressure. *Am J Cardiol*. 2013;111:731-736.

92. Eicken A, Pensl U, Sebening W, et al. The fate of systemic blood pressure in patients after effectively stented coarctation. *Eur Heart J*. 2006;27:1100-1105.

93. Hamdan MA, Maheshwari S, Fahey JT, Hellenbrand WE. Endovascular stents for coarctation of the aorta: initial results and intermediate-term follow-up. *J Am Coll Cardiol*. 2001;38:1518-1523.

94. Moltzer E, Mattace Raso FU, Karamermer Y, et al. Comparison of Candesartan versus Metoprolol for treatment of systemic hypertension after repaired aortic coarctation. *Am J Cardiol*. 2010;105:217-222.

95. Pelech AN, Kartodihardjo W, Balfe JA, Balfe JW, Olley PM, Leenen FH. Exercise in children before and after coarctectomy: hemodynamic, echocardiographic, and biochemical assessment. *Am Heart J*. 1986;112:1263-1270.

96. Hanson E, Eriksson BO, Sorensen SE. Intra-arterial blood pressures at rest and during exercise after surgery for coarctation of the aorta. *Eur J Cardiol*. 1980;11:245-257.

97. Hauser M. Exercise blood pressure in congenital heart disease and in patients after coarctation repair. *Heart*. 2003;89:125-126.

98. Hauser M, Kuehn A, Wilson N. Abnormal responses for blood pressure in children and adults with surgically corrected aortic coarctation. *Cardiol Young*. 2000;10:353-357.

99. Vriend JW, van Montfrans GA, Romkes HH, et al. Relation between exercise-induced hypertension and sustained hypertension in adult patients after successful repair of aortic coarctation. *J Hypertens*. 2004;22:501-509.

100. Singh JP, Larson MG, Manolio TA, et al. Blood pressure response during treadmill testing as a risk factor for new-onset hypertension. The Framingham heart study. *Circulation.* 1999;99:1831-1836.

101. Allison TG, Cordeiro MA, Miller TD, Daida H, Squires RW, Gau GT. Prognostic significance of exercise-induced systemic hypertension in healthy subjects. *Am J Cardiol.* 1999;83:371-375.

102. Vlodaver Z, Neufeld HN. The coronary arteries in coarctation of the aorta. *Circulation.* 1968;37:449-454.

103. Cook SC, Ferketich AK, Raman SV. Myocardial ischemia in asymptomatic adults with repaired aortic coarctation. *Int J Cardiol.* 2009;133:95-101.

104. Meyer AA, Joharchi MS, Kundt G, Schuff-Werner P, Steinhoff G, Kienast W. Predicting the risk of early atherosclerotic disease development in children after repair of aortic coarctation. *Eur Heart J.* 2005;26:617-622.

105. Swan L, Kraidly M, Muhll IV, Collins P, Gatzoulis MA. Surveillance of cardiovascular risk in the normotensive patient with repaired aortic coarctation. *Int J Cardiol.* 2010;139:283-288.

106. Younoszai AK, Reddy VM, Hanley FL, Brook MM. Intermediate term follow-up of the end-to-side aortic anastomosis for coarctation of the aorta. *Ann Thorac Surg.* 2002;74:1631-1634.

107. von Kodolitsch Y, Aydin MA, Koschyk DH, et al. Predictors of aneurysmal formation after surgical correction of aortic coarctation. *J Am Coll Cardiol.* 2002;39:617-624.

108. Parks WJ, Ngo TD, Plauth WH, Jr., et al. Incidence of aneurysm formation after Dacron patch aortoplasty repair for coarctation of the aorta: long-term results and assessment utilizing magnetic resonance angiography with three-dimensional surface rendering. *J Am Coll Cardiol.* 1995;26:266-271.

109. Bromberg BI, Beekman RH, Rocchini AP, et al. Aortic aneurysm after patch aortoplasty repair of coarctation: a prospective analysis of prevalence, screening tests and risks. *J Am Coll Cardiol.* 1989;14:734-741.

110. Knyshov GV, Sitar LL, Glagola MD, Atamanyuk MY. Aortic aneurysms at the site of the repair of coarctation of the aorta: a review of 48 patients. *Ann Thorac Surg.* 1996;61:935-939.

111. Vriend JW, Drenthen W, Pieper PG, et al. Outcome of pregnancy in patients after repair of aortic coarctation. *Eur Heart J.* 2005;26:2173-2178.

112. Krieger EV, Landzberg MJ, Economy KE, Webb GD, Opotowsky AR. Comparison of risk of hypertensive complications of pregnancy among women with versus without coarctation of the aorta. *Am J Cardiol.* 2011;107:1529-1534.

113. Saidi AS, Bezold LI, Altman CA, Ayres NA, Bricker JT. Outcome of pregnancy following intervention for coarctation of the aorta. *Am J Cardiol.* 1998;82:786-788.

114. Roberts JM, Pearson GD, Cutler JA, Lindheimer MD. Summary of the NHLBI Working Group on Research on Hypertension During Pregnancy. *Hypertens Pregnancy.* 2003;22:109-127.

115. Ray JG, Burrows RF, Burrows EA, Vermeulen MJ. MOS HIP: McMaster outcome study of hypertension in pregnancy. *Early Hum Dev.* 2001;64:129-143.

116. Goodwin JF. Pregnancy and coarctation of the aorta. *Clin Obstet Gynecol.* 1961;4:645-664.

117. Goodwin JF. Pregnancy and coarctation of the aorta. *Lancet.* 1958;1:16-20.

118. Boissonnas CC, Davy C, Bornes M, et al. Careful cardiovascular screening and follow-up of women with Turner syndrome before and during pregnancy is necessary to prevent maternal mortality. *Fertil Steril.* 2009;91:929.e5-e7.

119. Karnis MF, Zimon AE, Lalwani SI, Timmreck LS, Klipstein S, Reindollar RH. Risk of death in pregnancy achieved through oocyte donation in patients with Turner syndrome: a national survey. *Fertil Steril.* 2003;80:498-501.

4 THE ADULT WITH REPAIRED TETRALOGY OF FALLOT

Scott Cohen, MD
Michael G. Earing, MD

PATIENT STORY

A 29-year-old man born with tetralogy of Fallot (TOF) underwent repair when he was 9 months of age. Repair consisted of creation of a right ventriculotomy, just inferior to the pulmonary valve. Through the ventriculotomy, the surgeon closed a large ventricular septal defect (VSD) and resected muscle in the subpulmonary area of the right ventricular outflow tract (RVOT). Upon completion, the surgeon placed a large transannular patch to repair the ventriculotomy.

Approximately 14 years later, he was found to have severe pulmonary valve regurgitation complicated by severe right ventricle (RV) dilation and dysfunction and subsequently underwent pulmonary valve (PV) replacement. At the age of 29, a cardiac magnetic resonance imaging (MRI) demonstrated severe RV dilation with an RV end-diastolic volume index (RVEDVI) of 200 mL/m^2, mildly decreased RV function, and severe pulmonary regurgitation (PR). His pulmonary arteries were confluent without stenosis, but he had mild tricuspid regurgitation and a dilated right atrium (RA). The left ventricle (LV) ejection fraction (EF) was low-normal (50%-55%) and his aorta was mildly dilated with mild aortic valve regurgitation. From an extracardiac standpoint, he was noted to have a left superior vena cava (SVC) draining to a dilated coronary sinus and had a right aortic arch.

Shortly after his MRI, he underwent a third surgical procedure consisting of PV replacement. Following surgery, his RV did positively remodel, but unfortunately the RV size and function did not completely normalize. One month following surgery, he developed atrial flutter. He underwent electrical cardioversion and was started on anticoagulation and antiarrhythmic therapy. Unfortunately 6 months after his last surgery, while running, he suddenly collapsed and died.

CASE EXPLANATION

- TOF is one of the most common cyanotic congenital heart lesions for which infants undergo palliative repair. There is excellent long-term survival but young adults can often suffer from multiple complications.

- This case demonstrates several long-term complications that are known to occur after TOF repair including severe pulmonary regurgitation, severe RV enlargement, and the occurrence of arrhythmias that can lead to sudden cardiac death.

EPIDEMIOLOGY

- TOF is the most common form of cyanotic congenital heart disease.

- About 3.5% of all infants born with congenital heart disease have TOF which corresponds to 0.28 out of every 1000 live births.[1]

- It affects males and females approximately equally.[1]

- Most cases are sporadic, however, the risk of recurrence in siblings is approximately 2% to 3%, and the risk of the offspring of a patient having TOF (in the absence of 22q.11.2 deletion) is 3% to 4%.[2,3]

- It has been suggested that for many countries there are now more adults living with TOF than children.[4]

ETIOLOGY

- Although the majority of TOF appears to occur sporadically, its increased recurrence in some pedigrees and in consanguineous populations implies a central role for genetics.[5]

- 22q11.2 deletion has been found to be present in up to 25% of patients with TOF,[6] and single gene mutations have been found in other patients. In up to 50% to 60% of TOF patients the casual mutation remains unknown.[4]

- TOF patients may be syndromic or nonsyndromic. Most common identified cause of syndromic TOF is the 22q11.2 microdeletion which has a prevalence of approximately 1 per 6 to 10,000 live births.[7] The 22q11.2 microdeletion is found in patients with DiGeorge syndrome or velocardiofacial syndrome.

- DiGeorge syndrome is characterized by conotruncal defects (TOF, pulmonary atresia with ventricular septal defect, persistent arterial trunk, interrupted aortic arch, isolated arch anomalies, and ventricular septal defect), immunodeficiency, neonatal hypocalcemia, developmental or psychiatric abnormalities, facial dysmorphisms, and palatal defects.

- In those TOF patients without an overt syndrome, the prevalence of 22q11.2 deletions has been estimated at 6%.[8] Major chromosomal abnormalities are responsible for the second most common cause of syndromic TOF. These include Down syndrome (trisomy 21), Edward syndrome (trisomy 18), and Patau syndrome (trisomy 13).[9]

- Smaller deletions, duplications, and single gene mutations have also been described in syndromic patients with TOF. These include mutations in the *TBX5* gene which causes Holt-Oram syndrome, and mutations in the *JAG1* and *NOTCH2* genes that cause Alagille syndrome.[10-12]

- There are 12 single genes that have been associated with nonsyndromic TOF patients.[4] Some studies have shown that these mutations can be inherited from a phenotypically normal parent suggesting either varying penetrance of the gene, or the possibility of a "multiple hit" model. However, evidence to support a multiple hit model is sparse.[4,13,14]

- Some environmental maternal exposures have been associated with an increased risk of TOF or other conotruncal defects; these include maternal pregestational diabetes, vitamin, febrile, or viral illnesses, and exposure to organic solvents.

ANATOMY

- TOF is the result of the 4 anatomic features: a ventricular septal defect, an overriding (rightward deviating) aorta, right ventricular outflow tract obstruction, and right ventricular hypertrophy (Figure 4-1).

- Many believe the anterocephald deviation of the outlet septum (the muscular structure that separates the subaortic from the subpulmonary outlets) is the primary pathologic event with the other features of TOF being sequelae[15-17] (Figure 4-2).

- The VSD is almost always large and unrestrictive, except rarely when its right ventricular margin is shielded by accessory tricuspid valve tissue or if septal hypertrophy narrows the defect. It is usually perimembranous in 80% of cases with most of the remainder having a posteroinferior rim.[15]

- Rarely there may be an absence, or near absence, of the infundibular septum. In this circumstance, the cusps of the aortic and pulmonic valves are in fibrous continuity forming the superior border of the VSD. This type of VSD is called doubly committed. There is debate regarding whether this should truly be called TOF because the outlet septum is absent or only present as a fibrous remnant or raphe. Postnatally, however, the anatomy does exhibit all 4 components of TOF as the free wall of the subpulmonary infundibulum can possess hypertrophied trabeculations and may be obstructive after the closure of the defect. Therefore, having a doubly committed VSD is commonly thought of as a variant of TOF.[15,18,19]

- The aorta will always be rightward malpositioned and clockwise rotated. The aorta may override the VSD by 15% to 95% which has led to some debate on whether hearts with an aorta overriding the VSD by greater than 50% should be considered double-outlet right ventricles. Those patients with a significant aortic override may require larger patches during repair to connect the left ventricle to the aorta.[1,15,20]

- Multilevel obstruction to pulmonary blood flow is almost universally seen in TOF patients, but with variability in the severity from patient to patient. Infundibular stenosis is present in almost all TOF patients which is likely due to the narrowed diameter of the infundibular region.[15,21] The anterocephalad deviation and hypertrophy of the septoparietal trabeculations likely play a role in this narrowing, as well as trabeculations of the anterior limb of the septomarginal band. Other levels of right ventricular outflow tract obstruction may include hypertrophy of the moderator band and apical trabeculations which may give an appearance of a double-chambered right ventricle (DCRV).[15]

- The pulmonary valve is usually thickened, bicuspid, and may cause valvular stenosis.[1] The main pulmonary artery and its branches are highly variable in their anatomy, but hypoplasia of the pulmonary arteries has been reported to be as frequent as 50%. Stenosis usually occurs at branch points from the bifurcation onward[15,22] (Figures 4-3A and 4-3B).

- TOF with pulmonary atresia is often considered an extreme variant of TOF with significant variability in pulmonary blood supply (some coming from aortopulmonary collaterals) and clinical presentation.[1] The absence of pulmonary valve leaflets occurs in approximately 3% to 6% of patients with TOF.[23,24] Despite the

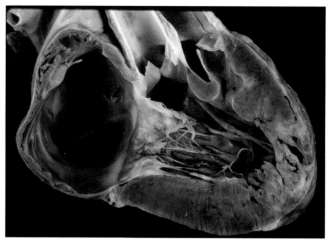

FIGURE 4-1 Anatomic specimen looking into the right atrium and right ventricle of a patient with tetralogy of Fallot. A membranous ventricular septal defect is seen with an overriding aorta. There is infundibular stenosis with right ventricular hypertrophy. (*Copyright © McGraw-Hill Education, Photographer: Dr. William Edwards.*)

Normal

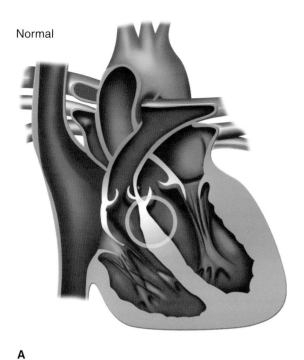

A

Tetralogy

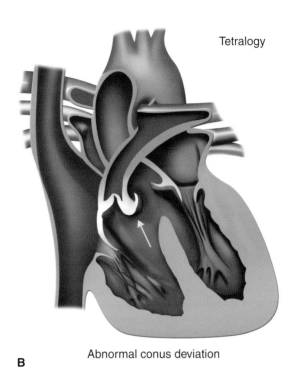

Abnormal conus deviation

B

FIGURE 4-2 Diagram demonstrating the anterior malalignment of the conus septum (outlet septum) thought to be the primary pathologic event that results in the 4 cardinal features seen in tetralogy of Fallot (ventricular septal defect, overriding aorta, right ventricular outflow tract obstruction, and right ventricular hypertrophy).

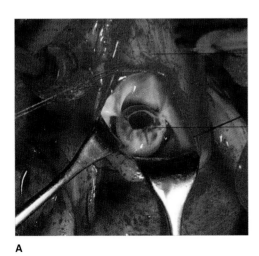

A

FIGURE 4-3A Intraoperative picture of a dysplastic pulmonary valve that resulted in pulmonary valve stenosis in a patient with tetralogy of Fallot.

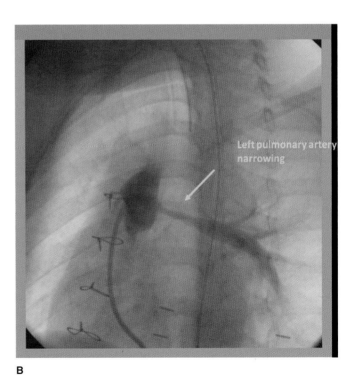

Left pulmonary artery narrowing

B

FIGURE 4-3B Left pulmonary artery angiography demonstrating left pulmonary artery narrowing in a child with tetralogy of Fallot.

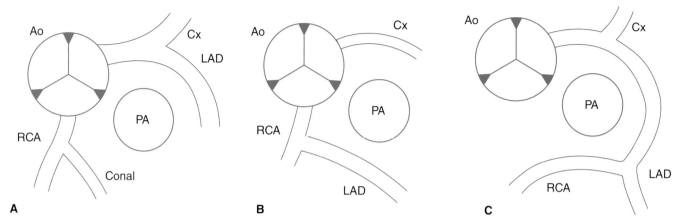

A   **B**   **C**

FIGURE 4-4 Diagram demonstrating the common coronary anomalies seen in tetralogy of Fallot. **A.** Normal coronary artery pattern with a conal branch crossing the right ventricular outflow tract. **B.** The left anterior descending (LAD) arising from the right coronary artery (RCA) and crossing the right ventricular outflow tract. **C.** A single coronary arising from the left sinus of Valsalva then splitting distal to a left circumflex takeoff into the LAD and RCA.

absence of leaflets there is still usually RVOT obstruction. This is often not caused by infundibular stenosis, but primarily by a ring of tissue at the level where the pulmonary valve leaflets would be expected. There is an association with an aneurysmal main and branch pulmonary arteries that may compromise airways and respiratory function.[25,26] In 50% of patients with this variant there is a right-sided aortic arch, and there is an association of an absent or aortic origin of a branch PA.[1]

- TOF with an atrioventricular septal defect (AVSD) should be excluded in patients with Down syndrome with an apparent isolated TOF. A primum component atrial septal defect may not be present, and the only manifestation of an AVSD may be a "cleft" left atrioventricular valve. The RVOT obstruction protects the pulmonary vasculature from overcirculation, and the patient from heart failure. Therefore, repair of an AVSD in this setting can usually be done later than those with an isolated AVSD and at the time of repair for the TOF.[1]

- Coronary artery abnormalities occur in approximately 5% to 7% of patients.[27] The most common being the left anterior descending artery coming from the right coronary artery which occurs in approximately 3% of patients (Figure 4-4). This becomes significant from a surgical standpoint if the anomalous artery crosses the RVOT as it may require the use of a change in surgical technique during repair to avoid transecting the anomalous artery.[15] A single coronary artery (usually from the left sinus) is the second most common coronary anomaly. This single artery usually divides early into a left and right branch, one of which may cross the RVOT[27] (Figure 4-5).

- In 20% to 25% of TOF patients there is right-sided aortic arch with mirror image branching[24,28] (Figure 4-6). In isolation this causes no additional morbidity, however, if there is a persistent left ligamentum arteriosum a complete vascular ring is formed. A patent foramen ovale, atrial septal defect, or a second muscular inlet VSD may also be seen in patients with TOF.[15]

PATHOPHYSIOLOGY

- The hemodynamics of tetralogy of Fallot depend on the degree of right ventricular (RV) outflow tract obstruction (RVOTO).

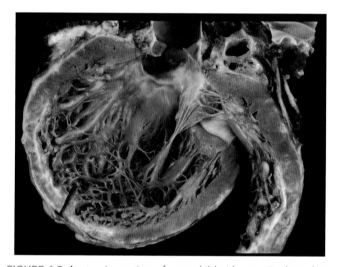

FIGURE 4-5 Anatomic specimen from a child with a repaired tetralogy of Fallot showing the left ventricular cavity with myocardial fibrosis in the anterior and apical wall segments from a left anterior descending infarction. (*Copyright © McGraw-Hill Education, Photographer: Dr. William Edwards.*)

- The VSD is usually nonrestrictive, and the RV and LV pressures are often equalized. If the obstruction is severe, the intracardiac shunt is from right to left, and pulmonary blood flow may be markedly diminished. In this instance, blood flow may depend on the patent ductus arteriosus (PDA) or bronchial collaterals.

- The wide range of clinical presentations of TOF is the result of a morphologic spectrum relating to the degree of right ventricular outflow tract obstruction. Although there is variability in the degree of RVOT obstruction, there seems to always be sufficient obstruction to protect the pulmonary vasculature from developing pulmonary vascular disease.

- Children that have severe obstruction have a large right-to-left shunt with little pulmonary blood flow, and severe cyanosis. These children usually require immediate intervention at the time of birth.

- Those children with little obstruction and adequate pulmonary blood flow may have minimal cyanosis at birth ("pink tets"), but can develop heart failure during the first few weeks or months of life as the pulmonary vascular resistance falls and they shunt more left to right.

- In addition, infundibular stenosis and RV hypertrophy typically worsen during the first 6 months of life resulting in increasing right-to-left shunting and the development of cyanosis at rest.[1]

DIAGNOSIS

- The majority of TOF patients present in infancy, but some patients can rarely present in adulthood if the RVOT obstruction is mild. In the current era, many patients with TOF are diagnosed during fetal life with a fetal echocardiogram.[2]

Physical Examination in the Unrepaired Infant With TOF

- If not found prenatally, many clinicians will suspect TOF based on the presence of cyanosis and the rest of the cardiac examination.

- The auscultatory findings in a newborn with TOF include a normal first heart sound, a single second heart sound, a loud systolic ejection murmur at the left lower sternal border that radiates to the back (due to flow across the narrowed RVOT not the nonrestrictive VSD).[1]

Electrocardiogram

- The electrocardiogram (ECG) findings in TOF patients typically show sinus rhythm with a normal or rightward axis and right ventricular hypertrophy. If an AVSD is present, there may be left-axis deviation. Because of disruption of the electrical conduction pathways during surgical repair, more than 90% of patients will have a right bundle branch block after surgical repair.[29]

- Over time, the QRS duration may increase if there are significant residual right-sided lesions leading to progressive RV dilation and associated RV dysfunction[1,30,31] (Figure 4-7).

Chest Radiography

- On chest radiograph, the typical normal cardiac size with an upturned apex (boot-shaped heart) may be seen. This is related

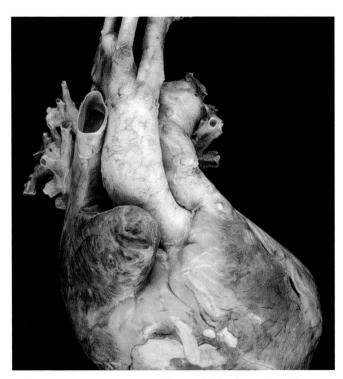

FIGURE 4-6 Anatomic specimen from a child with tetralogy of Fallot demonstrating a right aortic arch with mirror image branching. (*Copyright © McGraw-Hill Education, Photographer: Dr. William Edwards.*)

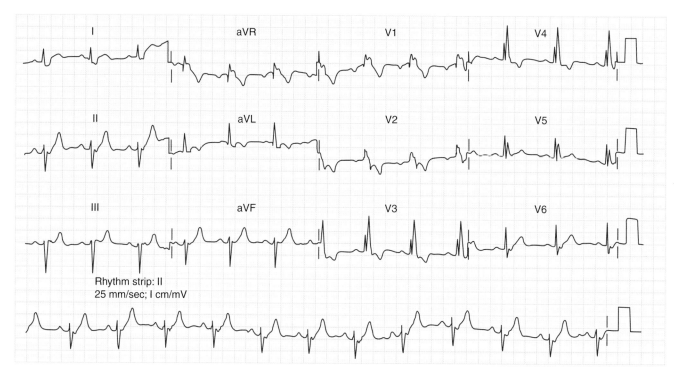

I   aVR   V1   V4

II   aVL   V2   V5

III   aVF   V3   V6

Rhythm strip: II
25 mm/sec; I cm/mV

FIGURE 4-7 An ECG from a child with tetralogy of Fallot demonstrating a sinus rhythm with a right bundle branch block and evidence of right ventricular hypertrophy.

to the RV hypertrophy, deficiency of the main PA segment, and reduced pulmonary vascularity.

- Currently, because many patients are repaired early, prior to acquiring significant RV hypertrophy, the typical "boot-shaped heart" is not seen as often. A right-sided aortic arch may be seen on the chest radiograph as a bulge to right of the upper mediastinum, and an impression to the right of the trachea, in addition to the absence of the usual left-sided aortic knuckle[1,32] (Figure 4-8).

Echocardiography

- Echocardiography is an important tool in diagnosing TOF. It is the best modality to assess for the anterior and cephalad deviation of the outlet septum, the position of the VSD, and the degree of RVOT obstruction.

- It is also a key instrument in looking for associated anomalies such as atrial septal defects, additional VSDs, a right-sided aortic arch, and coronary artery anomalies. It is of great use intraoperatively during primary repair to check the VSD closure and relief of RVOT obstruction.

- Echocardiography is routinely used in follow-up to assess ventricular size and function, atrioventricular valve competence, and to assess for long-term complications such as pulmonary regurgitation.

Cardiac MRI

- In the preoperative period, MRI is usually used for assessment of patients with vascular abnormalities such as major aortopulmonary collaterals.

- Postoperatively, it is useful in adults after repair to assess ventricular volumes and function (especially right ventricular sizes and

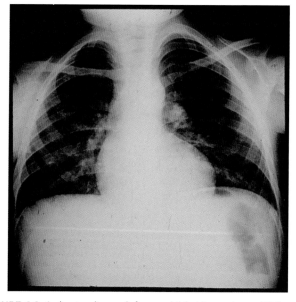

FIGURE 4-8 A chest radiograph from a child with tetralogy of Fallot demonstrating the typical "boot-shaped" heart.

function in the setting of pulmonary regurgitation), severity of pulmonary regurgitation, and pulmonary artery anatomy.

- The use of MRI is limited in patients with pacemakers or defibrillators and also in patients with arrhythmias or claustrophobia.[1]

Cardiac CT Angiogram/Cardiac Catheterization

- Invasive angiography has largely been replaced by other imaging techniques as a diagnostic tool for TOF. At times, however, it can be used to obtain hemodynamic data, such as shunt fractions and the degree of right ventricular outflow tract obstruction. Angiography may also be used to evaluate abnormal coronary arteries or peripheral pulmonary artery anatomy.

- High-resolution CT scans are a common noninvasive alternative to assess cardiovascular anatomy in patients with TOF.

MANAGEMENT

- Surgical repair TOF has been evolving over the past 60 to 70 years. In the 1960s a staged approach was frequently performed. This consisted of an aortopulmonary shunt (ie, Blalock-Taussig shunt, Potts shunt, or a Waterston shunt) early in life to relieve significant cyanosis, followed by complete repair (consisting of closing the VSD and relieving the RVOT obstruction) at ages above 4 to 6 years.

- The development of deep hypothermic circulatory arrest improved operative mortality in patients undergoing corrective repair in the first year of life.[33,34] This encouraged more centers to abandon the staged approach, and to attempt early complete repair. Initial follow-up studies suggested that early complete repair may reduce RV hypertrophy and promote pulmonary blood vessel growth.[35,36]

- Early complete repair avoided the known complications of the staged approach such as long-lasting pressure overload of the right ventricle and persistent cyanosis that may contribute to cardiomyocytic degeneration and interstitial fibrosis.[37] However, early repair subjected the infant to aggressive outflow tract procedures, the adverse effects of early bypass surgery on the neonatal brain, and a potential long and complicated postoperative course.[2,38] Currently the age of optimum elective repair is between 3 and 6 months.[2,39]

- The use of palliative shunts are now generally reserved for those infants under the age of 3 months with severe RVOT obstruction, little pulmonary blood flow, and significant cyanosis.

- The technique of complete repair has also been evolving. In the earlier eras, repair was performed through a right ventriculotomy. The VSD would be closed and extensive muscle resection would be performed in the RVOT. Because residual pulmonary stenosis was one factor that was thought to influence postsurgical mortality, surgeons frequently tried to completely obliterate the RVOT obstruction with the use of transannular patches.[40]

- Because of the growing knowledge regarding the importance of maintaining the competence of the pulmonary valve in preventing significant pulmonary regurgitation, and the detrimental effects of the right ventriculotomy, a modified technique was developed. This combined a transatrial and transpulmonary approach involving closure of the VSD and relief of the RVOT obstruction through the right atrium and the pulmonary artery.[41,42] A limited RV incision

may be required for patch augmentation of the RVOT and/or the pulmonary valve annulus.[15]

- Figures 4-9A and 4-9B shows 2 heart specimens with the RV opened. These 2 specimens are reflective of 2 different eras of complete repair.

- It is now a well-accepted practice to make an effort to maintain the competence of the pulmonary valve, therefore, leaving mild-to-moderate residual RVOT obstruction in order to avoid placing a transannular patch.[43]

- The use of percutaneous stent placement across the RVOT to improve pulmonary blood flow has been described.[44,45] This technique, however, destroys the native pulmonary valve. Therefore, it is generally reserved for very young, premature, or small infants who would eventually need a transannular patch, or in patients whose pulmonary arteries are diminutive and have an increased surgical mortality or morbidity.[46]

- Today, after corrective repair, infants have a greater than 96% rate of survival to hospital discharge.[47] In childhood, approximately 5% of patients will require a repeat operation, and approximately 6% will require further catheter-based intervention.[48] Given the improved perioperative, short-term, and medium-term mortality there is now a growing number of patients with TOF reaching adulthood. The survival at 32 and 36 years has been shown to be 86% and 85%, respectively.[49,50]

- The mortality rate for TOF patients that are unrepaired is 70% by the age of 10, and 95% before the age of 40 years. These patients tend to suffer from progressive cyanosis, exercise intolerance, arrhythmia, thrombosis, and cerebral abscess. Long-standing RV hypertension resulting in congestive heart failure or sudden death likely due to arrhythmia are the mechanisms of mortality in this population.[15]

FOLLOW-UP AND LONG-TERM COMPLICATIONS

Pulmonary Regurgitation

- Pulmonary regurgitation (PR) is by far the most common long-term complication after complete repair of TOF. Because of the past belief that complete relief of the RVOT obstruction was of the highest importance, sacrificing a competent pulmonary valve and placing a transannular patch were common. This inevitably left the patient with free pulmonary insufficiency and at risk for the development of a RVOT aneurysm in the area of the patch (Figures 4-10A and 4-10B).

- What was once thought to be benign and well tolerated, long-standing severe pulmonary insufficiency has now been demonstrated to adversely impact a patient's hemodynamic and rhythmic status. Shimazaki et al, were the first to demonstrate the adverse effects of long-standing pulmonary insufficiency on the RV. In 72 patients with congenital pulmonary valve incompetence, 6% had symptoms develop within 20 years. This number climbed to 29% of patients within 40 years, and death followed the onset of symptoms at an average of 39 months in the 3 patients that died.[51]

Right Ventricular Dilation

- The effect that chronic, severe pulmonary insufficiency (PI) has on the RV in TOF patients is influenced by ventricular compliance,

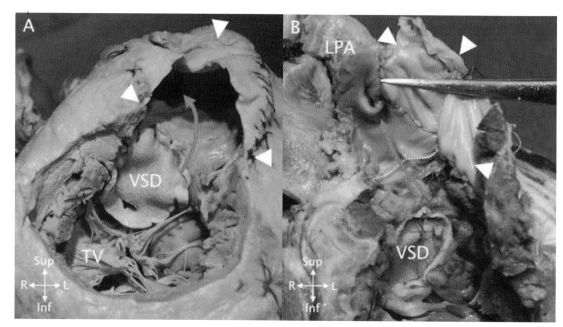

FIGURE 4-9 Two hearts after repair of TOF with the right ventricle opened. **A.** This heart was operated in an earlier era when wide patch plasty of the right ventricular outflow was the standard. Note the large patch defined by the arrowheads over the outflow (blue curved arrow). The ventricular septal defect patch (VSD) is seen between the tricuspid valve (TV) and the outflow. **B.** The outflow patch (arrowheads) is much smaller in a heart operated more recently. The patch crosses the pulmonary annulus (white dotted line) and extends onto the left pulmonary artery (LPA). (*Reproduced with permission from Stephen P. Sanders, MD, Professor of Pediatrics [Cardiology], Harvard Medical School; Director, Cardiac Registry, Departments of Cardiology, Pathology, and Cardiac Surgery, Children's Hospital Boston, Boston, Massachusetts.*)

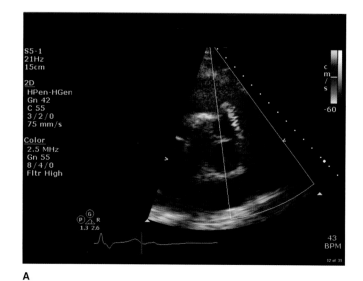

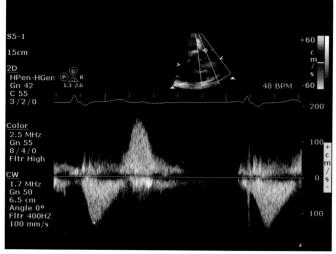

A   **B**

FIGURE 4-10A A still frame color Doppler image from the parasternal short-axis window at the base of the heart in an adult with tetralogy of Fallot and remote repair with a transannular patch. Flow reversal in the pulmonary artery is noted consistent with severe pulmonary regurgitation.

FIGURE 4-10B Spectral Doppler of severe pulmonary regurgitation in a patient with repaired tetralogy of Fallot with a transannular patch. Rapid return to baseline of the pulmonary regurgitant signal is seen consistent with early equalization of diastolic pressures between the pulmonary artery and right ventricle.

the degree and duration of the PI and particular characteristics of the pulmonary arteries (such as capacitance of the pulmonary arteries).[52,53] During childhood, at the time of TOF repair, the RV is hypertrophied and exhibits restrictive physiology, the PA is usually small with a low compliance, and diastole is usually short due to elevated heart rates.

- These factors limit the degree of PI. As the patient ages, however, the RV stroke volume increases leading to an increased diameter and capacitance of the PA. There is an increase in RV compliance and a longer duration of diastole as the heart rate decreases. Combined, these mechanisms lead to an increase in the degree of PI over time.[53] As the RV's compensatory mechanisms to handle the volume load imposed by long-standing PI fail, the RV progressively dilates (Figure 4-11).

- Progressive RV dilation has also been linked to other adverse events in TOF patients. Significant RV dilation can stretch the tricuspid annulus leading to poor coaptation of the tricuspid leaflets and progressive tricuspid regurgitation. The degree of PI has been shown to relate to RV size and exercise performance.[2,54] Both atrial and ventricular arrhythmias have been shown to be related to PI and the RV size in TOF patients. QRS duration relates to RV size and propensity to develop symptomatic arrhythmias and sudden cardiac death. A threshold of 180 ms was shown to relate to symptomatic ventricular tachycardia and sudden cardiac death.[30,55]

- In symptomatic patients (RV failure, exercise intolerance, and progressive atrial or ventricular arrhythmias), the benefits of pulmonary valve replacement (PVR) outweigh the operative risks. PVR has been shown to improve ventricular volumes,[56,57] improve New York Heart Association (NYHA) functional class,[56,57] stabilize the QRS duration, and in conjunction with intraoperative cryoablation, decrease the incidence of preexisting atrial and ventricular tachyarrhythmias.[58] However, at this point, there has been no study demonstrating improvement in survival after PVR.

Pulmonary Valve Replacement

- The timing of PVR in asymptomatic patients is the subject of great debate. Although there has been no evidence that PVR reduces mortality, the goal of PVR in the asymptomatic patient should be to prevent the comorbidities associated with the significant RV dilation seen with long-standing PI, and preserve a favorable quality of life.

- The optimal timing of PVR in the asymptomatic patient is a balance between allowing the RV to sustain irreversible damage making the likelihood of remodeling to a normal volume unlikely, the perioperative risks associated with PVR, as well as, subjecting the patient to future procedures once the prosthesis reaches its lifetime (Figure 4-12).

- The decision regarding the timing of PVR in the setting of severe pulmonary insufficiency must account for the risks of worsening morbidity and mortality that are inherent in living with chronic severe PI, the operative morbidity and mortality, and the possible need for future surgeries to replace a dysfunctional prosthetic valve.

- Cardiac MRI (CMR) is considered the gold standard for assessing RV volumes and function.[53] There have been numerous CMR studies investigating the size at which the RV will not remodel after

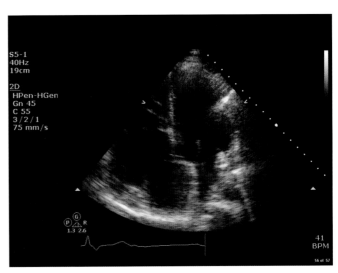

FIGURE 4-11 A still frame 2D echocardiographic image from the apical 4-chamber window at end-diastole in a patient with repaired tetralogy of Fallot and severe pulmonary regurgitation. The right ventricular cavity is noted to be larger than the left ventricular cavity consistent with severe right ventricular enlargement.

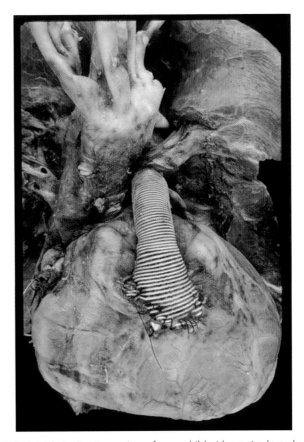

FIGURE 4-12 Anatomic specimen from a child with repaired tetralogy of Fallot demonstrating a right ventricular to pulmonary artery conduit. (*Copyright © McGraw-Hill Education, Photographer: Dr. William Edwards.*)

PVR. Therrien et al., demonstrated in 17 adults with repaired TOF evaluated by CMR before and after PVR that there was a significant decrease in the right ventricular end-diastolic volume index from 163 mL/m^2 prior to PVR to 107 mL/m^2 after PVR. It was also found that in no patient with a RVEDVI of greater than 170 mL/m^2, or a right ventricular end-systolic volume index (RVESVI) of greater than 85 mL/m^2 prior to PVR, did the RV volumes normalize after surgery.[59] In another study by Dave et al, 39 patients had a valved conduit placed when the RVEDVI on CMR exceeded 150 mL/m^2. Of these, 29 patients had a CMR 6 months postoperatively. Only 7 of the 21 patients had normalization of their RVEDVI. These 7 patients had significantly lower RVEDVI than the 14 patients who had improvement, but no normalization. They also demonstrated that the group that normalized their RVEDVI after PVR also improved their left ventricular ejection fraction (LVEF), whereas the group with the higher preoperative RVEDVI did not. This was thought due to improved LV filling by restoring the septal shift toward the RV.[60]

- These studies demonstrate the importance of monitoring preoperative RV volumes by CMR, as there is a RVEDVI and RVESVI threshold after which the RV has irreversible damage, and is less likely to normalize after PVR (Figures 4-13A and 4-13B).

- Percutaneous pulmonary valve implantation (PPVI) is a less invasive method of PVR than surgery, but its practice is currently limited due to availability and experience. It is used to replace dysfunctional RV to pulmonary artery conduits due to stenosis or PI. PPVI has been shown to decrease RV systolic pressure, RV outflow tract gradients, degree of PR, and improve RV volumes.[61]

Left Ventricular Dysfunction

- Although most think of TOF as a right heart disease, left ventricular dysfunction is common. In a study by Broberg et al, 511 adult

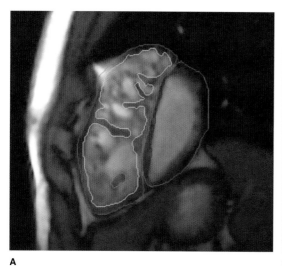
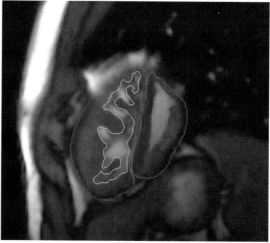

A   B

FIGURE 4-13A AND 4-13B A short-axis image of the right and left ventricles by magnetic resonance imaging (MRI) demonstrating epicardial and endocardial tracings of both ventricular cavities. There is predefined number of slices through the heart with a constant thickness. The volumes of the left and right ventricles in each slice are calculated and summed together in both end-diastole and end-systole to determine the total right and left ventricular volumes (Simpson's method).

patients with TOF repair had echocardiograms reanalyzed to assess LV systolic function. About 21% of patients were found to have some degree of LV dysfunction with 6.3% having moderate or severe LV dysfunction. Moderate-to-severe LV dysfunction was associated with male gender, LV enlargement, duration of shunt before repair, history of arrhythmia, QRS duration, implanted cardioverter-defibrillator (ICD), and moderate-to-severe RV dysfunction. After multivariate analysis, variables showing independent association with moderate-to-severe LV dysfunction were history of atrial flutter or fibrillation and placement of an ICD. However, after excluding ICDs from the model, independent variables were atrial arrhythmias, ventricular tachyarrhythmias, and shunt duration.[62]

• The mechanisms that cause LV dysfunction in repaired TOF are not entirely clear, but are likely multiple. These mechanisms potentially include adverse effects from the cyanosis prior to repair; perioperative insults (repeated bypass runs); long-term volume loading from palliative shunts; LV-RV mechanical, electrical, and neurohormonal interactions (abnormal septal contraction from a shared VSD patch, morphologic shape change of the LV due to progressive RV dilation, LV dyssynchrony related to a prolonged QRS duration, activation of the renin-angiotensin-aldosterone system from RV failure likely influencing LV shape and function), and adult-onset coronary disease.[1,62,63]

• The presence of moderate-to-severe LV dysfunction also has a significant impact on morbidity and mortality. Samman et al, found that both RV and LV dysfunction (measured by MPI) are associated with diminished exercise capacity in adults with repaired TOF.[64] Ghai et al, demonstrated that moderate-to-severe LV dysfunction was significantly more common in patients who suffered from sudden cardiac death long after TOF repair than in a control group of repaired TOF patients with a positive predictive value of 29%. The presence of both moderate or severe LV systolic dysfunction and a QRS of greater than 180 ms had a positive and negative predictive value for sudden cardiac death of 66% and 93%, respectively.[65]

Arrhythmias

• Nonsustained ventricular tachycardia (NSVT) can be seen on Holter monitoring in up to 60% of TOF patients.[15] Studies have failed to show an increased risk of sudden cardiac death in TOF patients with NSVT on a Holter monitor;[30,66] therefore, prophylactic antiarrhythmic therapy is not warranted.

• Sustained monomorphic ventricular tachycardia is uncommon, but when it does occur is usually due to a reentry circuit in the RVOT in the area of the previous infundibulectomy or VSD closure.[30] RV dilation plays a role in the creation of reentry circuits by slowing ventricular activation, and is associated with widening of the QRS complex. A QRS duration of 180 ms or greater is a sensitive, and relatively specific, marker for sustained ventricular tachycardia and sudden cardiac death in adult patients with prior TOF repair.[55] A measured QT dispersion (the difference between the shortest and longest QT interval in any of the 12 leads of a surface ECG), a marker of inhomogeneous repolarization, of greater than 60 ms has been shown to be predictive of sustained monomorphic ventricular tachycardia in patients late after TOF repair.[67]

• The incidence of sudden cardiac death is low in patients after TOF repair (0.5%-6%),[30,49] however, it accounts for approximately 33% to 50% of late deaths. The incidence of sudden death increases with age (1.2% and 2.2% at 10 years and 20 years after repair, respectively, and 4% and 6% at 25 and 35 years after repair, respectively.[50] Risk factors for sudden death include older age at repair, relative postoperative RV hypertension (compared with LV pressure),[49] accelerated rate of QRS prolongation (a likely surrogate for progressive RV dilation in the setting of long-standing PI),[30] and LV dysfunction.[65]

• Abnormal right-sided hemodynamics due to PI are very common in patients presenting with sustained ventricular tachycardia.[30] In treating ventricular arrhythmias in this population it is most important to correct any underlying hemodynamic derangement prior to proceeding with therapy directed toward the arrhythmia. Antiarrhythmic medications may be used for patients with symptoms, but their potential for proarrhythmic effects outweighs their benefit for use in patients with ventricular ectopy on Holter monitor. Transcatheter, or intraoperative ablation may be used if clinically indicated. ICD implantation is usually for secondary prevention in patients with sustained monomorphic ventricular tachycardia or an episode of sudden cardiac death.

• Supraventricular arrhythmias are more common than ventricular arrhythmias in patients late after TOF repair and a major cause of late morbidity in this population. Roos-Hesselink et al, found that up to 33% of adult patients will develop at least one episode of a supraventricular arrhythmia.[68] Risk factors for developing atrial fibrillation and atrial flutter include long-lasting systemic to pulmonary artery shunts (causing persistent volume overload) and the need for early reoperation for residual hemodynamic lesions, older age at repair, and moderate-to-severe tricuspid regurgitation.[30,68]

• Patients that develop atrial fibrillation or atrial flutter should generally be treated with systemic anticoagulation. Radiofrequency ablation, antiarrhythmic mediation, and new-generation atrial antitachycardia pacemakers are possible therapeutic options.[15]

Aortic Root Dilation

• Aortic root dilation is commonly seen in patients after TOF repair. Depending on the study, age of subjects, and location of measurement, the prevalence of aortic root dilation in patients after TOF repair ranges from 15% to 88%[69-72] (Figure 4-14).

• The mechanism behind aortic root dilation is likely related to the increased blood volume that must flow through the aorta prior to complete repair. This physiology persists even after palliation with aortopulmonary shunts.[73] Histopathologic changes have also been demonstrated in the aortic media in repaired TOF patients which also likely play a role in the high incidence of root dilation in these patients.[69]

• Although fairly uncommon, progressive aortic root dilation may lead to significant aortic insufficiency. The freedom from aortic insufficiency has been shown to be 95.1% at 20 years (84.3% in patients with pulmonary atresia vs 96.5% in classic TOF). The majority of patients with aortic insufficiency will only have a mild degree, with the prevalence of more than mild being 6.6% 15 years postrepair.[74]

- Aortic dissection is very uncommon, but there have been 2 reported cases. In both of these cases the ascending aorta measured greater than 7 cm.[75,76] Currently, there is no strict guideline dictating at what dimension the aortic root should be replaced, but 55 mm is commonly accepted as the dimension to intervene,[71] or 50 mm if surgery is being performed for aortic valve replacement or PVR.[73]

Pregnancy

- In the repaired TOF patient the risk to the mother and fetus during pregnancy, labor and delivery are related to the mother's underlying hemodynamic state. Those that have "good" hemodynamics generally have a cardiovascular risk equal to the general population.

- However, because of the increase in circulating blood volume during pregnancy, women who have significant hemodynamic abnormalities at baseline are at an increased risk for cardiovascular complications and adverse fetal outcomes. These hemodynamic disturbances include severe PI, RV dysfunction, RV hypertension, significant pulmonary hypertension (> three-fourths systemic pressure), and LV dysfunction. The adverse maternal cardiovascular outcomes include pulmonary edema, RV failure, arrhythmias and death; and the neonatal outcomes include spontaneous abortion, low birth weight, and prematurity.[77-80] Recent studies have suggested that the effects of the increased volume load on LV function (systolic and diastolic) in patients with structural heart disease, and RV volumes in patients with TOF, may persist after delivery.[81,82]

- Unrepaired TOF patients generally are at significant risk for both maternal cardiovascular complications including death and fetal complications. The elevated risk relates not only to the hemodynamic abnormalities mentioned earlier, but to the degree of baseline cyanosis. Because of the decreasing systemic vascular resistance seen with pregnancy the degree of right-to-left shunting can increase causing worsening cyanosis. In a study by Presbitero et al, 96 pregnancies in 44 women with cyanotic heart disease were studied. The majority of the women had baseline arterial saturations less than 90%. There were 41 live births (43%), 49 spontaneous abortions, and 6 stillbirths. In women with TOF or pulmonary atresia with aortopulmonary collaterals, 33% of the pregnancies resulted in live births, and 67% of pregnancies resulted in spontaneous abortions or stillbirths. Maternal hemoglobin and arterial saturation had the strongest relationship to birth.[83] Pregnant women with cyanotic congenital heart disease have a mortality reported at 4% to 15%,[15] and an increased risk for thrombotic events and clotting abnormalities.

- Vaginal delivery is the preferred method of delivery unless cesarean section is indicated for obstetrical reasons. All women of child-bearing age with TOF should receive individual preconception counseling regarding the risks pregnancy brings to both the mother and the fetus. Expectant mothers require diligent follow-up during pregnancy to assess for potential complications. A fetal echocardiogram in the second trimester and screening for the 22q11 deletion should both be offered.

Activity Restrictions

- Activity restrictions should be individualized to each patient, and typically depends on the hemodynamic and arrhythmia status of the patient. Patients who have been repaired and have good or mild

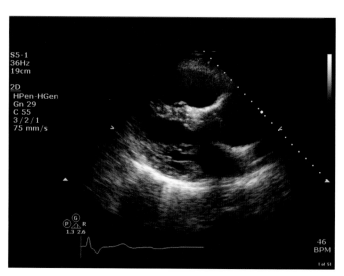

FIGURE 4-14 A still frame 2D echocardiographic image from the parasternal long-axis window demonstrating a severely enlarged aortic root (5.4 cm) in a 45-year-old patient with repair tetralogy of Fallot.

hemodynamic abnormalities can participate in various activities without restrictions.

- Those with moderate-to-severe residual hemodynamic abnormalities such as severe PI and an RV systolic pressure of one-half to two-thirds systemic with normal biventricular function can participate in light or low-intensity exercise. Those that have RV dilation and require reintervention can increase their activity once intervened upon and rehabilitation is completed.

- Those patients with significant biventricular dysfunction, exercise-induced life-threatening arrhythmias, or severe ascending aorta dilation should avoid competitive sports, isometric exercise, and limit them to low-intensity activity.[2,15]

CONCLUSION

- Tetralogy of Fallot (TOF) is a cyanotic congenital heart disorder that encompasses 4 anatomic features: right ventricular hypertrophy, ventricular septal defect (VSD), overriding aorta, and right ventricular (RV) outflow obstruction.

- Although TOF typically occurs sporadically without other anomalies, it can be present as part of a known syndrome or genetic disorder, such as Downs syndrome. TOF accounts for 7% to 10% of congenital heart disease.

- In the unrepaired infant with TOF, the pathophysiologic effects of TOF are largely dependent on the degree of RV outflow obstruction. The direction of blood flow across the VSD is determined by the path of least resistance for blood flow and not by the size of the VSD.

- The clinical presentation in the unrepaired infant with TOF, is dependent on the degree of RV outflow obstruction and determines whether there is a left-to-right (acyanotic) or right-to-left shunting.

- Surgical management for patients with TOF include several palliative shunt procedures (the Blalock-Thomas shunt) in infants who are not acceptable candidates for intracardiac repair.

- Whenever possible, patients will undergo complete intracardiac repair for all patients with TOF. Intracardiac repair consists of patch closure of the ventricular septal defect, and enlargement of the RVOT with relief of all sources of obstruction. Surgery is usually performed electively in the first year of life.

- Long-term outcome of patients after TOF repair is excellent, with estimated 20-year survival rates of over 90%. Long-term follow-up care includes monitoring and directed interventions for cardiac complications (eg, severe pulmonary regurgitation, right ventricular enlargement, and/or dysfunction and arrhythmias).

- Adult patients with repaired TOF, frequently undergo PVR (either surgical or via percutaneous techniques) with excellent results. More recently, the emphasis has shifted to preservation of pulmonary valve function as the late deleterious effects of chronic pulmonary regurgitation have become apparent.

REFERENCES

1. Shinebourne EA, Anderson RH. Fallots tetralogy. In: Anderson RH, Baker EJ, Macartney FJ, Rigby ML, Shinebourne EA, Tynan M, eds. *Paediatric Cardiology*. 2nd ed. London, UK: Churchill Livingstone; 2002:1213-1502.

2. Apitz C, Webb GD, Redington AN. Tetralogy of Fallot. *Lancet*. 2009;374:1462-1471.

3. Digilio MC, Marino B, Giannotti A, Toscano A, Dallapiccola B. Recurrence risk figures for isolated tetralogy of Fallot after screening for 22q11 microdeletion. *J Med Genet*. 1997;34:188-190.

4. Roche SL, Greenway SC, Redington AN. Tetralogy of Fallot with pulmonary stenosis and tetralogy of Fallot with absent pulmonary valve. In: Allen HD, Driscoll DJ, Shaddy RE, Feltes TF, eds. *Moss and Adams' Heart Disease in Infants, Children, and Adolescents: Including the Fetus and Young Adult*. 8th ed. Philadelphia, PA: Wolters Kluwer/Lippincott Williams & Wilkins; 2013:969-989.

5. Chehab G, Chedid P, Saliba Z, Bouvagnet P. Congenital cardiac disease and inbreeding: specific defects escape higher risk due to parental consanguinity. *Cardiol Young*. 2007;17:414-422.

6. Webber SA, Hatchwell E, Barber JC, et al. Importance of microdeletions of chromosomal region 22q11 as a cause of selected malformations of the ventricular outflow tracts and aortic arch: a three-year prospective study. *J Pediatr*. 1996;129:26-32.

7. Botto LD, May K, Fernhoff PM, et al. A population-based study of the 22q11.2 deletion: phenotype, incidence, and contribution to major birth defects in the population. *Pediatrics*. 2003;112:101-107.

8. Gioli-Pereira L, Pereira AC, Bergara D, Mesquita S, Lopes AA, Krieger JE. Frequency of 22q11.2 microdeletion in sporadic non-syndromic tetralogy of Fallot cases. *Int J Cardiol*. 2008;126:374-378.

9. Rauch R, Hofbeck M, Zweier C, et al. Comprehensive genotype-phenotype analysis in 230 patients with tetralogy of Fallot. *J Med Genet*. 2010;47:321-331.

10. Mori AD, Bruneau BG. TBX5 mutations and congenital heart disease: Holt-Oram syndrome revealed. *Curr Opin Cardiol*. 2004;19:211-215.

11. McDaniell R, Warthen DM, Sanchez-Lara PA, et al. NOTCH2 mutations cause Alagille syndrome, a heterogeneous disorder of the notch signaling pathway. *Am J Hum Genet*. 2006;79:169-173.

12. Li L, Krantz ID, Deng Y, et al. Alagille syndrome is caused by mutations in human Jagged1, which encodes a ligand for Notch1. *Nat Genet*. 1997;16:243-251.

13. Burn J, Brennan P, Little J, et al. Recurrence risks in offspring of adults with major heart defects: results from first cohort of British collaborative study. *Lancet*. 1998;351:311-316.

14. Nora JJ. Multifactorial inheritance hypothesis for the etiology of congenital heart diseases. The genetic-environmental interaction. *Circulation*. 1968;38:604-617.

15. Babu-Narayan SV, Gatzoulis MA. Tetralogy of Fallot. In: Gatzoulis MA WG, Daubeney PEF, eds. *Diagnosis and Management of Adult Congenital Heart Disease*. 2nd ed. Philadelphia, PA: Elsevier Saunders; 2011:316-327.

16. Anderson RH, Weinberg PM. The clinical anatomy of tetralogy of fallot. *Cardiol Young*. 2005;15:38-47.

17. Anderson RH, Jacobs ML. The anatomy of tetralogy of Fallot with pulmonary stenosis. *Cardiol Young*. 2008;18:12-21.

18. Griffin ML, Sullivan ID, Anderson RH, Macartney FJ. Doubly committed subarterial ventricular septal defect: new morphological criteria with echocardiographic and angiocardiographic correlation. *Br Heart J*. 1988;59:474-479.

19. Jacobs ML. Congenital Heart Surgery Nomenclature and Database Project: tetralogy of Fallot. *Ann Thorac Surg*. 2000;69:S77-S82.

20. Anderson RH, Allwork SP, Ho SY, Lenox CC, Zuberbuhler JR. Surgical anatomy of tetralogy of Fallot. *J Thorac Cardiovasc Surg*. 1981;81:887-896.

21. Van Praagh R, Van Praagh S, Nebesar RA, Muster AJ, Sinha SN, Paul MH. Tetralogy of Fallot: underdevelopment of the pulmonary infundibulum and its sequelae. *Am J Cardiol*. 1970;26:25-33.

22. Saeed S, Hyder SN, Sadiq M. Anatomical variations of pulmonary artery and associated cardiac defects in Tetralogy of Fallot. *J Coll Physicians Surg Pak*. 2009;19:211-214.

23. Lev M, Eckner FA. The pathologic anatomy of tetralogy of Fallot and its variations. *Dis Chest*. 1964;45:251-261.

24. Nagao GI, Daoud GI, McAdams AJ, Schwartz DC, Kaplan S. Cardiovascular anomalies associated with tetralogy of Fallot. *Am J Cardiol*. 1967;20:206-215.

25. Donofrio MT, Jacobs ML, Rychik J. Tetralogy of Fallot with absent pulmonary valve: echocardiographic morphometric features of the right-sided structures and their relationship to presentation and outcome. *J Am Soc Echocardiogr*. 1997;10:556-561.

26. Lakier JB, Stanger P, Heymann MA, Hoffman JI, Rudolph AM. Tetralogy of Fallot with absent pulmonary valve. Natural history and hemodynamic considerations. *Circulation*. 1974;50:167-175.

27. Gupta D, Saxena A, Kothari SS, et al. Detection of coronary artery anomalies in tetralogy of Fallot using a specific angiographic protocol. *Am J Cardiol*. 2001;87:241-244, A249.

28. Dabizzi RP, Teodori G, Barletta GA, Caprioli G, Baldrighi G, Baldrighi V. Associated coronary and cardiac anomalies in the tetralogy of Fallot. An angiographic study. *Eur Heart J*. 1990;11:692-704.

29. Wolff GS, Rowland TW, Ellison RC. Surgically induced right bundle-branch block with left anterior hemiblock. An ominous sign in postoperative tetralogy of Fallot. *Circulation*. 1972;46:587-594.

30. Gatzoulis MA, Balaji S, Webber SA, et al. Risk factors for arrhythmia and sudden cardiac death late after repair of tetralogy of Fallot: a multicentre study. *Lancet*. 2000;356:975-981.

31. Wall K, Oddsson H, Ternestedt BM, Jonzon A, Nylander E, Schollin J. Thirty-year electrocardiographic follow-up after repair of tetralogy of Fallot or atrial septal defect. *J Electrocardiol*. 2007;40:214-217.

32. Johnson C. Fallot's tetralogy—a review of the radiological appearances in thirty-three cases. *Clin Radiol*. 1965;16:199-210.

33. Hikasa Y, Shirotani H, Mori C, Kamiya T, Asawa Y. Open heart surgery in infants with an aid of hypothermic anesthesia. *Nihon Geka Hokan*. 1967;36:495-508.

34. Okamoto Y. Clinical studies on open heart surgery in infants with profound hypothermia. *Nihon Geka Hokan*. 1969;38:188-207.

35. Norwood WI, Rosenthal A, Castaneda AR. Tetralogy of Fallot with acquired pulmonary atresia and hypoplasia of pulmonary arteries. Report of surgical management in infancy. *J Thorac Cardiovasc Surg*. 1976;72:454-457.

36. Rabinovitch M, Herrera-deLeon V, Castaneda AR, Reid L. Growth and development of the pulmonary vascular bed in patients with tetralogy of Fallot with or without pulmonary atresia. *Circulation*. 1981;64:1234-1249.

37. Chowdhury UK, Sathia S, Ray R, Singh R, Pradeep KK, Venugopal P. Histopathology of the right ventricular outflow tract and its relationship to clinical outcomes and arrhythmias in patients with tetralogy of Fallot. *J Thorac Cardiovasc Surg*. 2006;132:270-277.

38. Zeltser I, Jarvik GP, Bernbaum J, et al. Genetic factors are important determinants of neurodevelopmental outcome after repair of tetralogy of Fallot. *J Thorac Cardiovasc Surg*. 2008;135:91-97.

39. Van Arsdell GS, Maharaj GS, Tom J, et al. What is the optimal age for repair of tetralogy of Fallot? *Circulation*. 2000;102:III123-III129.

40. Kirklin JW, Payne WS, Theye RA, Dushane JW. Factors affecting survival after open operation for tetralogy of Fallot. *Ann Surg*. 1960;152:485-493.

41. Giannopoulos NM, Chatzis AK, Karros P, et al. Early results after transatrial/transpulmonary repair of tetralogy of Fallot. *Eur J Cardio-thorac Surg*. 2002;22:582-586.

42. Karl TR, Sano S, Pornviliwan S, Mee RB. Tetralogy of Fallot: favorable outcome of nonneonatal transatrial, transpulmonary repair. *Ann Thorac Surg*. 1992;54:903-907.

43. Van Arsdell G, Yun TJ. An apology for primary repair of tetralogy of Fallot. *Semin Thorac Cardiovasc Surg Pediatr Card Surg Annu*. 2005;128-131.

44. Dohlen G, Chaturvedi RR, Benson LN, et al. Stenting of the right ventricular outflow tract in the symptomatic infant with tetralogy of Fallot. *Heart*. 2009;95:142-147.

45. Gibbs JL, Uzun O, Blackburn ME, Parsons JM, Dickinson DF. Right ventricular outflow stent implantation: an alternative to palliative surgical reliefof infundibular pulmonary stenosis. *Heart*. 1997;77:176-179.

46. Fraisse A. Stenting the paediatric heart. *Heart*. 2009;95:100-101.

47. Parry AJ, McElhinney DB, Kung GC, Reddy VM, Brook MM, Hanley FL. Elective primary repair of acyanotic tetralogy of Fallot in early infancy: overall outcome and impact on the pulmonary valve. *J Am Coll Cardiol*. 2000;36:2279-2283.

48. Ooi A, Moorjani N, Baliulis G, et al. Medium term outcome for infant repair in tetralogy of Fallot: indicators for timing of surgery. *Eur J Cardiothorac Surg*. 2006;30:917-922.

49. Murphy JG, Gersh BJ, Mair DD, et al. Long-term outcome in patients undergoing surgical repair of tetralogy of Fallot. *N Engl J Med*. 1993;329:593-599.

50. Nollert G, Fischlein T, Bouterwek S, Bohmer C, Klinner W, Reichart B. Long-term survival in patients with repair of tetralogy of Fallot: 36-year follow-up of 490 survivors of the first year after surgical repair. *J Am Coll Cardiol*. 1997;30:1374-1383.

51. Shimazaki Y, Blackstone EH, Kirklin JW. The natural history of isolated congenital pulmonary valve incompetence: surgical implications. *Thorac Cardiovasc Surg*. 1984;32:257-259.

52. Bouzas B, Kilner PJ, Gatzoulis MA. Pulmonary regurgitation: not a benign lesion. *Eur Heart J*. 2005;26:433-439.

53. Geva T. Indications and timing of pulmonary valve replacement after tetralogy of Fallot repair. *Semin Thorac Cardiovasc Surg Pediatr Card Surg Annu*. 2006:11-22.

54. Gatzoulis MA, Clark AL, Cullen S, Newman CG, Redington AN. Right ventricular diastolic function 15 to 35 years after repair of tetralogy of Fallot. Restrictive physiology predicts superior exercise performance. *Circulation*. 1995;91:1775-1781.

55. Gatzoulis MA, Till JA, Somerville J, Redington AN. Mechano-electrical interaction in tetralogy of Fallot. QRS prolongation relates to right ventricular size and predicts malignant ventricular arrhythmias and sudden death. *Circulation*. 1995;92:231-237.

56. Frigiola A, Tsang V, Bull C, et al. Biventricular response after pulmonary valve replacement for right ventricular outflow tract dysfunction: is age a predictor of outcome? *Circulation*. 2008;118:S182-S190.

57. Gengsakul A, Harris L, Bradley TJ, et al. The impact of pulmonary valve replacement after tetralogy of Fallot repair: a matched comparison. *Eur J Cardiothorac Surg*. 2007;32:462-468.

58. Therrien J, Siu SC, Harris L, et al. Impact of pulmonary valve replacement on arrhythmia propensity late after repair of tetralogy of Fallot. *Circulation*. 2001;103:2489-2494.

59. Therrien J, Provost Y, Merchant N, Williams W, Colman J, Webb G. Optimal timing for pulmonary valve replacement in adults after tetralogy of Fallot repair. *Am J Cardiol*. 2005;95:779-782.

60. Dave HH, Buechel ER, Dodge-Khatami A, et al. Early insertion of a pulmonary valve for chronic regurgitation helps restoration of ventricular dimensions. *Ann Thorac Surg*. 2005;80:1615-1620; discussion 1620-1611.

61. Khambadkone S, Coats L, Taylor A, et al. Percutaneous pulmonary valve implantation in humans: results in 59 consecutive patients. *Circulation*. 2005;112:1189-1197.

62. Broberg CS, Aboulhosn J, Mongeon FP, et al. Prevalence of left ventricular systolic dysfunction in adults with repaired tetralogy of fallot. *Am J Cardiol*. 2011;107:1215-1220.

63. Trojnarska O, Siwinska A, Mularek-Kubzdela T, Szyszka A, Cieslinski A. Aortic regurgitation in adults after surgical repair of tetralogy of Fallot. *Kardiol Pol*. 2003;59:484-491.

64. Samman A, Schwerzmann M, Balint OH, et al. Exercise capacity and biventricular function in adult patients with repaired tetralogy of Fallot. *Am Heart J*. 2008;156:100-105.

65. Ghai A, Silversides C, Harris L, Webb GD, Siu SC, Therrien J. Left ventricular dysfunction is a risk factor for sudden cardiac death in adults late after repair of tetralogy of Fallot. *J Am Coll Cardiol*. 2002;40:1675-1680.

66. Cullen S, Celermajer DS, Franklin RC, Hallidie-Smith KA, Deanfield JE. Prognostic significance of ventricular arrhythmia after repair of tetralogy of Fallot: a 12-year prospective study. *J Am Coll Cardiol*. 1994;23:1151-1155.

67. Gatzoulis MA, Till JA, Redington AN. Depolarization-repolarization in homogeneity after repair of tetralogy of Fallot. The substrate for malignant ventricular tachycardia? *Circulation*. 1997;95:401-404.

68. Roos-Hesselink J, Perlroth MG, McGhie J, Spitaels S. Atrial arrhythmias in adults after repair of tetralogy of Fallot. Correlations with clinical, exercise, and echocardiographic findings. *Circulation*. 1995;91:2214-2219.

69. Niwa K, Siu SC, Webb GD, Gatzoulis MA. Progressive aortic root dilatation in adults late after repair of tetralogy of Fallot. *Circulation*. 2002;106:1374-1378.

70. Mongeon FP, Gurvitz MZ, Broberg CS, et al. Aortic root dilatation in adults with surgically repaired tetralogy of fallot: a multicenter cross-sectional study. *Circulation*. 2013;127:172-179.

71. Nagy CD, Alejo DE, Corretti MC, et al. Tetralogy of fallot and aortic root dilation: a long-term outlook. *Pediatr Cardiol*. 2013;34:809-816.

72. Chong WY, Wong WH, Chiu CS, Cheung YF. Aortic root dilation and aortic elastic properties in children after repair of tetralogy of Fallot. *Am J Cardiol*. 2006;97:905-909.

73. Warnes CA, Child JS. Aortic root dilatation after repair of tetralogy of Fallot: pathology from the past? *Circulation*. 2002;106:1310-1311.

74. Ishizaka T, Ichikawa H, Sawa Y, et al. Prevalence and optimal management strategy for aortic regurgitation in tetralogy of Fallot. *Eur J Cardiothorac Surg* 2004;26:1080-1086.

75. Kim WH, Seo JW, Kim SJ, Song J, Lee J, Na CY. Aortic dissection late after repair of tetralogy of Fallot. *Int J Cardiol*. 2005;101:515-516.

76. Rathi VK, Doyle M, Williams RB, Yamrozik J, Shannon RP, Biederman RW. Massive aortic aneurysm and dissection in repaired tetralogy of Fallot; diagnosis by cardiovascular magnetic resonance imaging. *Int J Cardiol*. 2005;101:169-170.

77. Veldtman GR, Connolly HM, Grogan M, Ammash NM, Warnes CA. Outcomes of pregnancy in women with tetralogy of Fallot. *J Am Coll Cardiol*. 2004;44:174-180.

78. Earing MG, Webb GD. Congenital heart disease and pregnancy: maternal and fetal risks. *Clin Perinatol*. 2005;32:913-919, viii-ix.

79. Siu SC, Sermer M, Colman JM, et al. Prospective multicenter study of pregnancy outcomes in women with heart disease. *Circulation*. 2001;104:515-521.

80. Khairy P, Ouyang DW, Fernandes SM, Lee-Parritz A, Economy KE, Landzberg MJ. Pregnancy outcomes in women with congenital heart disease. *Circulation*. 2006;113:517-524.

81. Cornette J, Ruys TP, Rossi A, et al. Hemodynamic adaptation to pregnancy in women with structural heart disease. *Int J Cardiol*. 2013;168:825-831.

82. Uebing A, Arvanitis P, Li W, et al. Effect of pregnancy on clinical status and ventricular function in women with heart disease. *Int J Cardiol*. 2010;139:50-59.

83. Presbitero P, Somerville J, Stone S, Aruta E, Spiegelhalter D, Rabajoli F. Pregnancy in cyanotic congenital heart disease. Outcome of mother and fetus. *Circulation*. 1994;89:2673-2676.

5 THE ADULT WITH D-TRANSPOSITION OF THE GREAT ARTERIES (D-TGA)

Marc G. Cribbs, MD, MS
Ali N. Zaidi, MD

PATIENT STORY

A 29-year-old man was born a "blue baby" and found to have d-transposition of the great arteries (D-TGA). A balloon atrial septostomy (BAS) was performed as an infant, followed by the Mustard (atrial baffle) procedure. He did well for several years and did not require further surgical or percutaneous interventions. He was lost to follow-up for several years and ultimately presented to a local emergency room at 24 years of age, with atrial flutter and a rapid ventricular rate. He was electrically cardioverted back to sinus rhythm. At the time, an echocardiogram demonstrated mild systemic (right ventricular) dysfunction and concerns for narrowing of the superior vena cava (SVC) limb of the systemic venous baffle. Cardiac magnetic resonance imaging (MRI) subsequently demonstrated a mildly dilated and hypertrophied systemic right ventricle (RV) with mild global systolic dysfunction (estimated RV ejection fraction [EF] of 43%). The thin-walled left ventricle (LV) had normal size and function (LVEF of 63%). He was taken to the cardiac catheterization laboratory where SVC baffle limb stenosis was confirmed. A 36-mm max LD stent expanded to 34 mm was deployed to relieve the baffle stenosis. An electrophysiology (EP) study was also performed and revealed both atrial flutter and ventricular tachycardia. Given this, a transvenous implantable cardioverter-defibrillator (ICD) was placed for primary prevention of sudden cardiac death (SCD). He did well from 24 to 29 years of age with no major concerns and maintained regular follow-up with the Adult Congenital Heart Disease (ACHD) clinic. He maintained a regular job, got married, had two children, and exercised regularly. Closer to his 29th birthday, he noted that he was becoming "fatigued" with running 2 to 3 miles. He had rare episodes of palpitations associated with lightheadedness though he never had frank syncope or an ICD discharge. A Cardio-Pulmonary Exercise Test (CPET) was done to screen for desaturations and arrhythmias with exercise. This revealed a baseline oxygen saturation of 92% on room air with significant desaturation to 86% while running. There were no rhythm concerns. A repeat echocardiogram was done that showed a systemic venous baffle leak. He underwent cardiac catheterization with removal of the ICD leads, placement of a covered stent to relieve the baffle leak, and ICD lead replacement. Since this procedure, he has been doing well. He remains fully saturated, continues to work, and exercises often with no concerns.

CASE EXPLANATION

- This case highlights several important concepts for the long-term complications and management of adult patients who have had surgical palliation for D-TGA as an infant/child.

- These include concerns for both atrial and ventricular arrhythmias including the need for ICD placement to prevent SCD.

- These patients can also undergo both baffle leak and stenosis for which directed transcatheter interventions can be successfully performed in the cardiac catheterization laboratory.

- Most importantly this case highlights the importance of long-term follow-up and management in patients with complex congenital heart disease like D-TGA, so they may continue to lead active lifestyles as manifested by this patient having a full time job, exercising, and spending quality time with his family.

EPIDEMIOLOGY

- Transposition of the great arteries (D-TGA) was first described by Scottish pathologist Matthew Baillie in 1797.

- It is one of the most common forms of cyanotic congenital heart disease (CHD) and accounts for 5% to 7% of cardiac malformations.

- There is a male preponderance of approximately 2:1 and a birth incidence of 20 to 30 per 100,000 live births.[1]

ETIOLOGY

- Inheritance is considered multifactorial. Like many other CHD lesions, there is no known clear genetic association.

- Embryology likely involves abnormal persistence of the subaortic conus with resorption or underdevelopment of the subpulmonary conus (infundibulum). This abnormality aligns the aorta anterior and superior with the right ventricle during cardiac development.

- D-TGA is an isolated defect in 90% of patients and is rarely associated with syndromes or extracardiac malformations.

- Associated cardiac anomalies are common and most frequently include atrial septal defect (ASD), ventricular septal defect (VSD), pulmonary stenosis (PS), and coronary anomalies. While extracardiac anomalies are less common in D-TGA than in other CHD, 30% of neonates die within the first week of life without treatment.[2]

ANATOMY

- The definition of D-TGA varies among surgeons and cardiologists alike, however, it is generally agreed that it is a malformation in which the aorta arises from the morphologic right ventricle and the pulmonary artery (PA) arises from the morphologic left ventricle.

- In the majority of patients, the anatomy is atrial situs solitus with atrioventricular concordance, d-looping of the ventricles, and ventriculoarterial discordance.[2]

- In 95% of patients, the aorta is positioned anterior and to the right of the pulmonary artery,[3] hence, the term "dextro" or "D-TGA" (Figure 5-1). As a result, the circulation is parallel instead of normal in series circulation.

- In the absence of an intercirculatory shunt, especially an ASD, blood entering the systemic circulation remains deoxygenated and the infant will not survive.

- In approximately one-third of patients with TGA, the coronary artery anatomy is abnormal, with a left circumflex coronary arising from the right coronary artery (22%), a single right coronary artery (9.5%), a single left coronary artery (3%), or inverted origin of the coronary arteries (3%) representing the most common variants.

- Following are the primary anatomic subtypes:
  ○ D-TGA with intact ventricular septum
  ○ D-TGA with a VSD
  ○ D-TGA with VSD and left ventricular outflow tract obstruction
  ○ D-TGA with VSD and pulmonary vascular obstructive disease

PATHOPHYSIOLOGY OF UNREPAIRED D-TGA

- The postnatal clinical features of D-TGA are based on the degree of mixing between the 2 parallel circulations and the presence of other cardiac anomalies.

- Although, most patients present with cyanosis during the newborn period, the severity is based on the amount of intercirculatory mixing, which is particularly affected by the presence and size of an ASD.

- The following are 3 common anatomic sites for mixing of oxygenated and deoxygenated blood in D-TGA:
  ○ Atrial septal defect (most important)
  ○ Ventricular septal defect
  ○ Patent ductus arteriosus (PDA)

- Oxygen saturations and the degree of hypoxemia are largely based on the amount of this intercirculatory mixing that occurs through the intracardiac and extracardiac connections.

- The goal of optimizing intercirculatory mixing is achieved by balancing the effective pulmonary and systemic blood flows. This mixing occurs most efficiently at the level of the atria (eg, ASD) as lower pressure differences allow for bidirectional flow across the atrial septum (eg, flow in both systole and diastole).

- Mixing at other sites (eg, VSD or PDA) is more limited due to the presence of larger pressure gradients, which typically direct blood in only one direction. Shunting of blood preferentially toward the systemic or pulmonary circulation tends to result in clinical deterioration.

- Rarely, infants with an intact atrial septum can develop cyanosis within the first hours of life. Patients with a VSD or a large PDA, on the other hand, may present between 4 and 8 weeks of life with symptoms of heart failure, such as tachycardia, tachypnea, diaphoresis, and poor feeding. Cyanosis is not affected by exertion (eg, crying or feeding) or the use of supplemental oxygen.

- Reverse differential cyanosis with higher postductal saturations than preductal saturations can be found in patients with pulmonary hypertension, coarctation of the aorta, or interruption of the aortic arch. This is due to the right-to-left ductal shunting of blood into

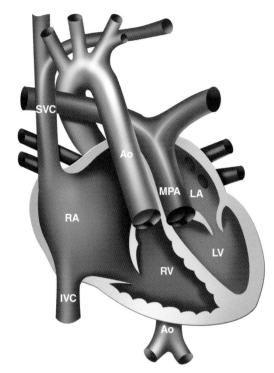

FIGURE 5-1 D-Transposition of the great arteries. Ao, aorta; IVC, inferior vena cava; LA, left atrium; LV, left ventricle; MPA, main pulmonary artery; RA, right atrium; RV, right ventricle; SVC, superior vena cava.

the descending aorta that is more fully saturated than that entering the ascending aorta.

- A small percentage of infants with D-TGA (often with a VSD) develop accelerated pulmonary vascular obstructive disease and progressive cyanosis despite surgical repair or palliation. Long-term survival in this subgroup is particularly poor.

- Without surgical treatment the majority of infants with D-TGA die by 1 year of age. Therefore, adult patients presenting to for long-term care have had corrective surgery in infancy or childhood or have had multiple surgical procedures during the course of their life.

MEDICAL MANAGEMENT OF THE INFANT WITH D-TGA

- From the time that a diagnosis of D-TGA is suspected, patients are managed with intravenous prostaglandin E_1 (PGE_1) in an effort to maintain or restore circulation between the 2 circuits.

- Side effects of PGE_1 include apnea, hyperthermia, muscular twitching, and flushing, especially with higher dosages.

- Once the oxygen saturation improves, the dosage of the PGE_1 can often be reduced.

TRANSCATHETER MANAGEMENT OF THE INFANT WITH D-TGA

- The Rashkind procedure (Figures 5-2A and 5-2B) was developed in the 1966 by William Rashkind for the initial management of the neonate with D-TGA and restrictive intra-atrial communication.[4] In this procedure, a catheter is introduced via femoral or hepatic venous access and positioned across the atrial septum into the left atrium. A balloon is then inflated and drawn back abruptly into the right atrium to create an atrial septostomy and improved circulation between the 2 circuits.

- As the trend toward earlier definitive repair has continued, Rashkind balloon atrial septostomy is now most often performed in infants with profound hypoxemia or in cases in which surgery must be delayed.[2,5]

- In 1950, American surgeons Alfred Blalock and C. Rollins Hanlon introduced the Blalock-Hanlon atrial septectomy in which an atrial septal defect was created by excising the posterior aspect of the interatrial septum.[6] Although a common palliative procedure in the past, it is now rarely performed.

SURGICAL MANAGEMENT: ATRIAL SWITCH OPERATION

- The first definitive surgeries for D-TGA were described by Åke Senning in 1959 and William Mustard in 1964 (Figure 5-3).[7,8]

- The "Senning" and "Mustard" procedures were considered "atrial switch operations" and allowed for blood to flow in series by baffling systemic venous blood to the left ventricle and pulmonary venous blood to the right ventricle (Figures 5-4A and 5-4B).

- The primary difference between the procedures is that the Senning procedure used the right atrial wall to create the baffle whereas the Mustard procedure employed autologous pericardium or synthetic material (eg, Dacron).

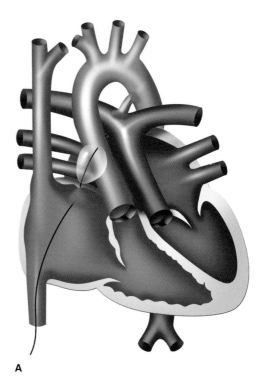

A

FIGURE 5-2A The Rashkind procedure. Via the femoral venous access, an angulated balloon-tipped Fogarty or Miller-Edwards catheter is positioned across the atrial septum.

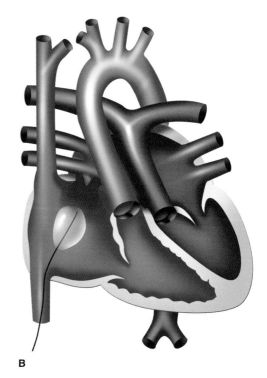

B

FIGURE 5-2B S/P balloon septostomy. Following balloon inflation with 1.8 to 4 mL of saline, the balloon is abruptly pulled back into the right atrium, thereby creating a balloon atrial septostomy.

- These operations were usually performed between 1 month and 1 year of life and, until the 1990s when the arterial switch repair became more widely used, had an operative mortality of as low as 1%.[9,10]

SURGICAL MANAGEMENT: ARTERIAL SWITCH OPERATION

- In 1975, Jatene et al successfully performed the first anatomic repair (arterial switch repair) of D-TGA.[11] This procedure involves transecting the aorta and pulmonary arteries at the level above the sinuses and positioning them above the left and right ventricle, respectively. The coronary arteries, along with a small area of surrounding tissue (called a "button"), are also detached from the aorta and sutured into place on the neoaorta (Figures 5-5A and 5-5B).

- Though technically challenging, the arterial switch operation (ASO) allows the left ventricle to become the systemic ventricle. Indeed, Mustard first conceived of, and attempted, the arterial switch for D-TGA in the early 1950s. His few attempts were unsuccessful owing to technical difficulties posed by the translocation of the coronary arteries, and the idea was abandoned.

- The ASO is now the most widely accepted operation for D-TGA and is typically performed within the first 2 weeks of life.[3]

SURGICAL MANAGEMENT: RASTELLI OPERATION

- The Rastelli operation was initially utilized for the repair of D-TGA with VSD and pulmonary stenosis by the Italian physician Giancarlo Rastelli. In this procedure, obstructive right ventricular muscle is excised and a large intraventricular baffle is sutured into place to effectively close the VSD while redirecting left ventricular outflow to the more anteriorly placed aortic valve. A valved homograft conduit is utilized to achieve right ventricular to pulmonary artery continuity (Figures 5-6A and 5-6B).

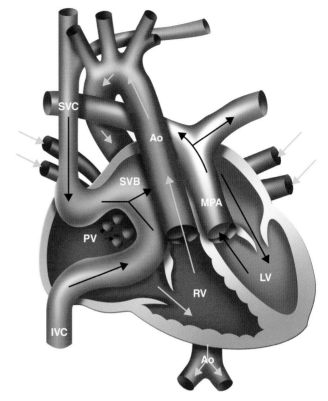

FIGURE 5-3 Atrial switch repair (Mustard procedure). Systemic venous blood (blue) returns from body and travels to the lungs (black arrows) via the LV. Pulmonary venous blood (red) returns from the pulmonary bed and travels to the systemic circulation (yellow arrows) via the RV. Ao, aorta; IVC, inferior vena cava; LA, left atrium; LV, left ventricle; MPA, main pulmonary artery; RA, right atrium; RV, right ventricle; SVC, superior vena cava SVB, systemic venous baffle.

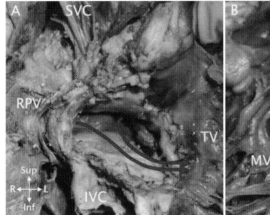
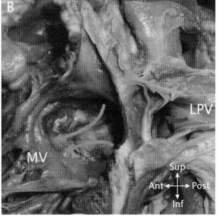

FIGURE 5-4A AND 5-4B Atrial switch repair (Mustard procedure). **A.** The opened pulmonary venous atrium in a heart after a Mustard atrial switch operation. The red curved arrows indicate flow from the right (RPV) and left pulmonary veins toward the tricuspid valve (TV) and right ventricle. The dashed blue curved arrows indicate flow from the superior vena cava (SVC) and inferior vena cava (IVC) behind the limbs of the baffle toward the mitral valve (MV) and left ventricle. **B.** The opened systemic venous atrium in the same heart showing the other side of the baffle with SVC and IVC flow (blue curved arrows) toward the mitral valve (MV). The left pulmonary veins (LPV) are seen posterior to the systemic venous atrium. (*Reproduced with permission from Stephen P. Sanders, MD, Professor of Pediatrics [Cardiology], Harvard Medical School; Director, Cardiac Registry, Departments of Cardiology, Pathology, and Cardiac Surgery, Children's Hospital Boston, Boston, Massachusetts.*)

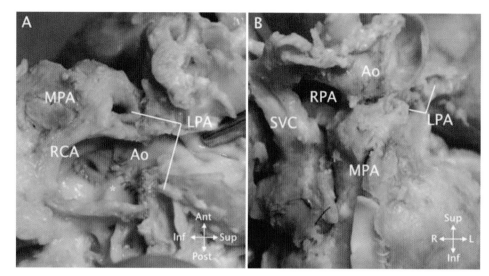

FIGURE 5-5A AND 5-5B Arterial switch operation (ASO). **A.** Left lateral view of the great arteries after an arterial switch operation. The main pulmonary artery (MPA) is anterior to the aorta (Ao). The left pulmonary artery (LPA) has been divided to show the inside of the aorta. The suture line (blue sutures) is evident between the ascending Ao and the pulmonary root (?). The right coronary artery ostium (RCA) with surrounding button of aortic wall is seen on the right side of the aorta. **B.** A frontal view of the same heart showing the MPA and branches. The right pulmonary artery (RPA) passes posteriorly between the Ao and the superior vena cava (SVC). The divided LPA is to the left of the Ao. (*Reproduced with permission from Stephen P. Sanders, MD, Professor of Pediatrics [Cardiology], Harvard Medical School; Director, Cardiac Registry, Departments of Cardiology, Pathology, and Cardiac Surgery, Children's Hospital Boston, Boston, Massachusetts.*)

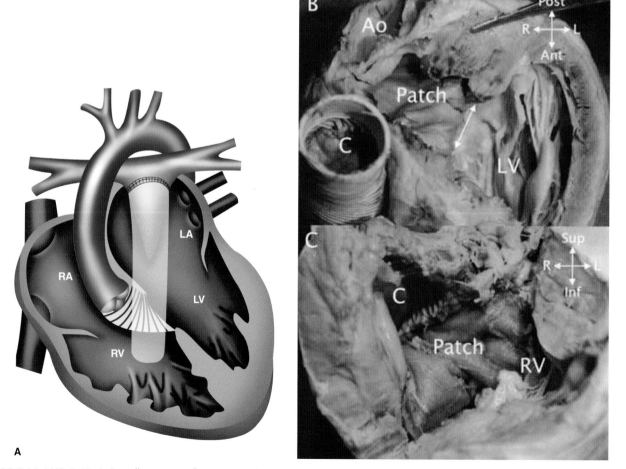

FIGURE 5-6A AND 5-6B **A.** Rastelli operation for D-TGA with ventricular septal defect. **B.** A heart specimen after a Rastelli operation shows the ventricular septal defect (double-headed arrow) and the patch (Patch) directing the LV to the aorta (Ao). The opened RV showing the other side of the patch (Patch) and the junction of the conduit (C) with the RV. (*Reproduced with permission from Stephen P. Sanders, MD, Professor of Pediatrics [Cardiology], Harvard Medical School; Director, Cardiac Registry, Departments of Cardiology, Pathology, and Cardiac Surgery, Children's Hospital Boston, Boston, Massachusetts.*)

- If the VSD is large and nonrestrictive and coronary artery anatomy makes an arterial switch operation inadvisable, a Rastelli-type intracardiac repair may be feasible.

- With the Rastelli-type procedure, waiting until the infant is older and larger may be preferred because of the need for a right ventricle–pulmonary artery conduit in the Rastelli operation.

- If the infant has excessive congestive heart failure, it may be advisable to either proceed with reparative surgery or, if not feasible, band/ligate the main pulmonary artery and place an aortopulmonary shunt during the newborn period to restrict pulmonary blood flow.

- In patients with D-TGA, with VSD and left ventricular outflow tract obstruction (LVOTO), an arterial switch operation may not be feasible due to pulmonary (left ventricular outflow tract) stenosis or atresia. If the ventricular septal defect is nonrestrictive and not too remote from the aorta, a Rastelli intracardiac repair could be possible. In this case, placing an aortopulmonary shunt during the newborn period may be necessary to establish adequate pulmonary blood flow while waiting as the infant grows older, before proceeding with the Rastelli intracardiac repair with an RV to PA conduit.

DIAGNOSTIC EVALUATION FOR THE ADULT WITH D-TGA

Physical Examination in the Adult/Adolescent Status Post Atrial Switch Repair

- Most commonly, the adult patient status post atrial switch repair will have right ventricular parasternal lift, a normal S1 and a single loud S2 (P2 is often not heard because of its posterior location to the more anterior aorta).

- Often a holosystolic murmur of tricuspid insufficiency can also be auscultated.

- In later childhood or adolescence, a high-pitched, blowing, early decrescendo diastolic murmur of pulmonary insufficiency may be appreciated.

- A blowing apical murmur of mitral insufficiency is rarely heard.

Physical Examination in the Adult/Adolescent Status Post Arterial Switch Operation

- Patients who have undergone an ASO often appear normal on physical examination.

- Rarely a systolic ejection murmur over the upper left sternal border can be auscultated due to supravalvular pulmonary stenosis. A systolic murmur over the same area may be heard due to left pulmonary artery stenosis as well.

- A diastolic murmur of neoaortic regurgitation can rarely be heard.

DIAGNOTIC TESTING FOR THE ADULT WITH D-TGA

- In patients with repaired D-TGA, a detailed clinical evaluation is mandatory and often encompasses a baseline ECG, echocardiography, exercise testing, and ambulatory ECG monitoring.

- Invasive hemodynamic cardiac catheterization with directed interventions may be indicated as well (eg, evidence of baffle stenosis or baffle leak).

- In patients with an atrial baffle procedure, comprehensive echocardiographic imaging should be performed in a regional ACHD center to evaluate the anatomy and hemodynamics.

- Additional imaging (as appropriate) with transesophageal echocardiography (TEE), cardiac computed tomography (CT), or cardiac MRI should also be performed in a regional ACHD center. Indications include further evaluation of the great arteries and veins as well as ventricular function.

- In patients s/p Mustard/Senning procedure or the Rastelli procedure, cardiac catheterization may be considered to delineate the coronary artery anatomy prior to intervention on right ventricular outflow tract (RVOT) obstruction. Direct assessment for residual VSD, the presence of pulmonary artery hypertension (PAH) (with or without vasodilator testing), subaortic obstruction across the left ventricle–to–aorta tunnel, baffle leaks or obstructions, myocardial ischemia, or systemic RV dysfunction can also be performed.[12]

- For adults with D-TGA s/p ASO, interventional catheterization can be beneficial to assist in dilation or stenting of supravalvular and branch pulmonary artery stenosis.[12]

- For adults with D-TGA, VSD, and PS, after Rastelli-type repair, interventional catheterization can be beneficial for dilation (with or without stent implantation) of conduit obstruction (RV pressure >50% of systemic levels, or peak-to-peak gradient greater than 30 mm Hg); these indications may be lessened in the setting of RV dysfunction.[12]

LONG-TERM FOLLOW-UP AND COMPLICATIONS IN ADULTS WITH D-TGA S/P SURGICAL REPAIR: SENNING AND MUSTARD PROCEDURES

- Prognosis depends on the specific anatomic substrate and type of surgical therapy used (arterial switch operation, atrial switch operation, or Rastelli procedure)[12-15] (Table 5-1).

- Long-term survival for the atrial switch operations is 75% to 80% at 25 years,[12] however, long-term morbidity associated with systemic (right) ventricular dilatation and failure, systemic atrioventricular (tricuspid) valve regurgitation, and atrial bradyarrhythmias and tachyarrhythmias is significant.[13,14]

- Despite excellent outcomes after atrial switch operation, there remains a concerning incidence of long-term complications in patients with D-TGA. These include arrhythmia, sinus node dysfunction, baffle leaks and obstruction, exercise intolerance, and right ventricular failure. In addition, sudden death has been documented in 6% to 17% of patients[15] (Table 5-1).

Arrhythmias

- Patients who have undergone the Senning or Mustard repair are at risk for brady- and tachyarrhythmias and the prevalence of these complications seems to increase with age.[16,17]

- Sinus node dysfunction is the most common cardiac dysrhythmia with up to 39% of patients displaying loss of sinus rhythm at 10 years.[18]

- Sinus node dysfunction is closely related to exercise tolerance. In fact, the maximal heart rate with exercise has been shown to

Table 5-1 Comparison of Corrective Surgery for D-TGA

Type of Surgery	Era	Early Mortality	Late Survival	Major Complications and Incidence	Reoperations
Arterial switch[14]	1980	3.8%	88% (10 and 15 years)	Pulmonary stenosis (3.9%)	4.5%-18%
				Aortic regurgitation (3.8%)	
				Coronary lesions (2%)	
Atrial switch (Mustard/ Senning)[14]	1960	16.5%	77.7% at 10 years	Arrhythmia (47.6%-64.3%)	5.1%
			67.2% at 30 years	Tricuspid regurgitation (34.9%)	
				Systemic ventricular dysfunction (11.5%-14.6%)	
				Baffle-related problems (5.6%)	
Rastelli[14]	1969	7%	80% at 10 years	RVOTO (65%)	44%
				Arrhythmias (24%)	
				LVOTO (16%)	

LVOTO, left ventricular outflow tract obstruction; RVOTO, right ventricular outflow tract obstruction.
(*Reproduced with permission from Stephen P. Sanders, MD, Professor of Pediatrics [Cardiology], Harvard Medical School; Director, Cardiac Registry, Departments of Cardiology, Pathology, and Cardiac Surgery, Children's Hospital Boston, Boston, Massachusetts.*)

be the most important predictor of exercise capacity in these patients.[3] As a result, pacemaker implantation is often necessary (Figures 5-7A and 5-7B), both for sinus node dysfunction, atrioventricular (AV) block, or to allow for medical therapy of tachyarrhythmias.

- The most common tachyarrhythmia is intra-atrial reentrant tachycardia (IART or "atypical atrial flutter") with an incidence of up to 22%.[19] In a study by Kammeraad et al, 47 adults with a history Mustard or Senning operation died suddenly. The risk factor for sudden death in this population was history of documented atrial flutter or atrial fibrillation.[20]

- Atrial arrhythmias have also been shown to have an association with deteriorating right ventricular function.[19]

- Because of the proarrhythmic potential and the lack of long-term success of antiarrhythmic medications, radiofrequency catheter ablation has become the primary mode of therapy for supraventricular arrhythmias in patients following Mustard procedure.[21] It should be noted, however, that successful ablation requires a detailed knowledge of the complex anatomy and the ability to access the pulmonary venous atrium.

Baffle Obstructions

- Up to 20% of patients with a Mustard or Senning repair will require one or more major reoperations or interventional catheterization procedures, most commonly repair of leaking or obstructed baffles. The latter has been associated with sudden death.[16] Baffle obstruction is a relatively uncommon but important late complication. It occurs most often in the superior or SVC limb of the systemic venous baffle with an incidence of 5% to 10% (Figures 5-8A and 5-8B), and 1% to 2% in the inferior limb.[3]

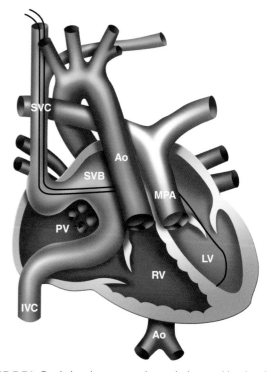

FIGURE 5-7A Dual-chamber pacemaker with the atrial lead in the left atrium and ventricular lead in the left ventricle (subpulmonic ventricle). Ao, aorta; IVC, inferior vena cava; LA, left atrium; LV, left ventricle; MPA, main pulmonary artery; RA, right atrium; RV, right ventricle; SVC, superior vena cava SVB, systemic venous baffle.

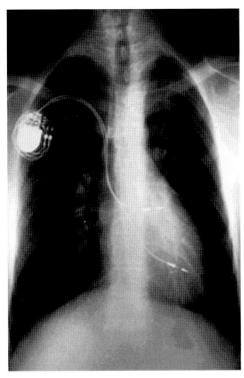

FIGURE 5-7B Chest radiograph showing the atrial lead in the left atrium and the ventricular lead in the left ventricle (subpulmonic ventricle).

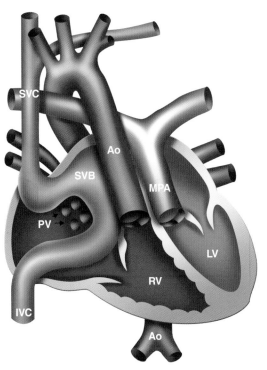

FIGURE 5-8A Baffle obstruction in the superior limb of the systemic venous baffle. Ao, aorta; IVC, inferior vena cava; LA, left atrium; LV, left ventricle; MPA, main pulmonary artery; RA, right atrium; RV, right ventricle; SVC, superior vena cava SVB, systemic venous baffle.

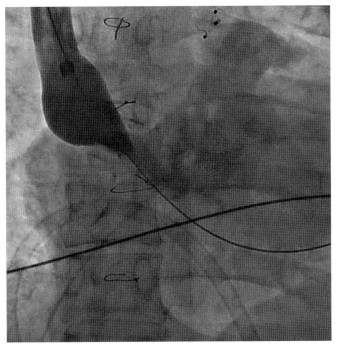

B

FIGURE 5-8B Angiography of a 21-year-old man with history of D-TGA, Mustard procedure, and superior baffle limb stenosis.

- Pulmonary venous baffle obstruction is also uncommon though the effects can be devastating and lead to the development of pulmonary edema and pulmonary hypertension. While echocardiography usually suggests the presence of baffle obstruction by a venous flow disturbance, complete occlusion can be missed by this modality. Whereas balloon angioplasty is ineffective in producing long-term relief of baffle obstruction, stent implantation appears to be safe and effective (Figure 5-8C). Cardiac MRI or computed tomography is more commonly utilized when baffle obstruction is suspected as they provide excellent anatomic resolution (Figure 5-9).

Baffle Leaks

- Baffle leaks are more common than baffle obstructions. They occur most often along the suture line of the superior limb (Figures 5-10A and 5-10B) but can be located in the inferior limb as well.
- While most are hemodynamically insignificant, the resultant left-to-right or right-to-left shunt can result in RV volume overload or systemic desaturation, respectively.
- More concerning is the risk of paradoxical embolism and stroke.
- Percutaneous intervention has been shown to be successful in most cases of baffle leaks. In rare cases, however, surgery is required.[22,23]

Heart Failure/Ventricular Dysfunction

- Systemic (right) ventricular enlargement and dysfunction is the primary long-term concern in patients with a history of atrial switch operation (Figures 5-11A and 5-11B). As shown by a study from the Netherlands, the incidence appears to increase with time.[24] In this study, all patients had normal or only mildly reduced RV function 14 years after repair. By 25 years, however, the percentage of patients with moderate or severe dysfunction had increased to 61%. Right ventricular dysfunction can lead to exercise intolerance, a decrease in New York Heart Association (NYHA) functional class, as well as atrial arrhythmias.[19]
- More importantly, congestive heart failure is now known to be the most common cause of death in patients with TGA.[25]
- Risk factors for RV dysfunction is a topic of intense research and, to date, no clear relationships have been shown. One proposed mechanism is right ventricular hypertrophy (RVH) as those with severe RVH seem to have decreased RV function compared to those without.[3] Another is the finding of RV myocardial perfusion abnormalities as shown by Millane et al.[26] Therefore, progressive deterioration in systemic right ventricular function may be related to "mismatch" between myocardial oxygen supply and demand.
- As with patients with congestive heart failure and structurally normal hearts, angiotensin-converting enzyme (ACE) inhibitors have been used in the medical management of RV dysfunction in TGA. To date, however, studies have not consistently shown significant differences before and after ACE inhibitor therapy.[27-29] It should be noted that these studies have included small numbers of patients and larger, prospective, multicenter studies are underway.

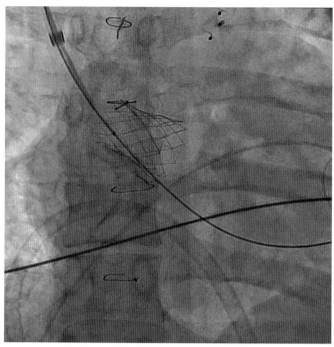

C

FIGURE 5-8C Angiography in the same patient, s/p stent implantation to relive the superior baffle limb stenosis.

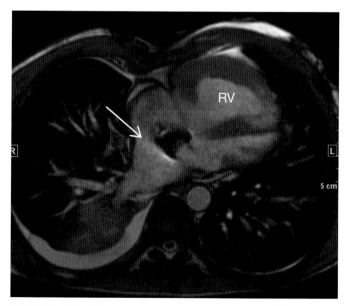

FIGURE 5-9 Cardiac magnetic resonance image (MRI) of the same patient reveals an unobstructed pulmonary venous baffle into the right ventricle, RV. (Arrow points to the pulmonary venous baffle.)

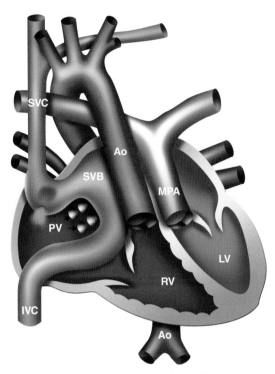

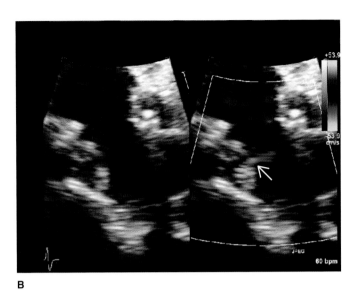

FIGURE 5-10B Still image from a transthoracic echocardiogram showing color flow across a leak in the systemic venous baffle (see arrow).

FIGURE 5-10A Baffle leak in the superior limb of the systemic venous baffle. Ao, aorta; IVC, inferior vena cava; LA, left atrium; LV, left ventricle; MPA, main pulmonary artery; RA, right atrium; RV, right ventricle; SVC, superior vena cava SVB, systemic venous baffle.

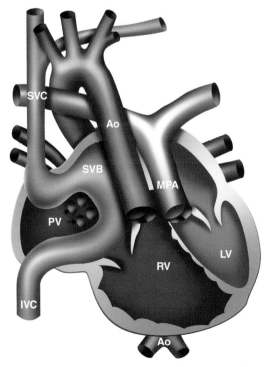

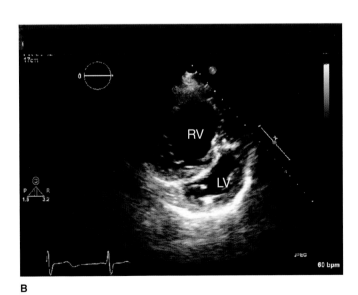

FIGURE 5-11A Systemic (right) ventricular enlargement. Ao, aorta; IVC, inferior vena cava; LA, left atrium; LV, left ventricle; MPA, main pulmonary artery; RA, right atrium; RV, right ventricle; SVC, superior vena cava SVB, systemic venous baffle.

FIGURE 5-11B Parasternal short-axis image from a transthoracic echocardiogram, showing a severely dilated systemic RV. The LV is much smaller in size. The interventricular septum has an abnormal configuration suggestive of elevated systemic pressures.

- Other modalities, including cardiac resynchronization therapy, repair of the tricuspid valve in patients with significant tricuspid insufficiency, and even late arterial switch after "retraining" left ventricle are also being evaluated. In general, the long-term prognosis is guarded and many often require cardiac transplantation.[24]

LONG-TERM COMPLICATIONS IN ADULTS WITH D-TGA S/P RASTELLI REPAIR

- Briefly, despite the good functional status reported in patients who have undergone the Rastelli procedure for D-TGA, these patients require close evaluation.

- Long-term survival (20 years) for the Rastelli operation in patients with D-TGA with a VSD or PS, has been disappointing at approximately 50%[12-14] (Table 5-1).

- Long-term complications of the Rastelli include conduit stenosis, left and right ventricular dysfunction, as well as arrhythmias and sudden cardiac death. There is a small of patients that can have left ventricular dysfunction in the presence of severe subaortic stenosis.

Long-Term Complications in Adults With D-TGA S/P Surgical Repair—Arterial Switch Operation

- In the next decade, a large number of patients who underwent the neonatal ASO will reach adolescence and young adulthood. The long-term effects of this surgical procedure are not yet fully known.

- The late survival is higher for the ASO compared with the atrial switch procedures, with fewer long-term complications[12-14] (Table 5-1).

- Early and mid-term complications include coronary stenosis of the reimplanted coronary arteries, distortion of the pulmonary arteries, dilatation of the neoaortic root, and aortic regurgitation. Coronary ischemia is a recognized late complication after ASO, with myocardial ischemia or infarction reported in up to 8% of patients after ASO. These complications are thought to be due to reimplantation of the coronary arteries (eg, coronary "buttons") during surgery.[30]

CONCLUSION

- Transposition of the great arteries (D-TGA) is one of the more common cyanotic congenital heart lesions and is characterized by the aorta arising from the morphologic right ventricle and the pulmonary artery originating from the morphologic left ventricle (ventriculoarterial discordance).

- Surgical correction in infancy, utilizing the atrial switch procedures and the comparatively newer arterial switch operations, is recommended for all patients with D-TGA.

- Complications of the atrial switch procedures include systemic (right) ventricular failure, brady- and tachyarrhythmias, and baffle-associated complications (eg, baffle limb obstructions or leaks). Older patients who underwent atrial switch procedures are at an increased risk for atrial and ventricular arrhythmias and progressive heart failure, which are the major causes of death (Table 5-1).

- Complications of the arterial switch operation (ASO) include pulmonary artery stenosis, coronary artery insufficiency, neoaortic root dilation, and neoaortic regurgitation. It remains unknown what effect atherosclerotic disease of the coronaries will have on patients who underwent ASO and these patients require long-term follow-up (Table 5-1).

- Regardless of the type of surgery, the adult with D-TGA requires careful and thorough evaluation and long-term follow-up.

- As outlined earlier, a detailed history of prior surgical repairs is critical as each is associated with a unique collection of long-term complications.

- These patients should have at least an annual follow-up with a cardiologist who has expertise in the management of ACHD patients, with periodic echocardiographic imaging or additional cardiac imaging using TEE, cardiac CT, or cardiac MRI as deemed appropriate. Periodic electrocardiograms and ambulatory ECG monitoring to screen for atrial and ventricular arrhythmias should be employed, particularly following atrial-level switch operations.

- These patients may require directed transcatheter or surgical interventions as needed for complications that may arise including, but certainly not limited to, systemic (right) ventricular failure, brady- and tachyarrhythmias, and baffle-associated complications including stenosis or leaks.

- Patients with worsening systemic RV dysfunction and CHF often have to be listed for cardiac transplantation.

REFERENCES

1. Fulton DR, Fyler DC. Transposition of the reat arteries. In: Keane JF, Lock JE, Fyler DC, eds. *Nadas Pediatric Cardiology*. 2nd ed. Philadelphia, PA: Hanley & Belfus, Inc.; 1992.

2. Wernovsky G. Transposition of the great arteries. In: Allen HD, Shaddy RE, Feltes TF, eds. *Moss and Adams' Heart Disease in Infants, Children, and Adolescents: Including the Fetus and Young Adult*. 7th ed. Philadelphia, PA: Lippincott Williams & Wilkins; 2008:1038-1087.

3. Hornung T. Transposition of the great arteries. In: Gatzoulis M, ed. *Diagnosis and Management of Adult Congenital Heart Disease*. Philadelphia, PA: Elsevier Saunders; 2011:347-357.

4. Rashkind WJ, Miller WW. Creation of an atrial septal defect without thoracotomy. A palliative approach to complete transposition of the great arteries. *JAMA*. 1966;196:991-992.

5. McQuillen PS, Hamrick SE, Perez MJ, et al. Balloon atrial septostomy is associated with preoperative stroke in neonates with transposition of the great arteries. *Circulation*. 2006;113:280-285.

6. Cooley DA HG. *Surgical Treatment of Congenital Heart Disease*. Philadelphia, PA: Lea & Febiger; 1966.

7. Mustard WT. Successful two-stage correction of transposition of the great vessels. *Surgery*. 1964;55:469-472.

8. Senning A. Surgical correction of transposition of the great vessels. *Surgery*. 1959;45:966-980.

9. Castaneda AR, Trusler GA, Paul MH, Blackstone EH, Kirklin JW. The early results of treatment of simple transposition in the current era. *J Thorac Cardiovasc Surg*. 1988;95:14-28.

10. Kirklin J. Complete transposition of the great arteries. In: *Cardiac Surgery*. White Plains, NY: White Plains; 1993:1383-1467.

11. Jatene AD, Fontes VF, Paulista PP, et al. Anatomic correction of transposition of the great vessels. *J Thorac Cardiovasc Surg*. 1976;72:364-370.

12. Warnes CA, Williams RG, Bashore TM, et al. ACC/AHA 2008 guidelines for the management of adults with congenital heart disease: a report of the American College of Cardiology/American Heart Association Task Force on Practice Guidelines (Writing Committee to Develop Guidelines on the Management of Adults With Congenital Heart Disease). Developed in Collaboration With the American Society of Echocardiography, Heart Rhythm Society, International Society for Adult Congenital Heart Disease, Society for Cardiovascular Angiography and Interventions, and Society of Thoracic Surgeons. *J Am Coll Cardiol*. 2008;52:e143-e263.

13. Romfh A, Pluchinotta FR, Porayette P, Valente AM, Sanders SP. Congenital Heart Defects in Adults: A Field Guide for Cardiologists. *J Clin Exp Cardiolog*. 2012;(suppl 8). pii:007.

14. Martins P, Castela E. Transposition of the great arteries. *Orphanet J Rare Dis*. 2008;3:27.

15. Wilson NJ, Clarkson PM, Barratt-Boyes BG, et al. Long-term outcome after the mustard repair for simple transposition of the great arteries. 28-year follow-up. *J Am Coll Cardiol*. 1998;32:758-765.

16. Gewillig M, Cullen S, Mertens B, Lesaffre E, Deanfield J. Risk factors for arrhythmia and death after Mustard operation for simple transposition of the great arteries. *Circulation*. 1991;84:III187-192.

17. Puley G, Siu S, Connelly M, et al. Arrhythmia and survival in patients >18 years of age after the mustard procedure for complete transposition of the great arteries. *Am J Cardiol*. 1999;83:1080-1084.

18. Gelatt M, Hamilton RM, McCrindle BW, et al. Arrhythmia and mortality after the Mustard procedure: a 30-year single-center experience. *J Am Coll Cardiol*. 1997;29:194-201.

19. Gatzoulis MA, Walters J, McLaughlin PR, Merchant N, Webb GD, Liu P. Late arrhythmia in adults with the mustard procedure for transposition of great arteries: a surrogate marker for right ventricular dysfunction? *Heart*. 2000;84:409-415.

20. Kammeraad JA, van Deurzen CH, Sreeram N, et al. Predictors of sudden cardiac death after Mustard or Senning repair for transposition of the great arteries. *J Am Coll Cardiol*. 2004;44:1095-1102.

21. Van Hare GF, Lesh MD, Ross BA, Perry JC, Dorostkar PC. Mapping and radiofrequency ablation of intraatrial reentrant tachycardia after the Senning or Mustard procedure for transposition of the great arteries. *Am J Cardiol*. 1996;77:985-991.

22. Balzer DT, Johnson M, Sharkey AM, Kort H. Transcatheter occlusion of baffle leaks following atrial switch procedures for transposition of the great vessels (d-TGV). *Catheter Cardiovasc Interv*. 2004;61:259-263.

23. Williams WG, McCrindle BW, Ashburn DA, et al. Outcomes of 829 neonates with complete transposition of the great arteries 12-17 years after repair. *Eur J Cardiothorac Surg*. 2003;24:1-9; discussion 9-10.

24. Roos-Hesselink JW, Meijboom FJ, Spitaels SE, et al. Decline in ventricular function and clinical condition after Mustard repair for transposition of the great arteries (a prospective study of 22-29 years). *Eur Heart J*. 2004;25:1264-1270.

25. Oechslin EN, Harrison DA, Connelly MS, Webb GD, Siu SC. Mode of death in adults with congenital heart disease. *Am J Cardiol*. 2000;86:1111-1116.

26. Millane T, Bernard EJ, Jaeggi E, et al. Role of ischemia and infarction in late right ventricular dysfunction after atrial repair of transposition of the great arteries. *J Am Coll Cardiol*. 2000;35:1661-1668.

27. Hechter SJ, Fredriksen PM, Liu P, et al. Angiotensin-converting enzyme inhibitors in adults after the Mustard procedure. *Am J Cardiol*. 2001;87:660-663.

28. Lester SJ, McElhinney DB, Viloria E, et al. Effects of losartan in patients with a systemically functioning morphologic right ventricle after atrial repair of transposition of the great arteries. *Am J Cardiol*. 2001;88:1314-1316.

29. Robinson B, Heise CT, Moore JW, Anella J, Sokoloski M, Eshaghpour E. Afterload reduction therapy in patients following intraatrial baffle operation for transposition of the great arteries. *Pediatr Cardiol*. 2002;23:618-623.

30. Losay J, Touchot A, Serraf A, et al. Late outcome after arterial switch operation for transposition of the great arteries. *Circulation*. 2001;104:1121-1126.

6 THE ADULT WITH CONGENITALLY CORRECTED TRANSPOSITION OF THE GREAT ARTERIES: (CC-TGA OR L-TGA)

Amber Khanna, MD

PATIENT STORY 1

A 45-year-old woman is referred to cardiology for a murmur and abnormal echocardiogram. She had overall a healthy life. She had 3 uncomplicated pregnancies. Although she does not exercise regularly, she had always been able to keep up with her peers. She denied chest pain, shortness of breath or palpitations. At her most recent annual physical examination, her primary care physician auscultated a holosystolic murmur at the apex and at the left sternal border. He referred her for an echocardiogram and subsequently to cardiology for further evaluation. Her past medical history included an appendectomy and well-controlled hypertension with a single drug (thiazide diuretic). She has been a lifelong nonsmoker, works as a second-grade teacher, lives with her husband and has a youngest child in college. Her physical examination revealed a blood pressure of 126/80 mm Hg, heart rate 65 bpm with normal saturations on room air. She had a diffuse apical impulse, 2/6 holosystolic murmur at the apex, radiating to the left sternal border, normal pulses, and no edema on her cardiovascular examination. There were clear lungs and no jugular venous distension. There was no evidence of hepatosplenomegaly on abdominal examination. Echocardiography revealed congenitally corrected transposition of the great arteries (CC-TGA) (with ventricular inversion) with moderate systemic atrioventricular valve regurgitation.

PATIENT STORY 2

A 2-month old infant presents for a routine visit. He was born at term to a G1, now P1 mother. His mother reported difficulty and diaphoresis with feeds. His birth weight was 7 lb 4 oz. Current weight was 8 lb 14 oz (<3 percentile). His pediatrician auscultated a murmur and refers to pediatric cardiology for further evaluation. On physical examination the infant appears to be thin, mildly ill-appearing infant but in no acute distress. O_2 saturations were 88% on room air. On cardiovascular examination, the infant had a soft holosystolic murmur at left lower sternal border and a harsh systolic ejection murmur at the right upper sternal border. The liver was 3 cm below the right costal margin. He had normal pulses and clear lungs. Echocardiography revealed the underlying diagnosis of CC-TGA with a ventricular septal defect and pulmonary valve stenosis.

CASE EXPLANATION

- These 2 cases represent the extremes at which CC-TGA, also known as L-TGA or ventricular inversion, can present.
- Patients with isolated CC-TGA are frequently diagnosed due to an abnormal chest x-ray (CXR), electrocardiography (ECG), development of a murmur, or rarely with the development of complete heart block.
- Presentation in middle age or beyond is not uncommon, and overall prognosis in these patients is excellent.
- Patients who have other associated cardiac anomalies, such as the infant in Case 2 with a ventricular septal defect and pulmonary stenosis, present at a younger age with a much more variable course.
- Management of the entire spectrum of CC-TGA is complicated by a lack of quality data to guide appropriate therapeutic options.

EPIDEMIOLOGY

- CC-TGA occurs in approximately 1 in 13,000 live births.
- Male to female ratio is approximately 1.5:1.
- Typically, CC-TGA occurs in situs solitus, which means the apex of the heart points to the left, the liver is on the right, and the stomach is on the left.
- Prior studies have suggested 90-99% of patients have coexisting cardiac malformations, including ventricular septal defect, pulmonary stenosis, and malformations of the systemic atrioventricular (AV) (tricuspid) valve.[1]
- Complete heart block is thought to occur at a rate of 2% per year.

ANATOMY AND PATHOPHYSIOLOGY

- To understand CC-TGA, and its complications, it is necessary to completely understand the anatomy.
- In congenital heart disease, the labels of "left" and "right" ventricle more commonly describe their morphology rather than position in a particular patient.
  - The "left" ventricle is a thick-walled, cone-shaped structure.
  - The "right" ventricle is thin-walled, banana-shaped structure that wraps around the left ventricle (LV) which is often not well suited to heavy work-loads.
  - The mitral valve is always associated with the left ventricle.
  - The tricuspid valve (TV) is always associated with the right ventricle (RV).

- In a normal heart, blood flows from the body to the right atrium, across the tricuspid valve, through the right ventricle and out to the lungs (Figure 6-1A). After becoming oxygenated, blood returns to the left atrium, crosses the mitral valve, through the left ventricle and out the aorta back to the body.

- In CC-TGA, there is atrioventricular discordance and ventricular arterial discordance (Figure 6-1B).
  - Deoxygenated blood from the body enters the right atrium normally; however, because of the atrioventricular discordance, it crosses the mitral valve into the left ventricle.
  - The ventricular arterial discordance means that the blood is pumped from the left ventricle to the pulmonary artery.
  - After becoming oxygenated, the blood returns to the left atrium.
  - Again the atrioventricular discordance means the blood crosses a tricuspid valve into the right ventricle.
  - Because of the ventricular arterial discordance, the blood is then pumped from the right ventricle to the aorta.

- The aorta and pulmonary artery are roughly parallel as they depart the heart. The aorta is anterior and leftward.

- The conduction system consists of inverted bundle branches and an anomalous anterior atrioventricular node with a bundle that penetrates the atrioventricular fibrous annulus. This bundle is well formed in young children, but replaced by fibrous tissue beginning in adolescence. The sinus node is positioned normally but the anatomic situation precludes normal conduction because the AV conduction tissue is profoundly abnormal. The normal AV node cannot give rise to the penetrating AV bundle. An anomalous second AV node is the functional AV conduction system in many patients, generally located beneath the opening of the right atrial appendage at the lateral margin between the pulmonic valve and the mitral valve; thus, the node has an anterior position and gives rise to the AV bundle immediately underneath the right anterior pulmonic valve leaflet. This accessory node is not always present and may be hypoplastic or nonfunctional.[2]

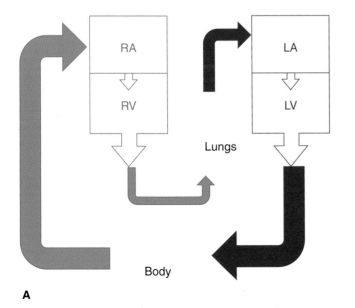 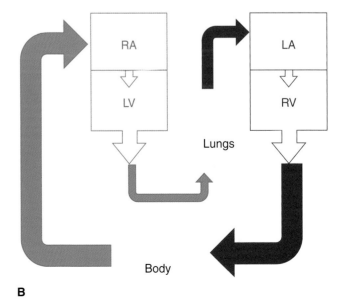

A   **B**

FIGURE 6-1 **A.** Normal connections between heart, lungs, and body. **B.** CCTGA demonstrates the primary abnormality of "ventricular inversion" where the morphologic left ventricle is pumping to the lungs and the morphologic right ventricle is pumping to the body. In the absence of associated anomalies, the patients are not cyanotic.

- Left ventricular outflow tract obstruction (pulmonary outflow tract) occurs in 30% to 50% of patients and is typically associated with a ventricular septal defect, with approximately one-third of patients also having tricuspid valve deformities.[3]

- The most common anatomic associations include the presence of a ventricular septal defect (VSD), which may be observed in almost 80% of cases (Figure 6-2) and the presence of pulmonary stenosis, which has been reported in approximately 50% of cases. The presence of a VSD causes a systemic-to-pulmonary shunt; however, this is usually balanced because of the protective effect of coexisting pulmonic stenosis.[2]

- Abnormal tricuspid valve morphology with an incidence as high as 90% in autopsy series, but clinically relevant abnormalities are less common and include dysplasia (malformed or imperforate leaflets), apical displacement of the septal leaflet (Ebstein-like malformation), or straddling and overriding of an inlet ventricular septal defect.

- Rarely coarctation and interrupted aortic arch have also been frequently reported, but subvalvular and valvular aortic stenosis are quite uncommon.

- In general, the coronary arteries follow the morphologic ventricle. A single right coronary artery supplies the systemic right ventricle. The left main, circumflex and left anterior descending artery supply the subpulmonary left ventricle. Anomalies are very common with many patients having a single sinus origin of the 2 main coronaries or from a single stem.

- CC-TGA is called "congenitally corrected" TGA because of the normal physiologic movement of blood from the body to the heart to the lungs and back to the heart. In the absence of associated defects, the patients are not cyanotic. It is a misnomer, because these patients are not completely corrected and have lifelong risks of complications from their congenital heart disease.

- The term L-TGA is frequently encountered. The L-loop indicates a left (levo) bend in the embryonic heart tube. In a completely formed heart, it refers to the inlet portion of the right ventricle. In L-TGA (CC-TGA) the right ventricle is on the left. In normally looped hearts, including d-transposition of the great arteries (D-TGA) (see Chapter 5 on D-TGA) the right ventricle is on the right (dextro).

- Because the morphologic right ventricle is on the left, and the morphologic left ventricle is on the right, this lesion is also sometimes called ventricular inversion.

- The most recent adult congenital heart disease (ACHD) guidelines use the term congenitally corrected TGA (CC-TGA). Because this term is used by most recent research publications, it is the term that is used in this chapter.

DIAGNOSIS

Clinical Presentation/History

- Prenatally diagnosed CC-TGA is rare:
  - In the absence of associated anomalies, it requires high degree of suspicion.
  - Parallel great vessels are a typical clue.

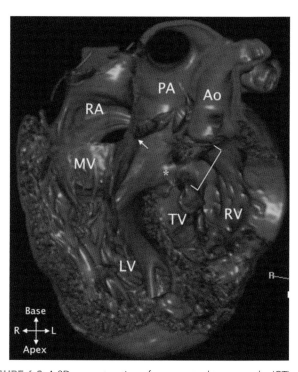

FIGURE 6-2 A 3D reconstruction of a computed tomography (CT) scan of a waxed heart specimen with CC-TGA and ventricular septal defect. The right-sided right atrium (RA) is aligned with the right-sided left ventricle (LV) via the mitral valve (MV) and the left-sided left atrium with the right ventricle (RV) through the tricuspid valve (TV). The pulmonary artery (PA) is aligned with the LV and there is mitral pulmonary fibrous continuity (white arrow). The aorta (Ao) is aligned with the RV and is separated from the tricuspid valve by subaortic conus (bracket). There is a large ventricular septal defect (*) in this specimen.

- Heart failure
  - Infants may present with heart failure if they have significant associated defects.
  - Older patients may present chronic systemic right ventricular failure. The right ventricle is not structurally well suited for systemic pressures and can fail over time.
  - Chronic tricuspid (systemic atrioventricular) regurgitation can also lead to heart failure.
- Heart block
  - Patients may present with new-onset fatigue and/or exercise intolerance due to the presence of heart block.

Physical Examination

- Cyanosis is present if there is a large VSD and either pulmonary stenosis or pulmonary vascular disease. Otherwise, patients are not cyanotic.[1]
- Jugular venous pulsation may give clue to conduction abnormalities:
  - 2:1 block will have twice as many A waves and V waves.
  - Complete heart block can give rise to cannon A waves when the atria contract against a closed atrioventricular valve.
- Palpation may be nearly normal:
  - Because of the "banana" shape of the right ventricle, the apical impulse may be diffuse.
  - Closure of the aortic valve may be palpated due to its anterior location.
  - Thrills may be felt due to a ventricular septal defect or pulmonary stenosis.
- Auscultation
  - The first heart sound may be soft or of varying intensity if there is conduction system disease.
  - Second heart sound is loud because of its anterior location. Pulmonary component of the second heart sound is soft because of its more posterior location.
  - Ventricular septal defect murmur is similar to patients without CC-TGA—holosystolic and may be absent if shunt is reversed.
  - Pulmonary stenosis murmur is softer than degree of obstruction compared to patients without CC TGA because of the posterior location of the pulmonary valve. It is located at the third left intercostal space and radiates upward and to the right.
  - Left atrioventricular (tricuspid) valve regurgitation murmur is similar to patients without CC-TGA with mitral regurgitation. It is an apical, holosystolic murmur.

Diagnostic Testing

Electrocardiography

- An ECG can provide the most significant clue of this condition with the presence of Q waves over the right precordium due to reverse septal depolarization with absent Q waves over the lateral precordium with lack of other criteria for right ventricular hypertrophy.
- Q waves also common in lead III and aVF (inferior myocardial infarction [MI] pattern).
- PR interval is frequently prolonged (Figure 6-3). 2:1 block and complete heart block may be present.

- P waves typically normal, unless severe tricuspid regurgitation (left atrial enlargement—broad, notched P waves) or pulmonary stenosis (right atrial enlargement—tall, peaked P waves)
- Bundle branches are inverted, so septal activation is right to left.
- T waves usually upright in V1 to V6.

Chest x-ray

- Often the findings can be subtle.
- Vascular pedicle is narrow.
- Left-sided heart border has a "humped" appearance.
- Severe left-sided atrioventricular (tricuspid) valve regurgitation can lead to cardiomegaly.

Echocardiography

- Goals of echocardiography are as follows:
  - Confirm diagnosis.
  - Evaluate right ventricular size and function.
  - Evaluate morphology of left atrioventricular (tricuspid) valve and degree of regurgitation.
  - Assess for left ventricular outflow tract (LVOT) obstruction or pulmonary stenosis.
  - Assess for a ventricular septal defect.
- Several characteristic features that are well identified on echocardiography are given below:
  - In parasternal long axis (Figure 6-4), aorta is anterior. There is lack of typical fibrous continuity between aortic and mitral valves. The great vessels are parallel to each other (Figure 6-5).
  - In parasternal short axis (Figure 6-6), aortic valve is anterior and leftward, pulmonary valve is posterior and rightward.
  - In apical 4-chamber view (Figure 6-7), left-sided AV valve (tricuspid valve) is apically displaced, there are chordal attachments to the septum. A moderator band may be visualized.
  - Associated anomalies may also be seen, such as ventricular septal defect or pulmonary stenosis.

Cardiac MRI

- Provides detailed anatomic and functional assessment (Figures 6-8 through 6-10).
- Requires experienced provider to accurately assess systemic right ventricular function due to complex shape of right ventricle and prominent trabeculations.
- Able to identify myocardial scarring on delayed gadolinium enhancement.
- Unable to obtain images in patients with traditional pacemakers.
- Safety of cardiac magnetic resonance imaging (MRI) in patients with MRI-compatible pacemakers is not well established.

Cardiac CT angiography

- Angiocardiography is now rarely required since imaging techniques can provide definitive diagnosis without subjecting the patient to an invasive procedure and radiation.
- Computed tomography (CT) angiography can be used to define segmental anatomy (Figures 6-11A and 6-11B) and to identify coronary artery anatomy.

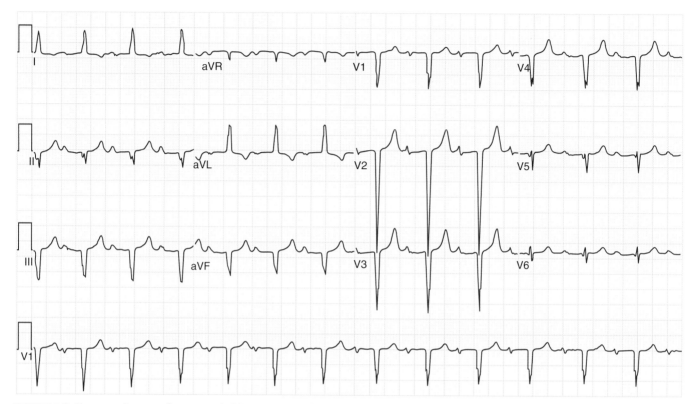

FIGURE 6-3 Electrocardiogram of patient with CC-TGA. Notice the prolonged first-degree AV block, Q waves in the anterior and inferior leads.

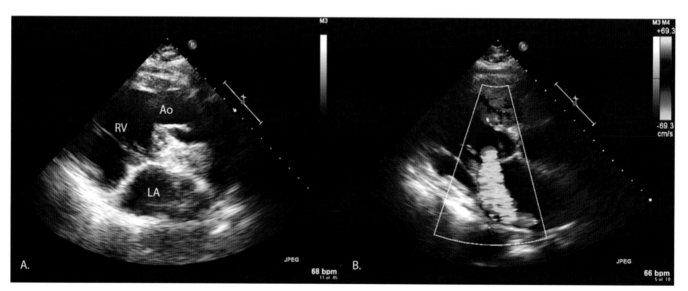

FIGURE 6-4 A. In the parasternal long-axis view, the aortic valve (Ao) is anterior. There is lack of fibrous continuity between the atrioventricular valve and the aortic valve. LA, left atrium; RV, right ventricle. **B.** There is significant atrioventricular valve regurgitation as noted by the broad color jet.

Nuclear Scintigraphy

- Useful to quantitate systemic right ventricular function.
- Evaluate for ischemia, which can be seen in older patients with late diagnosis of CC-TGA.

Cardiac catheterization

- There remains a real danger of causing complete heart block because the atrioventricular (AV) bundle is located on the left ventricular side of the septum, and because the left ventricle is connected to the right atrium, it is in the direct path of a catheter in a right heart catheterization.
- The morphologic left ventricle is supplied by a left main artery that branches into the circumflex and left anterior descending artery (Figure 6-12A). The morphologic right ventricle is supplied by the

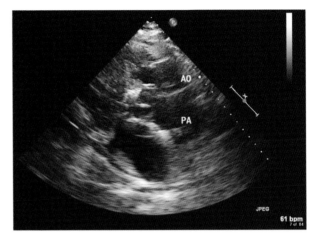

FIGURE 6-5 In the parasternal long-axis view, the aorta (Ao) and pulmonary artery (PA) are parallel to each other.

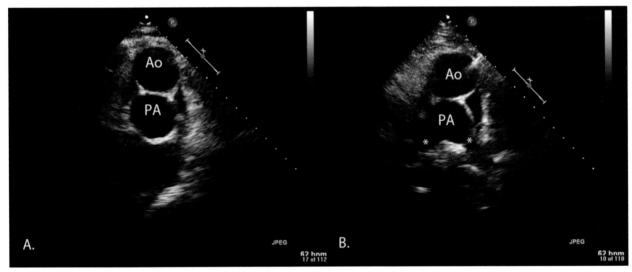

FIGURE 6-6 **A.** In the parasternal short-axis view, the aortic valve (Ao) is anterior and somewhat rightward to the pulmonary valve (PA). **B.** In a more superior view, the branches of the pulmonary artery are visualized (*).

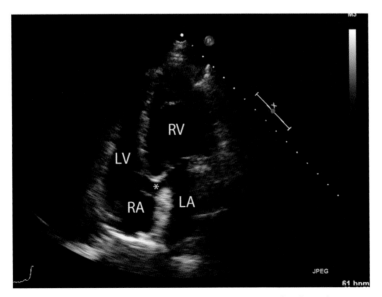

FIGURE 6-7 In the apical 4-chamber view, the anatomy is well visualized. On the patient's right, the right atrium (RA) and morphologic left ventricle (LV) are seen. On the patient's left, the left atrium (LA) and morphologic right ventricle (RV) are seen. The left-sided atrioventricular valve, the tricuspid valve, is apically displaced relative to the right atrioventricular valve (*). A bright moderator band is also visualized in the RV.

right coronary artery (Figure 6-12B). Because the right ventricle is hypertrophied, the right coronary artery is enlarged compared to the left system.

- Identifies coronary artery anomalies.

- Right ventriculogram can confirm degree of tricuspid regurgitation.

- Evaluate pulmonary pressures, particularly in presence of LVOT obstruction and/or VSD.

- Document degree of shunting with accurate assessment of Qp:Qs ratio.

- Directed percutaneous interventions, such as pulmonary artery or conduit dilation or stenting are possible.

Cardiac exercise testing

- Essential in evaluation of functional capacity of patient. Patients frequently do not realize how limited they are compared to their peers.

- Used in prepregnancy assessment.

- Used to follow patients over time to identify early deterioration in function or after intervention such as pacemaker or tricuspid valve surgery.

DIFFERENTIAL DIAGNOSIS

- Noncompaction: Prominent trabeculations are seen in both patients with CC-TGA and noncompaction. Clues to CC-TGA include apical displacement of tricuspid valve, septal attachments of the atrioventricular valve, moderator band, and discontinuity between atrioventricular valve and aortic valve.

- Patients with D-TGA after atrial level switch (Mustard or Sennig procedure) also have a systemic right ventricle, but they are easily differentiated from CC-TGA because in D-TGA, the morphologic right ventricle is on the right and the morphologic left ventricle is on the left (see Chapter 5 on D-TGA).

MEDICAL MANAGEMENT

Medical and Surgical Therapy

ACEI/ARB

- Angiotensin-enzyme inhibitors (ACEIs)/angiotensin receptor blockers (ARBs) and beta-blockers are the mainstays of medical management of left ventricular systolic dysfunction, but their benefit is unproven in CC-TGA.

- In 2 randomized trials of patients with systemic right ventricles (CC-TGA or D-TGA status post atrial switch), ARBs were not associated with improvement in right ventricular ejection fraction or exercise duration.[4]

- No specific harm was associated with ACEIs or ARBs. Although their routine use is probably not justified, it is reasonable, especially if the patient has hypertension.

Beta-blocker

- Beta-blockers have been shown to show modest improvement in ejection fraction with no significant improvement in oxygen consumption.[5]

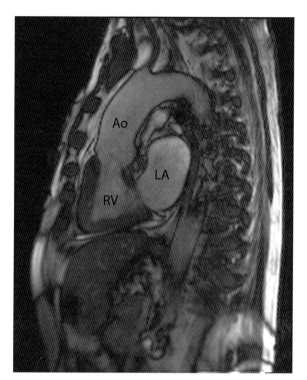

FIGURE 6-8 Magnetic resonance imaging (MRI) demonstrating the morphologic right ventricle (RV) with connections to the left atrium (LA) and aorta (Ao).

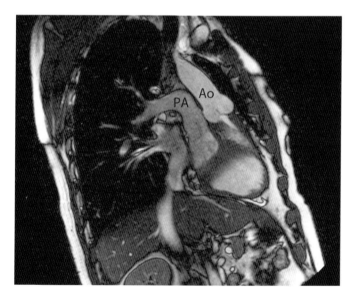

FIGURE 6-9 Magnetic resonance imaging (MRI) of the aorta (Ao) and the pulmonary artery (PA) in parallel.

- Potential benefit of beta-blockers must be weighed against effects on the AV node in patients at high risk of AV block.

Diuretics

- Diuretics have not been studied extensively, but remain essential in volume overloaded patients.

SURGICAL MANAGEMENT

- For patients that need surgery the type of operation will vary according to the associated defects.
- Possible surgical repair consists of the double-switch procedure (atrial and arterial level switches).
  - Venous return is redirected using a Mustard or Sennig procedure which uses baffles to shunt superior and inferior vena cava blood to the left atrium and shunts pulmonary venous return to the right atrium.
  - An arterial switch uses the Jatene procedure in which the aorta and pulmonary artery are transected and exchanged in position. The coronary arteries are reimplanted into the neoaorta.
  - The result of both switches is a right-sided, systemic left ventricle pumping to the body.
  - Surgery in infancy is associated with good long-term prognosis. It is not routinely done in adults due to higher complication rates. It can be considered in patients with significant, long-standing LVOT obstruction and the subpulmonary ventricle is "trained" against higher pressures.[6]

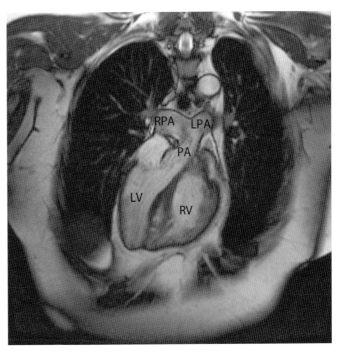

FIGURE 6-10 Magnetic resonance imaging (MRI) of the left ventricle (LV) with connection to the pulmonary artery (PA) and branch pulmonary arteries (LPA, left pulmonary artery; RPA, right pulmonary artery). The trabeculated morphologic right ventricle (RV) is also seen.

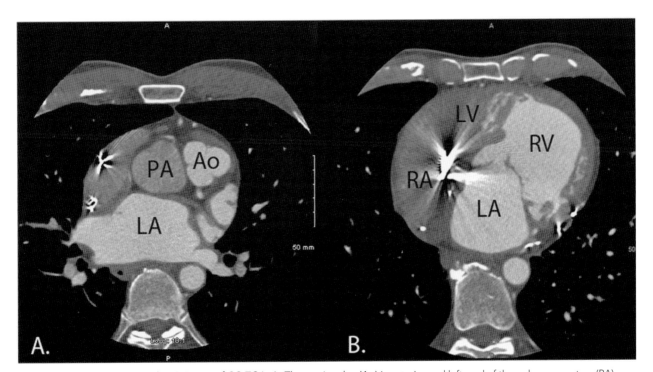

FIGURE 6-11 Computed tomography (CT) scan of CC-TGA. **A.** The aortic valve (Ao) is anterior and leftward of the pulmonary artery (PA). Pulmonary veins are draining into the left atrium (LA). **B.** The left ventricle (LV) is anterior to the right ventricle (RV). The artifact in the right atrium (RA) and LV is from pacing leads.

- Alternative surgery in patients with a ventricular septal defect and LVOT obstruction is a Rastelli procedure along with a Mustard/Sennig procedure (atrial switch). A Rastelli procedure involves an intraventricular baffle to shunt left ventricular blood flow across the ventricular septal defect and out the aorta. A right ventricle to pulmonary conduit is typically necessary. This procedure is associated with good long-term functional outcomes, but reoperations are common.

- In previously unrepaired adults, surgical interventions are focused on the systemic tricuspid valve.
  - In patients with progressive symptoms or right ventricular dysfunction, tricuspid valve disease should be aggressively evaluated. It can be underappreciated on echocardiography.
  - Similar to mitral valve regurgitation in patients with systemic left ventricles, surgery should be done before there is significant ventricular dysfunction.
  - Preoperative right ventricular function predicts outcomes. Surgery should be considered before the right ventricular ejection fraction falls below 40% to 45%.
  - In one retrospective review of 46 patients with congenitally corrected transposition who underwent tricuspid valve replacement for tricuspid regurgitation, the preoperative systemic ventricle ejection fraction (SVEF) was the only independent predictor of the postoperative SVEF after more than a year. The late SVEF was preserved (defined as ≥40%) in 63% of patients who underwent surgery with an SVEF greater than or equal to 40% compared with 10.5% of patients who underwent surgery with an SVEF less than 40%. Hence, the authors of this study suggested considering tricuspid valve replacement earlier while the SVEF is still above 40% and the subpulmonary ventricular pressure below 50 mm Hg.[7]

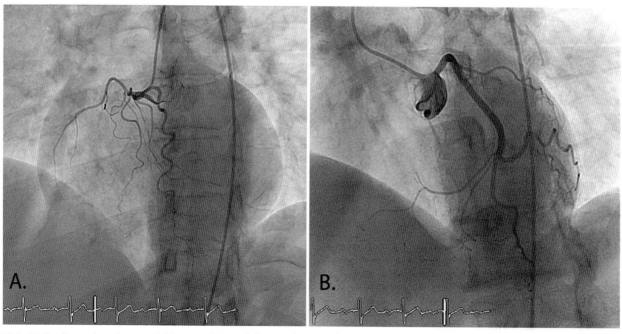

FIGURE 6-12 Cardiac catheterization. **A.** The morphologic left ventricle is supplied by a left main, left anterior descending and circumflex. **B.** The morphologic right ventricle is supplied by a right coronary artery.

- All surgery on patients with CC-TGA should be done by surgeons with experience in congenital heart disease, at adult congenital heart disease centers.

LONG-TERM COMPLICATIONS/FOLLOW-UP

- As the presentation of CC-TGA is variable, so is the long-term prognosis. The long-term outcomes for surgical repair for CC-TGA are outlined in Table 6-1.[8-13]
- Studies on long-term prognosis of uncomplicated CC-TGA are limited by referral bias.
- Survival to the seventh and eighth decade has been reported.
- Major postoperative residual complications include the following:
  - Complete heart block
  - Atrial or ventricular arrhythmias
  - Progressive tricuspid (systemic AV) regurgitation
  - Contractile dysfunction of the systemic right ventricle
  - Long-term postoperative conduit or homograft dysfunction

Heart Block/Arrhythmias

- Complete heart block occurs in 30% of patients and may be present at birth or develop at a rate of 2% per year. Other conduction disturbances described include sick sinus syndrome, atrial flutter, reentrant AV tachycardia due to an accessory pathway along the tricuspid valve annulus, and ventricular tachycardia. Surgical

Table 6-1 Outcomes for Surgical Repair for CTGA

Lead Author	Year	Patients	Outcomes
Lundstrom[9]	1990	111 patients from Hospital for Sick Children and National Heart of whom 51 underwent surgery	• Operative mortality: 11/51 (22%) • Dilated systemic ventricle is a risk factor for a poor outcome
Termignon[10]	1996	52 patients from Laennec Hospital, Paris	• Operative mortality: 15% • Survival: 83% at 1 year, 55% at 10 years (for patients with associated VSD/LVOTO) while those with only associated VSD had 71% survival at 10 years
van Son[11]	1995	40 patients from Mayo Clinic	• Operative mortality 10% • Survival: 78% at 5 years, 61% at 10 years • RVEF >44% favored survival
Yeh[12]	1999	127 patients underwent surgery at Hospital for Sick Children, median age at operation was 8 years	• Operative mortality 6% • Survival: 48% at 20 years
Hraska[13]	2005	123 patients underwent surgery at Children's Hospital Boston, median age at operation was 7.9 years	• Survival: 84% at 1 year, 75% at 5 years, 68% at 10 years, and 61% at 15 years • In patients who underwent a two ventricle repair • Ebstein malformation of the tricuspid valve is a risk factor for RV dysfunction

LVOTO, left ventricular outflow tract obstruction; RV, right ventricle; RVEF, right ventricular ejection fraction; TVR, tricuspid valve replacement; V, ventricle; VSD, ventricular septal defect.

intervention also increases the risk of this condition because the conduction tissue is fragile and in an abnormal position.

- Traditional dual-chamber pacemakers have leads in the right atrium and subpulmonic left ventricle.

- Pacing in the left ventricle can lead to dyssynchrony of the systemic right ventricle leading to progressive right ventricular dysfunction.

- Some patients have had symptomatic improvement with biventricular pacing, although anomalies of the coronary sinus are common. Devices should be inserted in experienced centers though results for biventricular pacing have been equivocal at best.

- Sudden death has been reported and may be related to the onset of complete heart block or atrial or ventricular arrhythmias.

Systemic (Tricuspid) Atrioventricular Valve Regurgitation

- Although it appears that systemic atrioventricular valve (tricuspid) regurgitation plays a role in the determination of RV dysfunction and congestive heart failure (CHF), it is extremely difficult to estimate whether this abnormality plays a primary or a secondary role.

- Prieto and associates in a cohort of 40 patients with CC-TGA found tricuspid regurgitation to be a major risk factor for systemic ventricular dysfunction during a follow-up of 7 to 36 years (mean 20 years).[14]

- Although the timing of tricuspid valve surgery beyond adolescence is still a matter of debate, mortality is low after tricuspid surgery in adult patients with mild-to-moderate right ventricular dysfunction; both tricuspid valve function and functional class significantly improve after surgery. However, an increased risk of RV dysfunction and CHF after TV surgery has been reported, possibly related to an increase in afterload and/or difficulty in myocardial protection during surgery.

Right (Systemic) Ventricular Dysfunction

- The right ventricle is morphologically different from the left ventricle and, in normally formed hearts, only sustains pressures that are one-fourth to one-fifth of that of the systemic circulation.

- Right ventricular failure can develop over time. It is postulated that this may be related to coronary perfusion mismatch as the right ventricle is often supplied by a single coronary artery. There are also differences in right and left ventricular fiber orientation, geometry, and cellular structural features which may play a role in early failure of the right ventricle when functioning as the systemic ventricle.

- Poor prognostic indicators include cyanosis, polycythemia, pulmonary vascular obstructive disease, tricuspid regurgitation, younger age at surgery, larger preoperative shunt size, and lower right ventricular ejection fraction.

- A multicenter series of 182 patients found that 25% of patients with uncomplicated CC-TGA have evidence of congestive heart failure by age 45.

Pregnancy

- Women should consult with an experienced cardiologist and high-risk maternal fetal medicine provider prior to conception.

- Evaluation should include history, physical examination, assessment of right ventricular size and function, assessment of systemic tricuspid valve function, and an exercise test.

- Predictors of poor outcomes include right ventricular ejection fraction less than 40%, functional aerobic capacity less than 75% predicted, more than mild tricuspid regurgitation, and cyanosis.[1,3]

- Risks include arrhythmias, heart failure, progressive right ventricular dysfunction, progressive tricuspid regurgitation, small for gestational age infants.[15-18]

- The genetics of CC-TGA is not fully understood. One study identified one offspring out of 27 had congenital heart disease.[15] Another study found none out of 50 live offspring had congenital heart disease. It is reasonable to offer prenatal echocardiogram to pregnant women.[16]

CONCLUSION

- As the presentation of CC-TGA is variable, so is the long-term prognosis.

- Studies on long-term prognosis of uncomplicated CC-TGA are limited by referral bias.

- Although some patients with this congenital abnormality continue to do extremely well beyond age 60, this circumstance is the exception rather than the rule.

- Heart block, progressive right ventricular dysfunction, and tricuspid regurgitation become more common with increasing age.

- Systemic ventricular dysfunction and clinical CHF are common in middle-aged adults with CC-TGA.

- Aggressive medical treatment with afterload reduction would appear indicated for these patients with ventricular enlargement and early symptoms; however, the benefits of the prophylactic use of vasodilators are unproven, but deserve study in an attempt to delay or prevent systemic ventricular dysfunction.

- Patients with favorable anatomy, depressed RV function, and normal LV function should be considered for the double-switch operation by centers with experience and expertise in this procedure.[19]

- Patients may have been given exercise restrictions in the past, however, regular aerobic physical activity is likely to be helpful.[20]

- All patients should be followed regularly by cardiologists with training and expertise in adult congenital heart disease.

REFERENCES

1. Hornung TS, Calder L. Congenitally corrected transposition of the great arteries. *Heart*. 2010;96:1154-1161.

2. Perloff JK. Congenitally corrected transposition of the great arteries. In: Perloff JK, ed. *The Clinical Recognition of Congenital Heart Disease*. 5th ed. Philadelphia, PA: Elsevier; 2003:62-80.

3. Graham TP, Markham LW. Congenitally corrected transposition of the great arteries. In: Gatzoulis MA, Webb GD, Daubeney

PEF, eds. *Diagnosis and Management of Adult Congenital Heart Disease*. 2nd ed. Philadelphia, PA: Elsevier; 2011:371-377.

4. Dore A, Houde C, Chan KL, et al. Angiotensin receptor blockade and exercise capacity in adults with systemic right ventricles: a multicenter, randomized, placebo-controlled clinical trial. *Circulation*. 2005;112:2411-2416.

5. Giardini A, Lovato L, Donti A, et al. A pilot study on the effects of carvedilol on right ventricular remodelling and exercise tolerance in patients with systemic right ventricle. *Int J Cardiol*. 2007;114:241-246.

6. Hiramatsu T, Matsumura G, Konuma T, Yamazaki K, Kurosawa H, Imai Y. Long-term prognosis of double-switch operation for congenitally corrected transposition of the great arteries. *Eur J Cardiothorac Surg*. 2012;42:1004-1008.

7. Mongeon FP, Connolly HM, Dearani JA, Li Z, Warnes CA. Congenitally corrected transposition of the great arteries ventricular function at the time of systemic atrioventricular valve replacement predicts long-term ventricular function. *J Am Coll Cardiol*. 2011;57:2008-2017.

8. Romfh A, Pluchinotta FR, Porayette P, Valente AM, Sanders SP. Congenital Heart Defects in Adults: A Field Guide for Cardiologists. *J Clin Exp Cardiolog*. 2012;(suppl 8). pii:007.

9. Lundstrom U, Bull C, Wyse RK, Somerville J. The natural and "unnatural" history of congenitally corrected transposition. *Am J Cardiol*. 1990;65:1222-1229.

10. Termignon JL, Leca F, Vouhe PR, et al. "Classic" repair of congenitally corrected transposition and ventricular septal defect. *Ann Thorac Surg*. 1996;62:199-206.

11. van Son JA, Danielson GK, Huhta JC, et al. Late results of systemic atrioventricular valve replacement in corrected transposition. *J Thorac Cardiovasc Surg*. 1995;109:642-652; discussion 652-653.

12. Yeh T Jr, Connelly MS, Coles JG, et al. Atrioventricular discordance: results of repair in 127 patients. *J Thorac Cardiovasc Surg*. 1999;117:1190-1203.

13. Hraska V, Duncan BW, Mayer JE Jr, et al. Long-term outcome of surgically treated patients with corrected transposition of the great arteries. *J Thorac Cardiovasc Surg*. 2005;129:182-191.

14. Prieto LR, Hordof AJ, Secic M, Rosenbaum MS, Gersony WM. Progressive tricuspid valve disease in patients with congenitally corrected transposition of the great arteries. *Circulation*. 1998;98:997-1005.

15. Therrien J, Barnes I, Somerville J. Outcome of pregnancy in patients with congenitally corrected transposition of the great arteries. *Am J Cardiol*. 1999;84:820-824.

16. Connolly HM, Grogan M, Warnes CA. Pregnancy among women with congenitally corrected transposition of great arteries. *J Am Coll Cardiol*. 1999;33:1692-1695.

17. Gelson E, Curry R, Gatzoulis MA, et al. Pregnancy in women with a systemic right ventricle after surgically and congenitally corrected transposition of the great arteries. *Eur J Obstet Gynecol Reprod Biol*. 2011;155:146-149.

18. Bowater SE, Selman TJ, Hudsmith LE, Clift PF, Thompson PJ, Thorne SA. Long-term outcome following pregnancy in women with a systemic right ventricle: is the deterioration due to pregnancy or a consequence of time? *Congenit Heart Dis*. 2013;8:302-307.

19. Graham TP Jr, Bernard YD, Mellen BG, et al. Long-term outcome in congenitally corrected transposition of the great arteries: a multi-institutional study. *J Am Coll Cardiol*. 2000;36:255-261.

20. Winter MM, van der Bom T, de Vries LC, et al. Exercise training improves exercise capacity in adult patients with a systemic right ventricle: a randomized clinical trial. *Eur Heart J*. 2012;33:1378-1385.

7 THE ADULT WITH A SINGLE VENTRICLE AND FONTAN PALLIATION

Jennifer Huang, MD
Craig Broberg, MD

PATIENT STORY

A 20-year-old man with a single morphologic left ventricle due to tricuspid atresia and ventricular inversion with transposed great arteries, with transposed great arteries presents with stunted growth and maturation. He initially had a pulmonary artery band (Figure 7-1) placed when he was 2 months old with an atrial septectomy at 9 months. At age 3 years he underwent a surgical Fontan palliation, which involved redirection of the superior vena cava (SVC) and inferior vena cava (IVC), by way of a lateral tunnel, to the right pulmonary artery, confluent with the left. The main pulmonary artery (MPA) was excised. Therefore, systemic venous flow was redirected to passively flow to the right and left pulmonary vascular beds, bypassing the heart entirely (Figure 7-2). He had an uneventful recovery in early childhood until he was diagnosed with protein-losing enteropathy (PLE) at the age of 6 years. Subsequently, at age 10, further surgery was done to remove the lateral tunnel and replace this with an extracardiac conduit between the IVC and pulmonary artery. Despite surgical revision and medical therapy, he continued to have evidence of PLE complicated by a small stroke and evidence of mild liver fibrosis. He was started on warfarin. By age 12, he had evidence of delayed maturation and stunted growth (Figure 7-3), as a complication of PLE. He had chronic hypoproteinemia, hypocalcemia, and hyponatremia. Measured testosterone and growth hormone levels were normal. He was considered for heart transplantation, but instead medical therapy was continued, including subcutaneous heparin, testosterone, and spironolactone.

Now at age 20, he is asymptomatic with no limitations in exercise capacity or palpitations. He is attending college. His blood pressure is 86/60 mm Hg, heart rate is 87 bpm, and oxygen saturation is 94% on room air. He is 59-in tall and weighs 40 kg. His body surface area was only 1.29 m^2, < 3rd percentile. He appears prepubescent. He had a loud systolic murmur at the base of the heart. There was no ascites or edema. The lower extremities were hyperpigmented with varicosities, both visible and palpable. Measured hemoglobin was 17.0 g/dL, total protein was 3.8 g/dL, albumin was 1.6 g/dL. Liver and kidney function tests are normal. He is in normal sinus rhythm. An echocardiogram showed a single ventricle with normal systolic function. There was no mitral valve regurgitation. There was stenosis through the ventricular septal defect (VSD) (in essence subaortic stenosis since this is the flow pathway to the hypoplastic right ventricle and aorta) with a peak gradient of 3.2 m/s. Bone densitometry measured 0.53 g/cm^2 of the lumbar region and 0.47 g/cm^2 of the femur (T scores severely low, −5.1 and −3.7, respectively). Measured peak oxygen consumption with exercise was 20.4 mL/kg/min (43% of predicted), despite his self-expressed lack of symptoms.

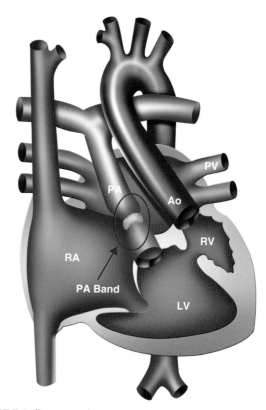

FIGURE 7-1 Illustration depicting a pulmonary band placed in the patient's anatomy of tricuspid atresia with transposed great arteries. Ao, aorta; LV, left ventricle; PA, pulmonary artery; PV, pulmonary vein; RA, right atrium; RV, right ventricle. (*Copyright © McGraw-Hill Education, Photographer: Dr. Laurie Armsby. Modified with permission from Dr. Laurie Armsby.*)

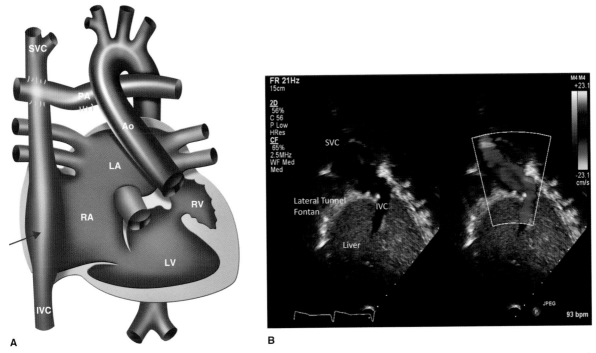

FIGURE 7-2 **A.** Illustration depicting a lateral tunnel Fontan connecting the inferior vena cava (IVC) and superior vena cava (SVC) to the pulmonary artery which has been disconnected from the pulmonary valve in the patient's anatomy of tricuspid atresia with transposed great arteries. Ao, aorta; LA, left atrium; LV, left ventricle; PA, pulmonary artery; PV, pulmonary vein; RA, right atrium; RV, right ventricle. **B.** Transthoracic echocardiogram showing a subcostal view of the inferior vena cava (IVC) being directed into the lateral tunnel through the right atrium. SVC, superior vena cava. (*Copyright © McGraw-Hill Education, Photographer: Dr. Laurie Armsby. Modified with permission from Dr. Laurie Armsby.*)

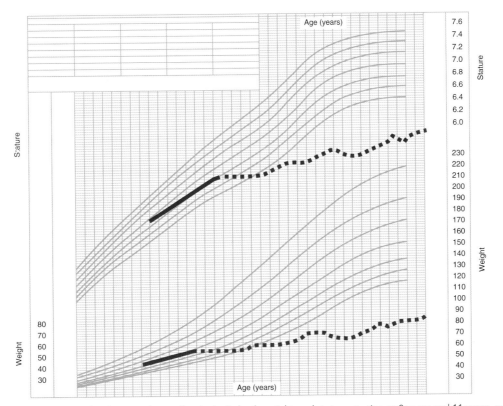

FIGURE 7-3 Growth chart depicting the decreased growth velocity in both weight and stature starting at 8 years and 11 years, respectively, and ultimately resulting in short stature.

Peak heart rate with exercise was 100 bpm, and peak oxygen saturation was 88%. Hepatic ultrasound showed no cirrhosis, but liver biopsy revealed mild centrilobular and portal fibrosis. By catheterization, his systemic venous pressure was 10 mm Hg, pulmonary capillary wedge pressure was 9 mm Hg. There was a 45-mm Hg systolic gradient between the left ventricle and the ascending aorta. His cardiac index was 2.3 L/min/m² (Figure 7-4).

CASE EXPLANATION

• For individuals born with complex congenital heart defects constituting a single ventricle, such as this patient, the Fontan procedure, a term referring to any variation of procedures used to surgically revise the circulation such that systemic venous drainage is directed to the pulmonary vasculature passively as opposed to via a cardiac pumping chamber, has revolutionized survival since its introduction in 1971. However, survival from the Fontan palliation and its many variations comes at a cost of long-term chronically elevated central venous pressure, with at times drastic multiorgan consequences.

• This young adult has what is considered to be a failing Fontan as evidenced by his complications of PLE, arrested growth, poor exercise capacity (objectively measured), and liver disease. The forward flow through his Fontan/pulmonary circuit is inadequate thereby resulting in passive venous congestion which is linked to PLE (enteric venous congestion) and liver disease. Venovenous collaterals form, bringing desaturated blood to the systemic ventricle. Furthermore, inadequate preload to his single ventricle limits cardiac output. Both these factors lower his resting oxygen saturation, and raise his hemoglobin.

• Surgical and interventional techniques in his case had been performed to alleviate any obstruction or excess flow through his Fontan circuit and promote forward flow, and medical therapy for PLE has also been extensive. However, these measures have not been able to prevent steady loss of protein with subsequent adverse effects including poor somatic growth, lack of sexual development, and bone disease. He continued to have moderate subvalvar aortic stenosis at the level of the bulboventricular foramen (Figure 7-5) which is difficult to address surgically given a perceived high operative risk given the above comorbidities.

• Medical therapies have been aimed at reducing his pulmonary vascular resistance and reducing afterload for his failing ventricle. Future options would include cardiac transplantation, which has a reported high mortality in the perioperative period, but could be curative of his PLE and offer favorable long-term survival.

• Such patients are often faced with a clinical dilemma; continue as he is doing in his fairly asymptomatic but limited state, or face high-risk transplantation in the hopes of favorable long-term outcome.

EPIDEMIOLOGY

• The true prevalence is unknown, but a rate reported in clinical studies was approximately 1.5%.

• The incidence of univentricular physiology is thought to be 0.05 to 0.1 per 1000 live births.[1]

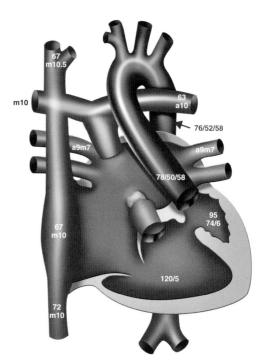

FIGURE 7-4 Diagram illustration hemodynamic measurements obtained at the time of the patient's cardiac catheterization. Of particular note is the 45-mm Hg systolic gradient between the left ventricle (120/5) and the right ventricle (74/6) demonstrating subaortic stenosis at the level of the bulboventricular foramen and the mildly elevated systemic venous pressure of 10 mm Hg. (Copyright © McGraw-Hill Education, Photographer: Dr. Laurie Armsby. Modified with permission from Dr. Laurie Armsby.)

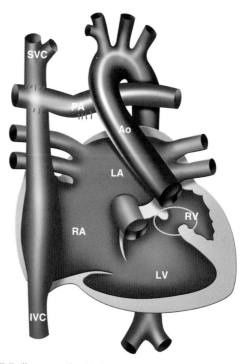

FIGURE 7-5 Illustration highlighting the restrictive bulboventricular foramen (yellow circle) that results in subaortic stenosis and outflow obstruction. Ao, aorta; IVC, inferior vena cava; LA, left atrium; LV, left ventricle; PA, pulmonary artery; RA, right atrium; RV, right ventricle; SVC, superior vena cava. (Copyright © McGraw-Hill Education, Photographer: Dr. Laurie Armsby. Modified with permission from Dr. Laurie Armsby.)

- No sex dominance is known: men and women are almost equally affected.

ETIOLOGY

There are many congenital cardiac anomalies that are palliated with multistage repair and ultimately the Fontan operation, which most commonly include (but not limited to) tricuspid atresia (22%), hypoplastic left heart syndrome (21%), and double inlet left ventricle (15%)[1-3] as listed below (Table 7-1).

PATHOPHYSIOLOGY

- In single ventricle physiology, there is complete mixing of pulmonary (desaturated) and systemic (saturated) blood resulting in cyanosis.

- Some very rare anatomies truly have 1 ventricle, whereas the majority of patients have 2 morphologically distinct ventricles though there is functionally only one chamber. This may result from 1 ventricle being hypoplastic or from the lack of a functional separation between the ventricles. Ultimately, some anatomies are not amenable to surgical separation (or septation) into 2 ventricles for various reasons and these patients are relegated to the surgical pathway of single ventricle palliation.

- There may be inadequate blood flow to the pulmonary or systemic circulations in unbalanced anatomies.

- Even with adequate blood flow to both circulations, in the absence of some degree of restriction to pulmonary blood flow, irreversible damage to the pulmonary vasculature with muscularization of pulmonary arterioles can lead to elevated pulmonary vascular resistance and Eisenmenger syndrome.

- Surgical palliation in the single ventricle is aimed toward separating the pulmonary and systemic circulations through a variety of staged surgeries resulting in what is commonly referred to as "Fontan" physiology.

DIAGNOSIS

- Most single ventricle anatomies are often readily detected before birth with fetal echocardiography.

- With the introduction of routine pulse oximetry of infants in recent years, some otherwise asymptomatic infants have been identified via screening.

- Ultimately the diagnosis is confirmed and refined using transthoracic echocardiography and cross-sectional imaging (computed tomography [CT] or magnetic resonance imaging [MRI]), which can provide useful supplemental information.

- On occasion, cardiac catheterization is needed to further define anatomy and for surgical planning during the diagnostic period. It is particularly helpful to determine pulmonary blood flow in patients with inadequate antegrade flow through the pulmonary valve or with pulmonary atresia. These hemodynamic data inform decisions about surgical intervention.

- Adult patients with single ventricular physiology should be followed by an adult congenital heart disease specialist with periodic visits

Table 7-1 Single Ventricle Anatomies

Anatomy	Incidence Rate (per 1000 live births)
Hypoplastic left heart syndrome	0.21-0.28
Pulmonary atresia	0.069-0.074
Tricuspid atresia	0.057
Unbalanced atrioventricular septal defect	Unknown
Double outlet right ventricle (unseptatable)	0.03-0.2
Double inlet left ventricle	Unknown
Heterotaxy	0.05
Miscellaneous unseptatable defects (multiple ventricular septal defects, straddling cords, etc)	Unknown

which should include symptom assessment with functional classification, growth charting when appropriate, weight and muscle mass assessment in adults, blood pressure, oxygen saturations, imaging, cardiac catheterization, and laboratory evaluation when needed.

DIAGNOSTIC TESTING

Exercise Testing

- It can be difficult to determine the important clinical marker of exercise tolerance in a patient chronically compensating for their single ventricle physiology. The case discussed earlier is exemplary—the patient has no subjective symptoms yet his measured oxygen consumption is very low.

- Particularly, it is known that patients who have undergone Fontan palliation have decreased exercise tolerance and therefore, exercise testing with measurement of oxygen consumption is a good objective clinical marker to follow in this patient population.[5,6]

Transthoracic Echocardiography

- Transthoracic echocardiography provides good information in this patient population. Key findings are patency and velocity of the Fontan and Glenn circuits, patency of the atrial septal defect, atrial size and presence of intracardiac thrombi, atrioventricular valve regurgitation, outflow tract obstruction, and ventricular size and function among other individual questions. These pathways are not always well visualized.

- Imaging often relies on knowledge of the specific surgical interventions performed in the individual being imaged.

Cardiac MRI or Cardiac CT

- Cross-sectional imaging such as cardiac MRI and cardiac CT provides useful information in single ventricle patients, particularly in those with anterior systemic ventricles that are difficult to image with echocardiography.

- MRI also provides useful information in quantifying ventricular volume, stroke volume, and ejection fraction (EF). New techniques which may be informative for this patient population in the future include fibrosis index and 4-dimensional flow imaging to determine caval blood flow distribution. As with echo, the best studies will be directed by an experienced imager with knowledge of the patient-specific procedures.

Cardiac Catheterization

- Cardiac catheterization provides hemodynamic assessment that is difficult or impossible to obtain via other techniques, particularly, diastolic pressure measurements, central venous pressures (Fontan circuit pressures), pulmonary vascular resistance, and the presence of right-to-left shunts.

- Also, interventions such as coiling of venovenous and aortopulmonary collaterals, dilation of branch pulmonary stenosis, re-coarctations, closure of baffle-leaks, and refenestration or closure of Fontan fenestration can be undertaken during catheterization to optimize the Fontan circuit.

Ambulatory ECG Monitoring

- Routine rhythm assessment may be useful to evaluate for the presence of clinically silent or symptomatic atrial or junctional rhythms, resting heart rate, and chronotropic response to exertion.

Thyroid Function

- Fontan patients on amiodarone are at increased risk for thyroid dysfunction. Furthermore, the myocardial depression or tachycardia, associated with hypo- or hyperthyroidism, respectively, are deleterious to single ventricle patients.

- Thyroid-stimulating hormone (TSH) and free thyroxine (T_4) should be followed intermittently, particularly in those patients who are symptomatic.

Hepatic Evaluation

- Poor forward flow through the Fontan circuit results in hepatic congestion from hepatic venous hypertension, inflammation/transaminitis, fibrosis, and ultimately dysfunction and failure. Therefore, assessing liver inflammation and function should be followed with serial liver profiles and coagulation panels as well as imaging.

- Some commercially available biomarker assays for fibrosis have been considered for longitudinal follow-up. Frequency and modality of liver imaging have not been routinely established.

- Liver biopsy should also be considered on occasion, and can often be combined in some institutions with cardiac catheterization.

Gastrointestinal Evaluation

- Fontan patients with PLE often have gastrointestinal fluid losses and may have symptoms of diarrhea and weight loss prior to complications of hypoproteinemia.

- Fecal α_1 antitrypsin is elevated in patients with PLE. Patients may also experience bloating, distention, and abdominal pain secondary to hepatic distention or ascites.

Hematologic Evaluation

- Routine complete blood counts and coagulation panels are prudent and particularly important in patients on antiplatelet and/or anticoagulation therapy.

Immunological Evaluation

- Patients with PLE also exhibit immune deficiencies primarily due to enteral losses of immunoglobulin. Serum immunoglobulin G (IgG) can be measured during routine screening and serially in patients with known PLE.

Metabolic Evaluation

- Single ventricle patients may have protein losses and malnutrition secondary to PLE as reflected in low albumin levels. They may also have increased bone turnover from chronic loop diuretic use and measures like alkaline phosphatase and bone mass densitometry may be appropriate in patients who have chronic diuretic use.

Renal

- Poor cardiac output and dysregulated renal flow in liver failure can both lead to renal injury in single ventricle patients. Blood urea nitrogen, electrolytes, and creatinine should be followed routinely, as well as trace elements. It is important to correct levels as much as possible.

SURGICAL MANAGEMENT

Provision of Adequate Pulmonary Blood Flow

- If pulmonary blood flow is inadequate or tenuous (ie, via a patent ductus arteriosus or small multiple aortopulmonary collateral arteries), it can be provided by either placement of an aortopulmonary shunt such as a Blalock-Taussig shunt (BT shunt) or a ventricular-to-pulmonary artery conduit such as a Sano (Table 7-2).
- The modified BT shunt uses a synthetic tube to connect the subclavian or carotid artery to the ipsilateral branch pulmonary artery (Figure 7-6). The Sano conduit is a synthetic homograft that connects the single ventricle directly to the pulmonary arteries (Figure 7-7).
- One of these 2 procedures is often used in conjunction with a Damus-Kaye-Stansel anastomosis (DKS, discussed below) such as in the Norwood procedure (Stage 1 palliation for hypoplastic left heart syndrome).

Table 7-2 Surgical Procedures Associated With Single Ventricles

Surgical Procedure	Brief Description	Figure
Blalock-Taussig shunt (BTS)	Subclavian artery connected to pulmonary artery to provide/augment pulmonary blood flow	7-6
Sano conduit	Synthetic homograft from the free wall of the single ventricle to the pulmonary artery	7-7
Damus-Kaye-Stansel (DKS) anastomosis	Creation of a neoaorta by anastomosing the pulmonary artery with the hypoplastic aorta	7-8
Pulmonary band	Restriction of pulmonary blood flow from a belt-like band around the main pulmonary artery	7-1
Bidirectional Glenn (BDG)	SVC connected directly to pulmonary artery to provide passive pulmonary blood flow	7-9
Atriopulmonary Connection (classic Fontan)	Right atrial appendage connected to the pulmonary artery to provide pulmonary blood flow	7-10
Lateral tunnel Fontan	Synthetic tunnel within the right atrium diverts systemic venous return directly to the pulmonary arteries bypassing the ventricle	7-11
Extracardiac total cavopulmonary anastomosis (ECC Fontan)	Synthetic conduit from the IVC to the pulmonary arteries bypasses the right atrium entirely	7-12
Kawashima	Glenn anastomosis in the setting of an interrupted IVC such that both SVC and IVC (excluding hepatic veins) flow to the pulmonary artery	7-13

ECC, extracardiac conduit; IVC, inferior vena cava; SVC, superior vena cava.

Provision of Adequate Systemic Blood Flow

- In patients with left heart hypoplasia particularly, there is often left outflow tract obstruction and the patient's native systemic outflow requires immediate augmentation. In some anatomies, this can be done either with coarctation repair alone or in more severe cases in conjunction with the DKS anastomosis (Figure 7-8).

- The DKS anastomosis creates a neoaorta by connecting the native pulmonary valve to the aorta, keeping the hypoplastic ascending aorta as a common coronary artery. As above, when performed with a BT shunt or Sano, the procedure is referred to as a Norwood procedure or Stage 1 palliation.

Protection of Pulmonary Vasculature

- In some patients with single ventricle physiologies, there is adequate blood flow to both the systemic and pulmonary circulations. However, because the pulmonary system inherently has a lower vascular resistance, and is exposed to the high pressures of a ventricle generating systemic pressures or high volumes of preferential blood flow, it is necessary to protect the pulmonary vascular bed from high pressure and flow, to prevent development of elevated pulmonary vascular resistance. This is particularly important in patients with single ventricle physiologies who will ultimately have

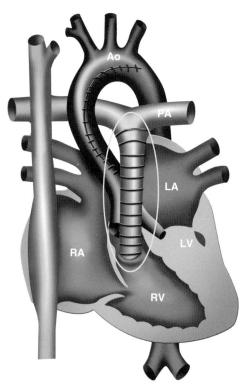

FIGURE 7-7 Illustration depicting a right ventricle to pulmonary artery conduit (Sano) in a hypoplastic left heart anatomy. Ao, aorta; LA, left atrium; LV, left ventricle; PA, pulmonary artery; RA, right atrium; RV, right ventricle. (*Copyright © McGraw-Hill Education, Photographer: Dr. Laurie Armsby. Modified with permission from Dr. Laurie Armsby.*)

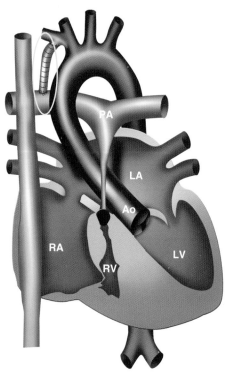

FIGURE 7-6 Illustration depicting a right-sided Blalock-Taussig shunt (yellow circle) connecting the right subclavian artery and the right pulmonary artery in a tricuspid atresia anatomy. Ao, aorta; LV, left ventricle; PA, pulmonary artery; RA, right atrium; RV, right ventricle. (*Copyright © McGraw-Hill Education, Photographer: Dr. Laurie Armsby. Modified with permission from Dr. Laurie Armsby.*)

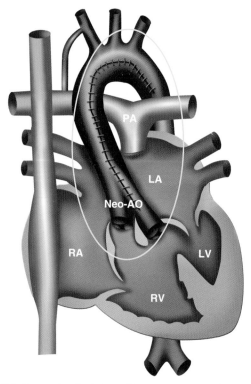

FIGURE 7-8 Illustration depicting a Damus-Kaye-Stansel (DKS) anastomosis in an unbalanced atrioventricular canal defect. LA, left atrium; LV, left ventricle; Neo-Ao, neoaorta; PA, pulmonary artery; RA, right atrium; RV, right ventricle. (*Copyright © McGraw-Hill Education, Photographer: Dr. Laurie Armsby. Modified with permission from Dr. Laurie Armsby.*)

Fontan physiology which is dependent on low pulmonary vascular resistance in order to be successful.

- Procedures to control and limit pulmonary blood flow include pulmonary artery banding, a belt-like band externally fixed to the main pulmonary artery to create pulmonary stenosis (Figure 7-1) and disconnection of the MPA with placement of a BT shunt.

Bidirectional Glenn Shunt/Palliation (BDG)

- This intermediate palliation is sometimes the first procedure performed in patients who have had adequate pulmonary and systemic blood flows and sufficient protection of their pulmonary vasculatures.
- During the BDG procedure, the SVC is connected directly to the pulmonary artery. Thereby the systemic venous return from the upper half of the body flows passively into the lungs and then back to the left heart (Figure 7-9).

Atriopulmonary Connections

- The principle of the Fontan operation is to connect both vena cavae to the pulmonary artery by bypassing the right ventricle. As Fontan originally described in 1971, it involved classic Glenn shunting (end-to-end SVC to right pulmonary artery anastomosis), a connection of the right atrium to the left pulmonary artery, and the interposition of 2 valved homografts (one between the IVC and the right atrium and one between the right atrium and the left pulmonary artery).[7] This type of anastomosis is rarely performed today (Figures 7-10A through 7-10D).

Lateral Tunnel Fontan

- The lateral tunnel, introduced in 1988, is a modification of the original Fontan technique that optimizes the hydrodynamic flow of the IVC return by channeling flow through a synthetic tunnel traversing the right atrium into the pulmonary artery. Still used today, the intra-atrial rerouting excludes most of the now redundant right atrium and streamlines flow (Figure 7-2).

Extracardiac Total Cavopulmonary Connection (TCPC)

- Often referred to as an extracardiac conduit, this Fontan modification was introduced in 1990 and is frequently used today. In this technique, the right atrium is bypassed altogether. The IVC blood flow is rerouted around the right atrium with a synthetic conduit that connects to the pulmonary artery.
- Often, a baffle fenestration is created between the conduit and the right atrium as a pop-off valve for blood to return to the right atrium and maintain cardiac output if higher venous pressure limits forward flow during the difficult postoperative transition period. In many patients, this fenestration can be closed with a device via cardiac catheterization up to several years later (Figure 7-11).

Kawashima Procedure

- The Kawashima procedure is a functional modification of the bidirectional Glenn. In terms of surgical technique it is essentially the same. However, in patients who have an interrupted inferior vena cava, the majority of blood from the lower body drains eventually

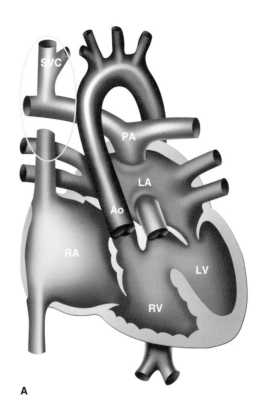

A

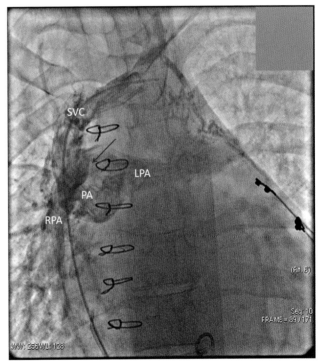

B

FIGURE 7-9 A. Illustration depicting a bidirectional Glenn anastomosis connecting the superior vena cava (SVC) directly to the pulmonary artery (PA) in transposition of the great arteries with discontinuous pulmonary arteries anatomy. **B.** Superior vena cava angiogram showing the bidirectional Glenn anastomosis with contrast filling the bilateral pulmonary arteries from the superior vena cava. The catheter runs up the inferior vena cava (IVC) through the lateral tunnel Fontan and into the superior vena cava. Ao, aorta; LA, left atrium; LPA, left pulmonary artery; LV, left ventricle; RA, right atrium; RPA, right pulmonary artery; RV, right ventricle. (*Copyright © McGraw-Hill Education, Photographer: Dr. Laurie Armsby. Modified with permission from Dr. Laurie Armsby.*)

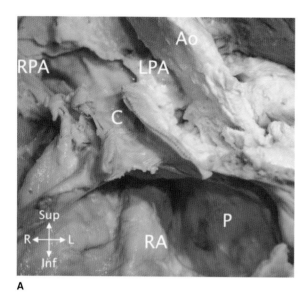

A

FIGURE 7-10 **A.** Frontal view of a heart after an atriopulmonary Fontan operation. A conduit (C) was used to join the right atrium (RA) and the pulmonary arteries. The right (RPA) and left (LPA) branches are seen arising from the junction with the conduit. The aorta (Ao) is anterior and leftward in this heart with double inlet left ventricle (DILV). There is a calcified patch (P) on the right atrioventricular (AV) valve to prevent flow of venous blood from the RA into the systemic ventricle. (*Reproduced with permission from Stephen P. Sanders, MD, Professor of Pediatrics (Cardiology), Harvard Medical School; Director, Cardiac Registry, Departments of Cardiology, Pathology, and Cardiac Surgery, Children's Hospital Boston, Boston, Massachusetts.*)

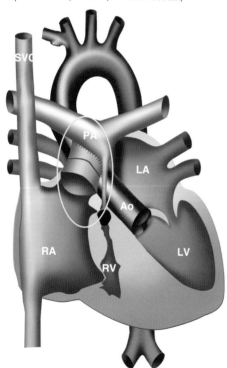

B

FIGURE 7-10 **B.** Illustration depicting an atriopulmonary connection directing blood from the right atrium (RA) through the right atrial appendage into the pulmonary artery (PA) in a hypoplastic left heart anatomy. Ao, aorta; IVC, inferior vena cava; LA, left atrium; LV, left ventricle; RV, right ventricle; SVC, superior vena cava. (*Copyright © McGraw-Hill Education, Photographer: Dr. Laurie Armsby. Modified with permission from Dr. Laurie Armsby.*)

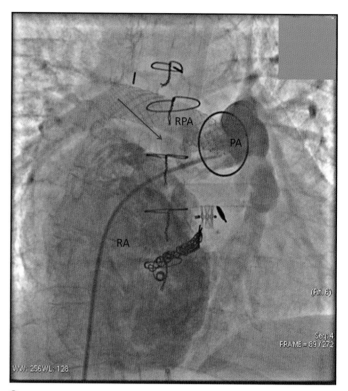

C

FIGURE 7-10 **C.** Pulmonary artery angiogram depicting reflux of contrast through the atriopulmonary connection back into the severely dilated right atrium (RA). A catheter is seen running from the inferior vena cava (IVC) through the right atrium and atriopulmonary connection into the main pulmonary artery (PA). A stent is seen in the right pulmonary artery (RPA) as well as multiple coils, a vascular plug, sternal wires, and a synthetic ring marking the pulmonary valve (PV).

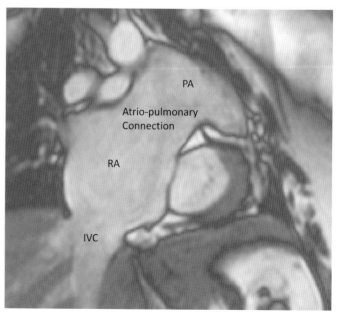

D

FIGURE 7-10 **D.** Magnetic resonance image of a classic atriopulmonary Fontan directing inferior vena cava (IVC) and hepatic venous blood flow to the pulmonary artery (PA). RA, right atrium.

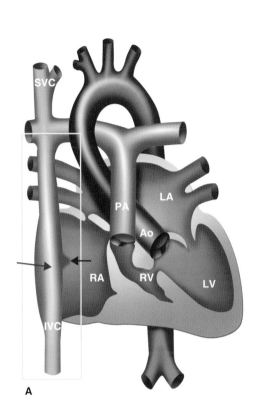

A

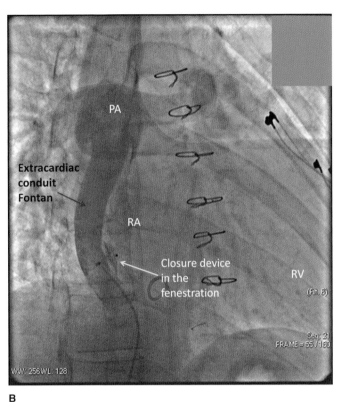

B

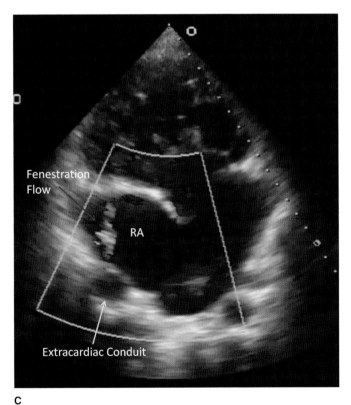

C

FIGURE 7-11 A. Illustration depicting the extracardiac total cavopulmonary anastomosis connecting the inferior vena cava (IVC) to the pulmonary artery (PA) (red arrow) and the fenestration (blue arrow) allowing some systemic venous return to enter the right atrium (RA). Ao, aorta; LA, left atrium; LV, left ventricle; RV, right ventricle; SVC, superior vena cava **B.** Inferior vena cava angiogram showing an extracardiac conduit with a device occluding the fenestration. Also seen are multiple coils, clips, and a stent placed in the ascending aorta. **C.** Transthoracic echocardiogram color Doppler showing flow through the fenestration. (*Copyright © McGraw-Hill Education, Photographer: Dr. Laurie Armsby. Modified with permission from Dr. Laurie Armsby.*)

into the superior vena cava system and therefore, the result is more systemic venous blood flow directed toward the pulmonary circulation (Figure 7-12).

- The hepatic veins draining the majority of the abdominal venous return, however, return to the right atrium directly, and hence from there to the systemic circulation. This is viewed as a disadvantage because of the perception of a "hepatic factor" which, if shunted away from the pulmonary vascular bed, leads to the formation of arteriovenous malformations. Therefore, these patients often need "completion" of their Fontan circulation to allow all venous flow to reach the lungs.

MEDICAL MANAGEMENT

Diuretics

- Diuretics can be used for both heart failure and for chronic accumulation of extracellular fluid such as with chronic pleural effusions and edema from hypoproteinemia in PLE.

- In case of long-term use they can have deleterious effects on bone metabolism exacerbating osteoporosis.

Anticoagulants

- There is debate on anticoagulation in patients with Fontan circulations. Most recent literature suggests this high-thrombosis risk population should be on anticoagulation though there has been no clear recommendation for aspirin or warfarin or a combination.

- A recent multicenter, randomized trial showed no difference in thrombotic complications in patients taking aspirin versus warfarin for thrombotic prophylaxis.[8]

ACE Inhibitors

- Angiotensin-converting enzyme (ACE) inhibitors are often used in Fontan patients in the setting of right ventricular (RV) morphology and AV valve regurgitation.

- They are used in failing Fontan physiology though no clear benefits exist in the literature.

Beta-blockade

- Like in patients with other etiologies of heart failure, patients with heart failure and a single ventricle may benefit from beta-blockade in reducing cardiothoracic ratio, and improving ejection fraction though no clear benefits exist in published literature.[9]

Pulmonary Vasodilators

- Sildenafil is increasingly used in patients with congenital heart disease to lower pulmonary arterial pressures. In Fontan patients, some recent studies have shown its effectiveness in managing patients with failing Fontans[10] and improving exercise tolerance.[11]

- A possible mechanism includes decreasing pulmonary vascular resistance (PVR) in pulmonary circulations uncoupled from ventricular pump mechanisms and thereby dependent on passive flow. Decreasing PVR results in improved pulmonary blood flow, increased cardiac filling, and thereby larger stroke volume resulting in improved cardiac output.

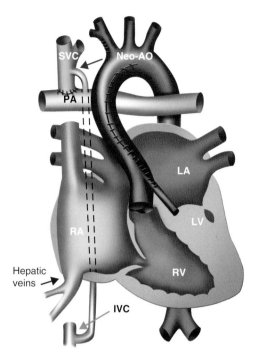

FIGURE 7-12 Illustration depicting a Kawashima palliation with the inferior vena cava flow (IVC) (green arrow) connecting via an azygous vein into the superior vena cava (SVC) (red arrow) which is anastomosed to the pulmonary artery (PA) as in a Glenn anastomosis. The hepatic veins (blue arrow) drain normally into the right atrium (RA). LA, left atrium; LV, left ventricle; Neo-Ao, neoaorta; RV, right ventricle. (*Copyright © McGraw-Hill Education, Photographer: Dr. Laurie Armsby. Modified with permission from Dr. Laurie Armsby.*)

LONG-TERM COMPLICATIONS

Decreased Exercise Tolerance

- Patients with Fontan palliation have decreased exercise tolerance as compared to the normal population as they have a decreased ability to increase cardiac output with exercise.

- Some studies project a 0.5% to 2% annual decline in maximal oxygen consumption in Fontan patients starting in adolescence.[4]

Growth Failure

- In general, the Fontan population has shorter stature than the general population.[12] However, some individuals have particularly stunted growth, as in the case discussed earlier.

- Failure of somatic growth is often secondary to poor cardiac output during childhood or PLE. Interventions to improve cardiac output are the most efficacious in improving growth velocity.

Atrial Arrhythmias

- While the incidence of atrial arrhythmias (Figure 7-13) has decreased some with the strategy of extracardiac Fontan (which exclude the right atrium), atrial arrhythmias are still common in Fontan patients occurring in 60% of patients with atriopulmonary anastomosis and 12% of patients with extracardiac total cavopulmonary connections.[11]

- Potential risk factors are atrial dilation from previous volume overload and commonly, atrioventricular valve regurgitation, atrial hypertension from ventricular dysfunction, and atrial scarring.

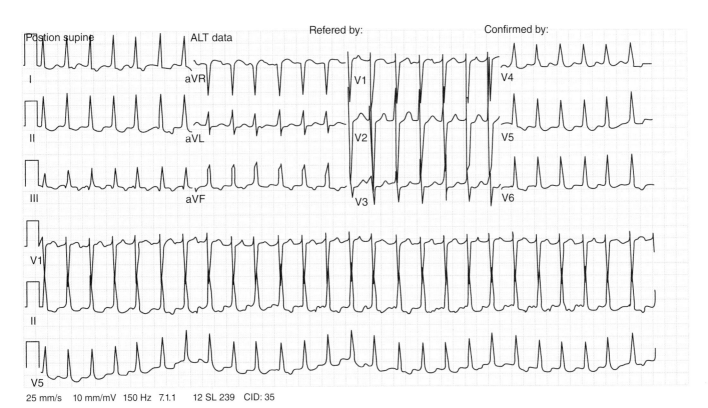

FIGURE 7-13 Electrocardiogram (ECG) showing fine atrial flutter with 2:1 atrioventricular node conduction in a 47-year-old patient with congenital tricuspid atresia status post atriopulmonary Fontan.

Other arrhythmias seen include sinus node dysfunction, predominant junctional rhythm, atrioventricular block, and ventricular arrhythmias.

- Long-term follow-up of these patients should include regular electrocardiographic assessment with ambulatory Holter monitors, event monitors, and exercise testing. Importantly in this patient population, atrial dysrhythmias can severely compromise cardiac output as the single ventricle relies greatly on atrioventricular synchrony.

- Even transient atrioventricular dyssynchrony and atrial tachycardia can result in elevation of atrial pressures which transmit retrograde to impede forward passive flow through the pulmonary circulation.

- Atrial arrhythmia, when found, should be treated expeditiously and aggressively. In addition, any arrhythmia should be seen as an invitation to reassess and optimize the patients' hemodynamics.

Protein Losing Enteropathy (PLE)

- The incidence of PLE in patients with Fontan palliation is 2%-13%.[13] The chronic high systemic venous pressure and subsequent chronic passive venous congestion inherent in the Fontan circulation result in lymphatic dysfunction resulting in third spacing in various tissues.

- This occurs markedly in the gastrointestinal system where it is hypothesized that chronic bowel edema results in protein loss which further exacerbates third spacing in various tissues manifesting with pleural effusions, diarrhea, immunodeficiencies from loss of immunoglobulins and lymphocytes, and coagulopathies.[14] However, high systemic venous pressures are not the only determinant of PLE as normal Fontan pressures on cardiac catheterization do not exclude this diagnosis. The diagnosis is made by elevated α_1 antitrypsin levels, low IgG and albumin levels.

- Diuretics, anti-inflammatories such as steroids, unfractionated heparin that stabilizes the proteoglycan membranes, particularly in the epithelial tight junctions, and maneuvers to improve overall cardiac output have all been used to improve PLE.[15]

- The only universal cure however is heart transplantation, although surgical risk is higher in individuals with PLE.

Plastic Bronchitis

- Plastic bronchitis is a rare complication of the Fontan procedure (with an incidence of <2%), which is also thought to be secondary to elevated systemic venous pressures and elevated PVR and like PLE is thought to be secondary to lymphatic dysfunction in the bronchioles. Symptoms include chronic cough, wheezing, and characteristically expectoration of bronchial casts (Figure 7-14).

Hepatic Failure

- Liver dysfunction is a common finding in late follow-up of Fontan patients. Elevated systemic venous pressure also increases sinusoidal pressures within the liver resulting in hepatic venous hypertension (Figure 7-15).

- Chronic exposure to these elevated pressures can result in liver fibrosis and subsequent liver dysfunction as evidenced by transaminitis, coagulation abnormalities, and impaired clearance of bilirubin. Ultimately, if severe and progressive, this passive congestion

can lead to frank cirrhosis. Hepatocellular carcinoma has also been described as a complication in Fontan patients.

Ventricular Systolic Dysfunction

- The incidence of ventricular systolic dysfunction in patients with Fontan palliation is 7%-10%.[13] The single ventricle undergoes many stressors before and after conversion to the final stage of palliation with the Fontan circuit. Prior to complete separation of the pulmonary and systemic circulations with the Fontan circuit, the single ventricle is volume-overloaded from both systemic-to-pulmonary artery shunting and, in many cases, atrioventricular or semilunar valve regurgitation (Figure 7-16).

- There may also be a pressure overload from persistent outflow tract obstruction, as in the case discussed herein. After conversion to the Fontan circulation, the dominant systemic ventricle may be hypertrophied and dilated from these previous insults which are early determinants of ventricular failure. Lastly, in those ventricles that are morphologic right ventricles, the myocardial fiber architecture is not well suited to supporting a systemic circulation and they often fail earlier than morphologic left ventricles.

Thromboembolic Complications (3%-33%)[16]

- Patients who have undergone Fontan palliation have an increased risk of thromboembolic complications including thrombus occluding or partially occluding their Fontan circuit (Figure 7-17), stroke, and pulmonary embolus. These phenomena have high associated morbidity and therefore most patients undergoing Fontan palliation are placed on antiplatelet or anticoagulation therapy.

- The risk remains the highest in the immediate post-operative period, however there remains a sustained long term risk for thromboembolic complications as well.

Neurologic

- Attention for potential cerebrovascular accidents is warranted given the increased risk in this patient population due to thromboembolic potential in the setting of liver dysfunction, PLE, atrial arrhythmias, and dilated intracardiac structures with potential areas of stagnant flow and synthetic material.

Psychiatric

- Patients who have undergone the Fontan procedure have a higher rate of depression than age-matched healthy counterparts.[17] Depression screening should be considered for all adult patients with univentricular physiology after the Fontan operation.

CONCLUSION

- The Fontan operation, first developed in 1971, is a palliative procedure for patients with functional univentricular physiology. As this complex cohort of patients continues to survive, these patients are often faced with life-threatening long-term complications.

- Concerns about the long-term functioning of a single ventricle remain.

- It is now evident that the Fontan operation remains an imperfect solution for a complex cardiovascular problem. Advances in heart

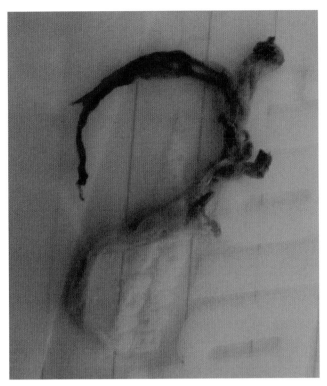

FIGURE 7-14 Photograph of a bronchial cast expectorated from a patient with plastic bronchitis. (*Copyright © McGraw-Hill Education, Photographer: Dr. G. Michael Silberbach.*)

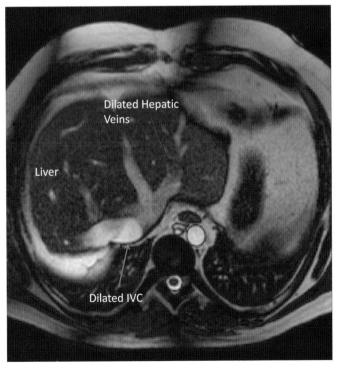

FIGURE 7-15 Magnetic resonance image of a congested liver with dilated hepatic veins and inferior vena cava (IVC) in a patient with a failing Fontan. Also seen is trace ascites.

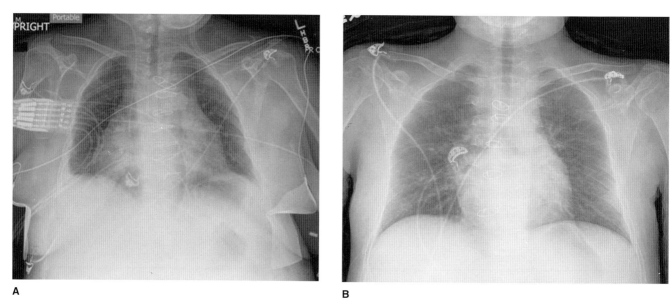

A   B

FIGURE 7-16 A. Portable chest x-ray image highlighting significant cardiomegaly and pulmonary vascular congestion in a 49-year-old woman with tricuspid atresia and ventricular systolic dysfunction. B. A similar image for comparison in a stable patient with Fontan physiology showing a small cardiac silhouette without increased pulmonary vascular markings.

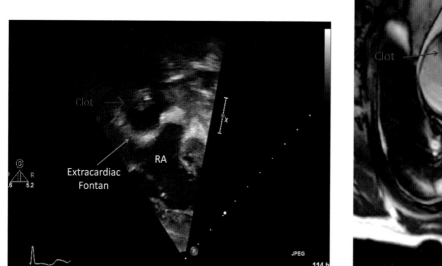

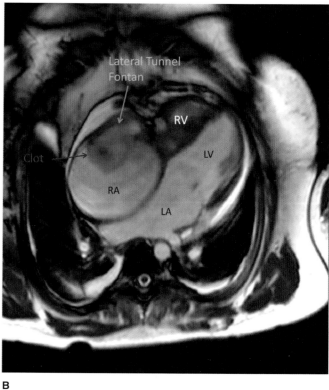

A   B

FIGURE 7-17 A. Transthoracic echocardiogram image of a thrombus partially occluding an extracardiac conduit in a patient with recurrent pleural effusions. B. Magnetic resonance image of a thrombus filling the lateral tunnel Fontan. LA, left atrium; LV, left ventricle; RA, right atrium; RV, right ventricle.

failure management along with newer medical and surgical techniques and therapies continue to emerge to address these long-term risks.

REFERENCES

1. Fyler DC, Buckley LP, Hellenbrand WE, et al. Report of the New England Regional Infant Cardiac Program. Pediatrics 1980;65(2):377-461.

2. Anderson PAW, Breitbart RE, McCrindle VW, et al. The Fontan patient: Inconsistencies in medication therapy across seven pediatric heart network centers. Pediatr Cardiol 2010;31:1219-1228.

3. Gewillig M. The Fontan Circulation. *Heart*. 2005;91:839-846.

4. Reller MD, Strickland MJ, Riehle-Colarusso T, et al. Prevalence of Congenital Heart Defects in Metropolitan Atlanta, 1998-2005. The J of Pediatrics 2008;153(6):807-13.

5. Diller GP, Giardini A, Dimopoulos A, et al. Predictors of morbidity and mortality in contemporary Fontan patients: results from a multicenter study including cardiopulmonary exercise testing in 321 patients. *Eur Heart J*. 2010;31:3073-3083.

6. Fernandez SM, McElhinney DB, Khairy P, et al. Serial cardiopulmonary exercise testing in patients with previous Fontan surgery. Pediatr Cardiol. 2010;31(2):175-80.

7. Fontan F, Baudet E. Surgical repair of tricuspid atresia. *Thorax*. 1971;26:240-248.

8. McCrindle BW, Manlhiot C, Cochrane A, et al. Factors associated with thrombotic complications after the Fontan procedure: A secondary analysis of a multicenter, randomized trial of primary prophylaxis for 2 years after the Fontan procedure. JACC 2013;61(3):346-53.

9. Ishibashi N, Park IS, Waragai T, et al. Effect of Carvedilol on heart failure in patients with a functionally univentricular heart. Circulation Jour 2011;75:1394-99.

10. Reinhardt Z, Uzun O, Bhole V, et al. Sildenafil in the management of the failing Fontan circulation. Cardiology in the Young 2010;20:522-25.

11. Goldberg DJ, French B, McBride MG, et al. Impact of oral sildenafil on exercise performance in children and young adults after the Fontan operation: a randomized, double-blind, placebo-controlled, crossover trial. Circulation 2011;123(11):1185-93.

12. Francois K, Bove T, Panzer J, et al. Univentricular heart and fontan staging: analysis of factors impacting body growth. Eur J Cardiothorac Surg 2012;41(6): e139-45.

13. Deal BJ, Jacobs ML. Management of the Failing Fontan. *Heart*. 2012;98:1098-1104.

14. Khambadkone S. The Fontan pathway: What's down the road? Annals of Pediatric Cardiology 2008;1(2):83-92.

15. Griffiths ER, Kaza AK, Wyler von Ballmoos MC, et al. Evaluating Failing Fontans for Heart Transplantation: Predictors of Mortality. *Ann Thorac Surg*. 2009;88(2):558-564.

16. Idorn L, Jensen AS, Juul K, et al. Thromboembolic complications in Fontan patients: Population-based prevalence and exploration of the etiology. Pediatr Cardiol. 2012. Epub ahead of print.

17. Pike NA, Evangelista LA, Doering LV, et al. Quality of Life, Health Status, and Depression: Comparison between adolescents and adults after the Fontan procedure with healthy counterparts. J Cardiovasc Nurs 2012;27(6):539-46.

8 THE ADULT WITH EBSTEIN'S ANOMALY OF THE TRICUSPID VALVE

W. Aaron Kay, MD
Sharon Roble, MD
Ali N. Zaidi, MD

PATIENT STORY

A 32-year-old woman presented for evaluation of decreasing exercise tolerance and a loud heart murmur. On physical examination, she had a fixed split second heart sound with a normal pulmonary component. She had a holosystolic murmur at the mid-left sternal border that did not radiate and increased with inspiration. An electrocardiogram (ECG) and echocardiogram were performed. ECG demonstrated right atrial enlargement and a right bundle branch block. Echocardiogram showed apical displacement of the septal and posterior leaflets of her tricuspid valve resulting in severe tricuspid regurgitation. Her clinical findings were consistent with Ebstein's anomaly. Further testing included a functional VO_2 exercise stress test. With exercise, she was found to have significant oxygen desaturation to the mid-80s on room air. A subsequent transesophageal echocardiogram showed a patent foramen ovale (PFO) with bidirectional shunting, severe tricuspid regurgitation, and an apically displaced septal leaflet of the tricuspid valve consistent with Ebstein's anomaly. Because of her significant hypoxia with exercise, she underwent a catheter-based closure of her PFO. A repeat exercise study following PFO closure showed normal oxygen saturations with exercise and improved exercise capacity. She was followed with serial imaging that continued to demonstrate the severe tricuspid regurgitation and gradual worsening in her functional capacity. She developed atrial flutter with rapid ventricular rate for which she needed to be cardioverted. She was managed with antiarrhythmic medications and has had no further arrhythmia recurrences. She finally underwent surgical management in the form of a tricuspid valve replacement with a bioprosthetic valve and plication of the atrialized ventricle. The patient had an uneventful postoperative recovery with significant improvement in her functional capacity.

CASE EXPLANATION

- This case highlights several important concepts for the long-term complications and management of adult patients with Ebstein's anomaly of the tricuspid valve.

- These include the concerns for atrial arrhythmias, atrial level shunting secondary to an interatrial communication, severity of tricuspid regurgitation, and declining functional capacity.

- Ebstein's anomaly is a rare congenital heart disorder (1 / 200,000 live births), accounting for about 0.3% to 0.7% of all cases of congenital heart disease (CHD), however this case highlights that Ebstein's anomaly can present later in life since patients can have a wide spectrum of symptoms that may prevent the underlying pathology from being discovered until adulthood.

- Such patients require regular long-term cardiac follow-up with an adult congenital cardiologist to prevent long-term cardiac complications.

EPIDEMIOLOGY

- Ebstein's anomaly is a rare congenital heart disease that consists of apical displacement of the septal leaflet of the tricuspid valve and atrialization of the right ventricle. The estimated risk of Ebstein's anomaly in the general population is 1 in 200,000 live births, with males and females being at equal risk.[1]

- Lithium use during pregnancy has been considered a risk factor for developing Ebstein in the fetus, although the classic case series of "Lithium babies" reported by Weinstein and Goldfield in 1975 showed an extremely high incidence of congenital heart disease in general, not limited to just Ebstein's anomaly.[2]

- The severity of the disease encompasses a wide spectrum of symptoms such that it may not be discovered until adulthood. The prognosis is extremely variable and can range from severe hydrops fetalis and fetal demise to simply an isolated murmur in an otherwise asymptomatic patient.

- Severe and often fatal cases occur in newborns with severe cardiomegaly and heart failure. These cases are often diagnosed prenatally on fetal echocardiography. Patients diagnosed in the neonatal period tend to have more severe disease and present with cyanosis whereas older children tend to present with a heart murmur. Adults present most frequently with atrial arrhythmias.[3]

- If unrepaired, about 25% of affected children die in the first 10 years of life, and over 70% will die before age 30.

ETIOLOGY AND PATHOPHYSIOLOGY

- The primary abnormality in Ebstein's anomaly occurs during embryonic development of the cardiovascular system; there is a failure of delamination of the posterior and septal leaflets of the tricuspid valve from the myocardium of the right ventricle resulting in the displacement of the attachment of the septal leaflet of the tricuspid valve into the body of the right ventricle, causing a large portion of the right ventricle to become "atrialized."

- The portion of the right ventricle that is "atrialized" does not contribute to right ventricular function and cardiac output. In severe cases, the nonatrialized part of the right ventricle is small and may consist of only the right ventricular outflow tract.

- In addition to the apical displacement of the tricuspid valve, the tricuspid valve leaflets themselves tend to be abnormal. The morphology of the tricuspid valve in Ebstein's anomaly is variable which may affect the severity of the clinical presentation. Typically, the tricuspid valve leaflets are partly attached to the fibrous tricuspid valve annulus as well as to the endocardium of the right ventricle. The anterior leaflet is the largest leaflet and is usually attached to the tricuspid valve annulus (Figure 8-1). Because of the large size of the anterior leaflet, it is often described as looking like a "sail" on echocardiography. The posterior and septal leaflets are often hypoplastic or even completely absent. These abnormalities result in varying degrees of tricuspid regurgitation.

- Forward flow through the right heart is reduced, with right-to-left shunting across the atrial septum and/or reduced systemic cardiac output. The tricuspid regurgitation reduces the forward stroke volume of the hypoplastic right ventricle. The atrialized portion of the right ventricle balloons out during atrial systole, acting as a passive reservoir rather than participating in coordinated atrial contraction, thus hindering coordinated atriosystolic filling of the right ventricle.

- Depending on the degree of valve displacement, the right ventricle can become dilated and/or dysfunctional. With severe right ventricular enlargement, the ventricular septum shifts leftward adversely affecting left ventricular (LV) filling and adversely affecting systemic cardiac output.

- Results of the anatomic derangement stemming from Ebstein's anomaly can include right ventricular dysfunction, right atrial dilation, atrial arrhythmias, and, in cases with an atrial communication, cyanosis due to right-to-left intracardiac shunting.

ANATOMIC CLASSIFICATION OF SEVERITY

- Given the varying severity of disease and clinical presentation, several different classification systems have been proposed. One system stratifies severity into mild, moderate, or severe disease based on the degree of apical displacement of the tricuspid valve leaflets as well as the severity of tricuspid valve regurgitation and resultant dilation and dysfunction of the right-sided cardiac chambers.

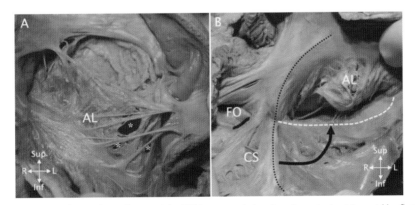

FIGURE 8-1 A heart with Ebstein's anomaly. **A.** The right ventricle (RV) is opened showing the anterior tricuspid leaflet (AL) with multiple small fenestrations (∗) and nearly continuous attachment of the anterior leaflet free edge to the RV wall. **B.** The right atrium and right ventricular inflow have been opened. The fossa ovalis (FO) and coronary sinus (CS) are seen in the right atrium. The black dotted line indicates the anatomic annulus of the tricuspid valve and the white dashed line the actual hinge point of the septal tricuspid leaflet. The space below the white line is the atrialized right ventricle. The black curved arrow indicates the superior rotation of the functional tricuspid annulus toward the RV outflow tract. (*Reproduced with permission from Stephen P. Sanders, MD, Professor of Pediatrics (Cardiology), Harvard Medical School; Director, Cardiac Registry, Departments of Cardiology, Pathology, and Cardiac Surgery, Children's Hospital Boston, Boston, Massachusetts.*)

- A more detailed classification includes anatomy of the tricuspid valve leaflets along with the Carpentier classification (A, B, C, D). This classification is based on anatomic findings found at the time of surgery with the following 4 grades of severity:[4]
  - Type I—The anterior tricuspid leaflet is large and mobile but the posterior and septal leaflets are apically displaced, dysplastic, or absent. The size of the atrialized portion of the right ventricle ranges from relatively small to large.
  - Type II—The anterior, posterior, and often septal leaflets are present, but are relatively small and displaced. A large portion of the ventricular chamber is atrialized.
  - Type III—The anterior leaflet has restricted motion with a shortened, fused, and tethered chordae. Papillary muscles might insert directly into the anterior leaflet. The posterior and septal leaflets are not generally repairable due to severe displacement or dysplasia. A large portion of the right ventricle is atrialized.
  - Type IV—All 3 tricuspid valve leaflets are severely deformed. Chordae are often absent and there may be direct insertions of papillary muscles into the leading edge of the valve. The posterior leaflet is typically dysplastic or absent. There is no true septal leaflet but rather a ridge of fibrous material descending apically from the membranous septum. Severe tricuspid valve tissue displacement may actually cause tricuspid stenosis. Nearly the entire right ventricle is atrialized. These patients typically present very early on in the neonatal period.

ASSOCIATED ANATOMIC LESIONS

Associated congenital heart lesions are common in Ebstein's anomaly. The most commonly seen lesions are the following:

- Patent foramen ovale (PFO) or atrial septal defects (ASD) occur in about 80% of patients with Ebstein's anomaly. An interatrial communication from a PFO or an ASD can allow right-to-left shunting, particularly during exercise, which can result in cyanosis as well as paradoxical embolism.
- Ventricular septal defect (VSD).
- Right ventricular outflow tract obstruction, which can be due to complete absence of the pulmonary valve (pulmonary atresia), structural pulmonary valve stenosis, or "functional" pulmonary atresia.
- Patent ductus arteriosus.
- Coarctation of the aorta.
- Accessory electrical pathways (Wolff-Parkinson-White [WPW] syndrome). These are seen in up to 20% of patients with Ebstein's anomaly and are most often right-sided pathways.

DIAGNOSIS

Clinical Features

- Clinical features of Ebstein's anomaly are dependent on the severity of the disease, including the degree of tricuspid regurgitation, right ventricular size and function, presence or absence of intracardiac shunting, and accessory pathways.
- Patients may be asymptomatic with just a murmur heard on examination or they may have more severe symptoms including cyanosis, arrhythmias, or heart failure, depending on the underlying anatomy.

Neonates with severe tricuspid regurgitation and hypoplastic right ventricles tend to present with cyanosis and heart failure early on, whereas patients with less severe disease may not present until adulthood.

- The most common presenting symptom in older adults is atrial arrhythmias which occur in 20% to 30% of patients.[3,5] Because of a strong association between Ebstein's anomaly and right-sided accessory pathways (Wolff-Parkinson-White syndrome), it is important to obtain a screening echocardiogram in patients who present with WPW to evaluate for the presence of underlying congenital heart disease.
- Female patients with Ebstein's anomaly may not present with symptoms until pregnancy, primarily during the second trimester, when there is significant increase in plasma blood volume.

Physical Examination

- Physical examination findings vary based on severity of disease. Mild cases may be clinically silent or present with an asymptomatic murmur and click, which may be mistaken for mitral valve prolapse.[3] In more severe forms, patients may have prominent "V-waves" depending on the severity of the tricuspid regurgitation. They may be cyanotic if there is significant tricuspid regurgitation and intracardiac right to left shunting at the atrial level. Many patients will also have a prominent right ventricular impulse which is not displaced.
- Heart sounds are frequently abnormal in patients with Ebstein's anomaly of the tricuspid valve. Splitting of the first heart sound is due to apical displacement of the tricuspid valve and the tricuspid and mitral valves closing out of sync with each other. Splitting of the second heart sound occurs in patients with a right bundle branch block which is commonly seen in patients with severe right-sided chamber enlargement. There may also be prominent third and/or fourth heart sounds giving the impression of multiple heart sounds (triple or quadruple gallop). There is often a holosystolic murmur of tricuspid regurgitation which should increase in intensity with inspiration.
- In cases of severe tricuspid regurgitation, a mid-diastolic rumble may be heard due to increased diastolic flow across the tricuspid annulus. In many cases of severe tricuspid regurgitation, the murmur may be soft or even absent due to lack of turbulence across the valve because of rapid equalization of pressures. In patients with severe tricuspid regurgitation, the liver can be enlarged and even pulsatile on palpation. Patients can rarely present with ascites and lower extremity edema.

Electrocardiogram

The electrocardiogram is usually abnormal in Ebstein's anomaly. Typical findings include the following:

- Right atrial hypertrophy with tall, broad ("Himalayan") P-waves (Figure 8-2).
- Right bundle branch block.
- First-degree atrioventricular (AV) block.
- Pre-excitation (Wolff-Parkinson-White pattern) is seen in about 20% of patients with Ebstein's anomaly. The accessory pathway generally is right-sided including a predominant S-wave in the right precordium.[6,7]
- Arrhythmias are common, including supraventricular tachycardia, atrial tachycardia, atrial flutter, and atrial fibrillation (Figure 8-3).

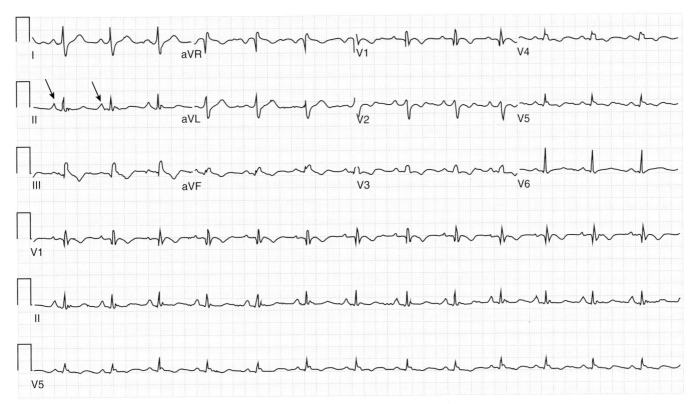

FIGURE 8-2 A 12-lead electrocardiogram with enlarged P-waves consistent with right atrial enlargement.

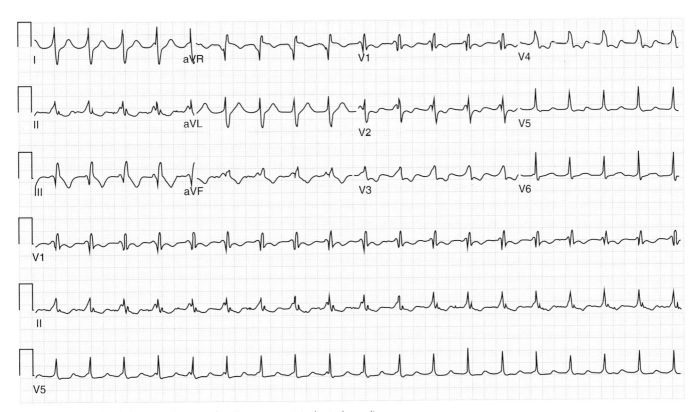

FIGURE 8-3 A 12-lead electrocardiogram showing supraventricular tachycardia.

Chest X-Ray

- In severe cases of Ebstein's anomaly, there can be cardiomegaly that may occupy nearly the entire cardiothoracic diameter. There may be diminished pulmonary vascularity. The right atrium (RA) is enlarged and the left heart border is often straight or convex due to the dilation of the right ventricle.

- In milder cases of Ebstein's anomaly, the chest x-ray can be within normal limits.

Echocardiography

- Key features that should lead to suspicion of Ebstein's anomaly are right-sided chamber enlargement with moderate to severe tricuspid regurgitation.

- Ebstein's anomaly is diagnosed when the septal and posterior leaflets of the tricuspid valves are significantly displaced toward the cardiac apex. To meet diagnostic criteria, the septal tricuspid valve leaflet must be apically displaced greater than or equal to 8 mm/m^2 of body surface area compared with the position of the mitral valve on the apical 4-chamber view[8,9] (Figure 8-4). This displacement leads to a small right ventricular cavity as well as a large atrium, including a large amount of "atrialized" right ventricle.

- The tricuspid valve can vary from being relatively normal to severely dysplastic resulting in variable degrees of tricuspid regurgitation (Figure 8-5). Patients with Ebstein's anomaly who are cyanotic generally have normal pulmonary arterial pressures, in contrast with other patients with cyanosis due to pulmonary arterial hypertension and the Eisenmenger syndrome.

- Transesophageal echocardiogram may be necessary when the transthoracic echocardiographic images inadequately evaluate structural and functional abnormalities.

Cardiac MRI and CT

- Magnetic resonance imaging (MRI) (Figure 8-6) or computed tomography (CT) can be useful in imaging Ebstein's anomaly. Cardiac MRI has the ability to accurately quantify ventricular volumes and ventricular ejection fractions which may be useful in surgical planning. However, distinguishing the "true" right ventricle (the portion of the ventricle below the tricuspid valve that maintains cardiac output) from the entire right ventricle (true right ventricle + atrialized portion of right ventricle) can be challenging (Figures 8-6 and 8-7).

- MRI can also be useful in patients who are obese or have other reasons for having poor acoustic windows. MRI is often superior at visualizing the posterior leaflet of the tricuspid valve, thus it may be useful in conjunction with echocardiography when planning surgical intervention.[10]

- Cardiac CT is primarily reserved for patients who have poor acoustic windows and also have a contraindication to undergoing MRI, such as a pacemaker, aneurysm clips or other metallic foreign bodies, severe claustrophobia, and other patient-specific factors.

Cardiac Catheterization

- The role of diagnostic cardiac catheterization is very limited in Ebstein's anomaly as echocardiography and other noninvasive imaging modalities have improved and are now the mainstays of diagnosing patients.

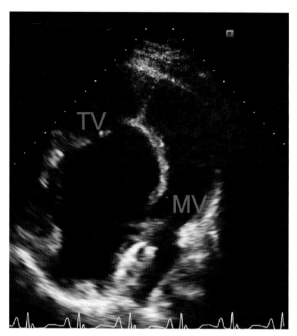

FIGURE 8-4 Two-dimensional echocardiogram of a 20-year old patient with Ebstein's anomaly of the great vessels. The tricuspid valve (TV) is markedly apically displaced compared with the normal location of the mitral valve (MV).

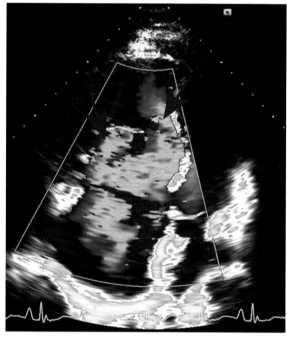

FIGURE 8-5 Two-dimensional echocardiogram of the same patient in Figure 8-1, with color Doppler. Two broad jets of tricuspid regurgitation can be seen consistent with severe tricuspid regurgitation.

- Rarely, some patients with Ebstein's anomaly may also have pulmonary hypertension, and in those cases, cardiac catheterization can be very useful in precisely quantifying pulmonary vascular resistance.

- Cardiac catheterization is currently indicated if there is a need to directly measure pulmonary artery pressures or to perform coronary angiography in preparation for surgical repair or replacement of the tricuspid valve.

- Coronary angiography is generally reserved for patients with suspected coronary disease or in the presurgical risk assessment for men greater than or equal to 35 years of age, premenopausal women greater than or equal to 35 years of age with coronary risk factors, and postmenopausal women.

- Cardiac catheterization may be indicated for percutaneous closure of an atrial septal defect or patent foramen ovale in patients who demonstrate exercise induced hypoxia but may not require surgical intervention for their tricuspid valve.

Exercise Testing

- Formal exercise testing, sometimes with direct measurement of oxygen consumption, can be helpful in quantifying functional limitation in patients who have an unclear history of symptoms or who have cardiomegaly with limited symptoms.

- Exercise testing is also useful to evaluate for intracardiac shunting which may result in exercise-induced hypoxia.

Laboratory Studies

- Most patients with Ebstein's anomaly have no specific laboratory abnormalities; however, patients with chronic cyanosis may have polycythemia.

MANAGEMENT

- Management largely depends on the physiologic consequences of the anatomic derangement. It is not uncommon for a patient with Ebstein's anomaly to be remarkably asymptomatic and live a long

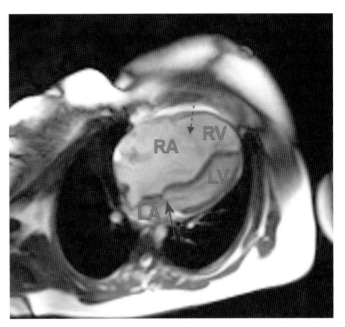

FIGURE 8-6 Horizontal long-axis steady-state free-precession cine loop of a cardiac MRI. Dotted arrow shows apical displacement of tricuspid valve between the right atrium (RA) and right ventricle (RV). Solid arrow points to location of normally positioned mitral valve between the left atrium (LA) and left ventricle (LV).

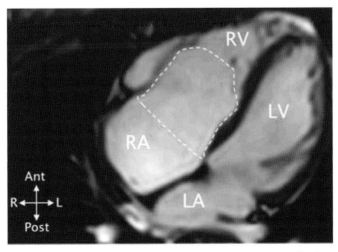

FIGURE 8-7 MRI cine SSFP 4-chamber projection in a patient with Ebstein's anomaly showing the offset between the mitral and tricuspid insertions. The dotted line indicates the atrialized right ventricle. The functional right ventricle (RV) is small. LA, left atrium; LV, left ventricle; RA, right atrium. (*Reproduced with permission from Stephen P. Sanders, MD, Professor of Pediatrics (Cardiology), Harvard Medical School; Director, Cardiac Registry, Departments of Cardiology, Pathology, and Cardiac Surgery, Children's Hospital Boston, Boston, Massachusetts.*)

and active life, requiring only medical therapy. Nearly all patients with Ebstein's anomaly have at least moderate, if not severe tricuspid regurgitation, and the amount of tricuspid regurgitation itself is not a good prognostic indicator.

- Development of heart failure symptoms and arrhythmias are the main concerns that might prompt intensifying medical therapy or perhaps referral to surgery for tricuspid valve repair or replacement.

- In many patients, the only invasive management necessary to control symptoms is to occlude residual atrial septal defects with right-to-left shunting, in cases of symptomatic cyanosis or stroke due to paradoxical embolism. In most patients, atrial septal defects can be closed nonsurgically in the interventional catheterization laboratory.

- Surgical techniques, mostly focused on repair of the tricuspid valve, can be used to control medically refractory heart failure symptoms or unloading of the right atrium in cases of medically uncontrollable arrhythmias. Several techniques exist to surgically repair Ebstein's anomaly of the tricuspid valve.

Medical Therapy

- Diuretics are the mainstays of treatment in patients with Ebstein's anomaly to control volume status in setting of tricuspid regurgitation and right-sided volume overload. Additional heart failure medications, such as beta-blockers, angiotensin-converting enzyme inhibitors (ACEIs), and digoxin may be useful although there has been limited evidence that these medications improve right ventricular function in patients with Ebstein's anomaly.

- Because patients with Ebstein's are at risk for atrial arrhythmias, antiarrhythmic therapy is frequently required. The type of treatment indicated is dependent on the origin and severity of the arrhythmia. Patients may be on beta-blockers or a number of antiarrhythmic agents including sotalol, mexiletine, and amiodarone. Frequently management of patients with Ebstein's anomaly will require the expertise of both an adult congenital heart disease specialist and an electrophysiologist with knowledge of congenital heart disease.

- Endocarditis prophylaxis prior to dental procedures only is recommended for patients who have underlying cyanosis, a residual shunt at the site of prior repair or a prosthetic heart valve.[11]

- Anticoagulation, with either aspirin or an oral vitamin K antagonist such as warfarin, is recommended in patients with atrial fibrillation, atrial flutter, residual right-to-left shunting with a history of paradoxical embolism, or a mechanical prosthetic valve.

- Newer oral anticoagulants such as dabigatran and oral factor Xa inhibitors have not been scientifically evaluated in patients with congenital heart disease, although they may be useful in selected patients.[12]

Electrophysiology and Radiofrequency Ablation of Arrhythmias

- The conduction system is often abnormal in patients with Ebstein's anomaly, with prolonged conduction in the enlarged RA. The right bundle is abnormally located in the majority of cases resulting in right bundle branch block. The AV node is usually located in the triangle of Koch, however, there is often discontinuity of the central fibrous body leaving accessory pathways often located on the same side as the malformed tricuspid valve.

- A variety of electrophysiologic ablations can be attempted, depending on the source of the arrhythmia. Radiofrequency catheter ablation or surgical ablation of atrioventricular accessory pathways is suggested in symptomatic patients, especially if the accessory pathway is capable of rapid conduction to the ventricle.[6,13,14]

- Success rates of electrophysiologic ablation largely depend on the degree of atrial dilation and location of the electrical pathway. Patients with severe volume overload may have multiple pathways and ultimately require surgical treatment to control arrhythmias.

Surgical Repair

- Approximately 80% of patients with Ebstein's anomaly will eventually require some type of surgical intervention.[3] Cardiac surgery for Ebstein's anomaly should be performed by surgeons with training and expertise in congenital heart disease. In selected cases, addition of a left-sided maze procedure during Ebstein's surgery may be beneficial at decreasing burden of atrial fibrillation.

- Surgical ablation of an accessory pathway should be performed if the pathway was unable to be ablated in the catheterization laboratory.

- Potential indications for surgical intervention include symptoms or worsening exercise capacity, cyanosis (oxygen saturation <90% on room air), paradoxical embolism, progressive right ventricular (RV) dilation, or deterioration of RV systolic function.

- Indications for reoperation following tricuspid valve repair include the following:

  ○ Worsening of symptoms to NYHA class III or IV symptoms
  ○ Redevelopment of severe tricuspid regurgitation accompanied by progressive RV dilation, worsening RV systolic function
  ○ Development or worsening of atrial and/or ventricular arrhythmias that are not amenable to medical management
  ○ Tricuspid stenosis with mean gradient greater than 12 mm Hg
  ○ Mixed tricuspid valve dysfunction with significant regurgitation and stenosis

SURGICAL TECHNIQUES

- Tricuspid valve repair is preferred over valve replacement in order to lower the risk of long-term complications.[15,16] When valve replacement is necessary, tissue valves are preferred to mechanical valves since right-sided mechanical valves have a high propensity for thromboembolic complications. In addition, it would be ideal to avoid warfarin in women of childbearing age due to the teratogenic effects of warfarin.[17] Types of tricuspid valve repairs include the following:

  ○ Danielson repair: Monocusp repair of the tricuspid valve using the anterior leaflet. In this repair, the hinge point of the anterior leaflet may be apical to the true annulus of the tricuspid valve. The RV is plicated vertically in selected cases, and a posterior annuloplasty is performed.[18]
  ○ Carpentier technique: The large sail-like anterior leaflet is excised free from the valve annulus and the posterior and septal leaflets are surgically separated from the RV endocardium. The leaflets are rotated clockwise to the coronary sinus to create a

monocusp valve. The hinge point of the monocusp anterior leaflet is at the level of the true annulus. The atrialized RV is plicated vertically.[19]

  ○ Cone reconstruction: This repair is the newest and most anatomically correct repair. All 3 leaflets are surgically delaminated from the myocardium. The anterior and posterior leaflets are rotated to meet the mobilized septal leaflet. As a result, there is a ring of valve tissue resembling a cone. The valves are then reanchored at the level of the true tricuspid annulus. The RV is vertically plicated.[20]

- In cases of a severely dysplastic right ventricle that may not be able to maintain cardiac output, a "ventricle and a half" repair may be pursued if the pulmonary vascular resistance is acceptably low. The advantage of this type of repair is to ensure adequate preload to the left ventricle. This procedure has been shown to reduce early mortality in some series and may be useful as an intraoperative "salvage" procedure or procedure to avoid the need for transplant in a very symptomatic patient.[21,22] Severe cases of Ebstein's anomaly that are not amenable to surgical intervention may require a heart transplant.

ATHLETIC PARTICIPATION

Some patients with Ebstein's anomaly are at risk of cardiac events, including sudden death, during sports participation. Recommendations for eligibility for participation in competitive athletics for patients with Ebstein's anomaly were outlined in 2005 at the 36th Bethesda Conference on Eligibility Recommendations for Competitive Athletes with Cardiovascular Abnormalities.[23]

- Athletes with mild Ebstein's anomaly (no cyanosis, normal size of the right ventricle, and no evidence of arrhythmias) may participate in all sports at all levels without restriction.

- Athletes with mild tricuspid regurgitation can participate in low-intensity competitive sports if they have no evidence of arrhythmia other than isolated premature atrial or ventricular contractions on Holter monitoring.

- Athletes with severe Ebstein's anomaly should not be allowed to participate in any competitive sports, unless surgically repaired, after which time they can participate in low-intensity sports. Patients with an excellent result from surgery may be allowed to participate in higher impact sports on a case-by-case basis.

PREGNANCY

- A majority of women with Ebstein's anomaly who survive to childbearing age tolerate pregnancy well; however, they do warrant close cardiovascular monitoring during pregnancy. The increase in plasma blood volume from pregnancy augments the degree of right ventricular volume overload in Ebstein's anomaly, sometimes resulting in heart failure symptoms. In addition, patients with atrial septal defects may develop new right-to-left shunting and cyanosis due to increases in right ventricular filling pressure during pregnancy.

- Right-to-left shunting increases the risk of stroke and other paradoxical emboli, and cyanosis can adversely affect fetal development. Because of the physiologic changes of pregnancy, the risk of arrhythmia is increased during pregnancy in patients with

Ebstein's anomaly. However, the majority of acyanotic Ebsteins patients tolerate pregnancy well, as long as arrhythmias are well controlled.[24-26]

- Ebstein's anomaly does portend some risk to the fetus. In one series, prematurity occurred in 22% of pregnancies and perinatal mortality occurred in 2.3%. The rate of congenital heart disease (of any type) in this series was 4%.

LONG-TERM COMPLICATIONS AND PROGNOSIS

- The prognosis of patients with Ebstein's anomaly is again dependent on the severity of the disease. In patients who are diagnosed with Ebstein's anomaly during adulthood, the prognosis is generally favorable. In a classic series of 220 patients seen between 1958 and 1991, 83% who presented in adulthood had no cardiac symptoms and 67% were not requiring cardiac medications.[3]

- Risk factors for poor outcomes in unoperated adult patients include an early age at diagnosis, male sex, severity of morbid anatomy, pulmonary outflow obstruction, and cardiothoracic ratio >0.65. Surprisingly, supraventricular arrhythmia does not appear to be associated with worse outcomes.[27,28]

- In patients who undergo tricuspid valve surgery, atrial tachyarrhythmias occur in one-third of postoperative patients.

- Recurrent hospitalizations are frequent, occurring in up to 65% of patients at 20 years postoperatively, with arrhythmia being the most common indication for readmission.[28]

- Sudden death is a rare late complication, occurring in about 2% of patients.[29]

- The overall freedom from late reoperation is 74% at 10 years and 46% at 20 years. Risk factors for reoperation include an arrhythmia procedure, wide complex tachycardia, at least moderate ventricular dysfunction, and age at surgery less than 12 years.[28]

- However, patients who do require surgery also have a relatively favorable prognosis as surgical outcomes have improved dramatically over the past few decades with refinements in technique and improvements in postoperative intensive care. In a series of 158 patients who underwent tricuspid valve replacement with a tissue valve, 10-year survival was 93% with freedom from valve re-replacement of 98% at 10 years and 81% at 15 years. The majority had no or minimal cardiac symptoms, and 94% were not requiring anticoagulation.[17]

CONCLUSION

- Ebstein's anomaly is a relatively rare congenital heart lesion consisting of apical displacement of the tricuspid valve which results in tricuspid valve regurgitation, "atrialization" of the right ventricle, and varying degrees of right ventricular hypoplasia and dysfunction. The severity of the disease is dependent on the severity of the degree of apical displacement and the morphology of the tricuspid valve.

- Patients with Ebstein's anomaly also may have evidence of atrial level shunting as manifested by either resting or exercise-induced hypoxemia. Atrial arrhythmias are also very common in patients with Ebstein's anomaly typically secondary to accessory pathways although other atrial arrhythmias such as atrial flutter/fibrillation, atrial tachycardia, and AV-nodal reentry tachycardia have been seen. With improving surgical techniques and a better understanding of the pathophysiology of the disease, the overall prognosis for these patients is good.

- However, severe cases may present in the neonatal period with severe cyanosis and death. Whenever possible, adult patients with Ebstein's anomaly should be followed by a cardiologist with special expertise in adult congenital heart disease. Patients should be monitored closely for development of atrial or ventricular tachyarrhythmias.

- Patients who undergo surgical intervention for their valvular disease are at risk for developing complete atrioventricular block during surgery and should be monitored for this complication postoperatively.

- Antibiotic prophylaxis should be provided to patients with cyanosis, a prosthetic valve or residual shunting at the site of prior repair.

REFERENCES

1. Correa-Villaseñor A, Ferencz C, Neill CA, et al. Ebstein's malformation of the tricuspid valve: genetic and environmental factors. The Baltimore-Washington Infant Study Group. *Teratology*. 1994;50:137-147.

2. Weinstein MR, Goldfield MD. Cardiovascular malformations with lithium use during pregnancy. *Am J Psychiatry*. 1975;132:529-531.

3. Celermajer DS, Bull C, Till JA, et al. Ebstein's anomaly: presentation and outcome from fetus to adult. *J Am Coll Cardiol*. 1994;23:170.

4. Dearani JA, Danielson GK. Congenital Heart Surgery Nomenclature and Database Project: Ebstein's anomaly and tricuspid valve disease. *Ann Thorac Surg*. 2000;69:S106.

5. Watson H. Natural history of Ebstein's anomaly of tricuspid valve in childhood and adolescence. An international co-operative study of 505 cases. *Br Heart J*. 1974;36:417.

6. Cappato R, Schluter M, Weiss C, et al. Radiofrequency current catheter ablation of accessory atrioventricular pathways in Ebstein's anomaly. *Circulation*. 1996;94:376.

7. Lev M, Gibson S, Miller RA. Ebstein's disease with Wolff-Parkinson-White syndrome: report of a case with a histopathologic study of possible conduction pathways. *Am Heart J*. 1955;49:724.

8. Shiina A, Seward JB, Edwards WD, et al. Two-dimensional echocardiographic spectrum of Ebstein's anomaly: detailed anatomic assessment. *J Am Coll Cardiol*. 1984;3:356.

9. Gussenhoven EJ, Stewart JB, Becker AE, et al. "Offsetting" of the septal tricuspid leaflet in normal hearts and hearts with Ebstein's anomaly. Anatomic and echographic correlation. *Am J Cardiol*. 1984;54:172.

10. Attenhofer Jost CH, Edmister WD, Julsrud PR, et al. Prospective comparison of echocardiography versus cardiac magnetic imaging in patients with Ebstein's anomaly. *Int J Cardiovasc Imaging*. 2012;28:1147.

11. Wilson W, Taubert KA, Gewitz M, et al. Prevention of infective endocarditis. Guidelines from the American Heart Association. A Guideline from the American Heart Association Rheumatic Fever, Endocarditis, and Kawasaki Disease Committee, Council on Cardiovascular Disease in the Young, and the Council on Clinical Cardiology, Council on Cardiovascular Surgery and Anesthesia, and the Quality of Care and Outcomes Research Interdisciplinary Working Group. *Circulation*. 2007;115 published online April 19, 2007. www.circ.ahajournals.org/cgi/reprint/CIRCULATIONAHA.106.183095v1.

12. Abadir S, Khairy P. Electrophysiology and adult congenital heart disease: advances and options. *Prog Cardiovasc Dis*. 2011;53:281-292.

13. Misaki T, Watanabe G, Iwa T, et al. Surgical treatment of patients with Wolff-Parkinson-White syndrome and associated Ebstein's anomaly. *J Thorac Cardiovasc Surg*. 1995;110:1702.

14. Reich JD, Auld D, Hulse E, Sullivan K, Campbell R. The Pediatric Radiofrequency Ablation Registry's experience with Ebstein's anomaly. Pediatric Electrophysiology Society. *J Cardiovasc Electrophysiol*. 1998;9:1370.

15. Augustin N, Schmidt-Habelmann P, Wottke M, et al. Results after surgical repair of Ebstein's anomaly. *Ann Thorac Surg*. 1997;63:1650.

16. Vargas FJ, Mengo G, Granja MA, et al. Tricuspid annuloplasty and ventricular plication for Ebstein's malformation. *Ann Thorac Surg*. 1998;65:1755.

17. Kiziltan HT, Theodoro DA, Warnes CA, et al. Late results of bioprosthetic tricuspid valve replacement in Ebstein's anomaly. *Ann Thorac Surg*. 1998;66:1539.

18. Danielson GK, Driscoll DJ, Mair DD, et al. Operative treatment of Ebstein's anomaly. *J Thorac Cardiovasc Surg*. 1992;104:1195.

19. Carpentier A, Chauvaud S, Macé L, et al. A new reconstructive operation for Ebstein's anomaly of the tricuspid valve. *J Thorac Cardiovasc Surg*. 1988;96:92.

20. da Silva JP, Baumgratz JF, da Fonseca L, et al. The cone reconstruction of the tricuspid valve in Ebstein's anomaly. The operation: early and midterm results. *J Thorac Cardiovasc Surg*. 2007;133:215.

21. Malhotra SP, Petrossian E, Reddy VM, et al. Selective right ventricular unloading and novel technical concepts in Ebstein's anomaly. *Ann Thorac Surg*. 2009;88:1975.

22. Quinonez LG, Dearani JA, Puga FJ, et al. Results of the 1.5-ventricle repair for Ebstein's anomaly and the failing right ventricle. *J Thorac Cardiovasc Surg*. 2007;133:1303.

23. Graham TP Jr, Driscoll DJ, Gersony WM, et al. Task Force 2: congenital heart disease. *J Am Coll Cardiol*. 2005;45:1326.

24. Connolly HM, Warnes CA. Ebstein's anomaly: outcome of pregnancy. *J Am Coll Cardiol*. 1994;23:1194.

25. Donnelly JE, Brown JM, Radford DJ. Pregnancy outcome and Ebstein's anomaly. *Br Heart J*. 1991;66:368.

26. Drenthen W, Pieper PG, Roos-Hesselink JW, et al. Outcome of pregnancy in women with congenital heart disease: a literature review. *J Am Coll Cardiol*. 2007;49:2303.

27. Attie F, Rosas M, Rijlaarsdam M, et al. The adult patient with Ebstein's anomaly. Outcome in 72 unoperated patients. *Medicine (Baltimore)*. 2000;79:27-36.

28. Brown ML, Dearani JA, Danielson GK, et al. The outcomes of operations for 539 patients with Ebstein's anomaly. *J Thorac Cardiovasc Surg*. 2008;135:1120-1136.

29. Watson H. Natural history of Ebstein's anomaly of tricuspid valve in childhood and adolescence. An international co-operative study of 505 cases. *Br Heart J*. 1974;36:417-427.

9 PULMONARY HYPERTENSION IN ADULTS WITH CONGENITAL HEART DISEASE

Alexander R. Opotowsky, MD

INTRODUCTION

- Pulmonary hypertension (PH) itself is not a disease and does not specify any unique pathophysiology. PH refers to elevated pulmonary artery (PA) pressure.

- The underlying physiology is variable with a major distinction between PH caused by elevated pulmonary venous (distal) pressure, elevated pulmonary vascular resistance (PVR), and high flow (Figure 9-1).[1]

- Pulmonary hypertension can be due to any combination of these 3 underlying physiologies in various types of congenital heart disease. Marked pulmonary vascular remodeling does not necessarily translate into elevated pulmonary artery pressure in the setting of low flow. The presence of dynamic shunting complicates interpretation. An acute increase in flow itself causes recruitment and dilation of pulmonary vessels, resulting in decreased pulmonary vascular resistance.

- While the equation for PVR (PVR = ΔP/CO) may suggest that PVR is equivalent at any flow (eg, if you double CO then ΔP will double and therefore PVR will remain stable), the relationship is not linear (Figure 9-2). While this phenomenon can be important in the absence of congenital heart disease (CHD), its appreciation is critical in interpretation of hemodynamic data in patients with shunting.

- Further, distinct underlying etiologies often produce equivalent physiology and indistinguishable pulmonary vascular pathology.

- Pulmonary arterial hypertension (PAH) is defined as PH with high PVR without pulmonary venous hypertension.[2]

- This chapter will review PH in adults with congenital heart disease from the perspective of the underlying physiology followed by several cases which highlight dynamic interplay between the component parts of "pulmonary pressure" and finally a discussion of special cases of right heart pathology requiring special consideration.

DIAGNOSTIC TESTING

- There are a number of approaches to determine the physiologic underpinning of elevated pulmonary artery pressure in a given patient with congenital heart disease.

- Complete understanding of the underlying defect and prior procedures is essential and this information alone usually provides a good sense of the most likely reason a patient has high PA pressure.

- However, many defects may be associated with high flow, high resistance, or high distal pressure. Atrial septal defect (ASD) is a

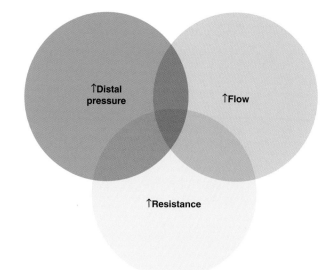

FIGURE 9-1 The hemodynamic underpinnings of elevated pulmonary artery pressure. Elevated left-sided filling (or distal) pressure is the most common reason for elevated pulmonary artery pressure in the general population, and is a contributor in a significant subset of patients with congenital heart disease. High pulmonary vascular resistance is the hemodynamic cause of elevated pulmonary pressure in pulmonary arterial hypertension (PAH) of various causes. Increased pulmonary flow is seen in patients with left-to-right shunting, and defining the extent of flow is critical in the assessment of shunt lesions. There is important overlap and the findings are flow-dependent and may be dynamic for a given patient depending on the context. That is, distal pressure and pulmonary vascular resistance may vary at different levels of pulmonary flow.

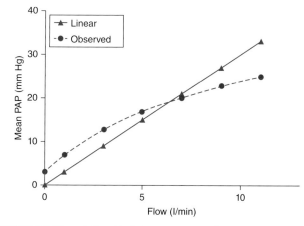

FIGURE 9-2 The relationship between mean pulmonary artery pressure and mean flow (ie, pulmonary vascular resistance) is not equivalent at all levels of flow as a result of vessel recruitment and distention with higher flow. Therefore, resistance (the ratio of pressure to flow) is lower at higher flow. PAP, pulmonary artery pressure.

common example where this distinction is critical and this chapter will review several cases of patients presenting with ASD and pulmonary hypertension, each of which constitutes a different clinical picture.

- Physical examination is helpful in exploring the cause of high PA pressure, as is the 12-lead electrocardiogram and chest radiograph. In the current era, however, it is rare that a patient does not undergo more technologically involved cardiac imaging and, sometimes, catheterization.

- While pulmonary function testing, cardiac magnetic resonance imaging (MRI), cardiac computed tomography (CT), and nuclear imaging have a role in evaluation in a subset of patients, the vast majority of clinically actionable data on pulmonary hypertension in adult congenital heart disease (ACHD) is derived from echocardiography and catheterization.

- These 2 common techniques will be reviewed in further depth.

ECHOCARDIOGRAPHIC EVALUATION FOR SUSPECTED PULMONARY HYPERTENSION

- An isolated unexpected finding of elevated PA systolic pressure on a transthoracic echocardiography is a common reason for the initial suspicion that a patient has PH.

- The PA systolic pressure is estimated using the modified simplified Bernoulli equation ($\Delta P = 4V^2$) from the systolic transtricuspid velocity adding a value for estimated right atrial (RA) pressure (whether a constant based on examination or the size and pattern of inferior vena cava [IVC] collapse) (Figure 9-3). This is the extent of the evaluation for many patients. This is unfortunate not only because pulmonary artery systolic pressure (PASP) is only moderately accurate by echocardiography,[3] but even more importantly because even when accurate, the PA pressure provides no information on why there is elevated pulmonary artery pressure.

- Also unfortunate, adequate tricuspid regurgitant jets are not present in all patients and the echocardiographic evaluation often does not extend beyond this single measurement.

- On a more positive note, there are several very simple variables that can be gleaned from clinically obtained echocardiograms that provide further insight.

- In addition to PA systolic pressure, PA diastolic and mean pressures can also be estimated using echocardiography. The most common, though not the only, method to estimate diastolic pressure uses the estimated gradient between main PA and right ventricular (RV) outflow tract by measuring transpulmonic valve end regurgitant velocity ($\Delta P \approx 4 \times V^2$). This value added to the estimated right atrial pressure approximates end-diastolic PA pressure. Mean PA pressure can be estimated using the equation in Table 9-1.

- Right ventricular geometry is complex, and RV volume and function are difficult to assess precisely with 2-dimensional echocardiography. Nevertheless, there are several simple parameters that provide relatively robust estimates of RV function in patients without for sake of uniformity-should congenital heart disease be CHD through the chapter (after the first time its used), though these must be used with caution in CHD patients. Tricuspid annular plane systolic excursion (TAPSE) describes the distance traveled by the tricuspid annulus toward the probe during systole

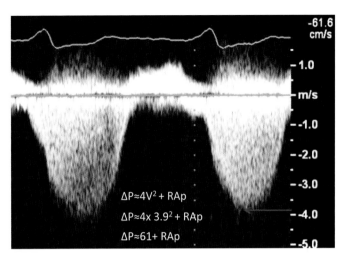

FIGURE 9-3 Continuous-wave Doppler across the tricuspid valve, measuring systolic transtricuspid velocity. This velocity is used to estimate pulmonary artery (or right ventricular) systolic pressure using the modified simplified Bernoulli equation as outlined on the figure.

using M-mode or 2D imaging. A low value (eg, <1.8 cm) argues for right ventricular dysfunction.

- In patients with CHD with the real potential to have unappreciated RV dyssynchrony (eg, those with repaired tetralogy of Fallot who have had a prior right ventriculotomy and/or transannular patch placement), any single variable is likely to be misleading.

- Late systolic flattening of the ventricular septum (quantified by the eccentricity index) is often reported as "RV pressure overload."[4] This is an excellent marker of elevated impedance to RV ejection, but may give a false impression that peak systolic RV pressure must be approximating left ventricular (LV) pressure to be able to "push the septum back" toward the LV. In fact, late systolic flattening is a relatively early sign of elevated pulmonary vascular impedance and is related to delayed and prolonged RV systolic time compared with the left ventricle.[5,6]

- There are also echocardiographic signs indicated adverse ventricular interaction in patients with a volume-loaded right ventricle, such as with atrial septal defect, but with normal pulmonary vascular resistance.[7]

- There are more complex quantitative methods to estimate RV size or function such as fractional area change, but these are little used in clinical practice. The advent of 3-dimensional imaging promises improvements in echocardiographic RV quantification.

- It is equally important to assess for evidence of elevated left atrial (LA) pressure or characteristics that predispose to left atrial pressure.[8] Left atrial size, left ventricular hypertrophy, and abnormal diastolic indices are the most common. The presence of a dilated left atrium strongly suggests long-standing left atrial hypertension.

- Note that "grade 1" diastolic dysfunction (reversed E:A) is often present in pulmonary arterial hypertension because of ventricular interaction and actually argues quite strongly against elevated LA pressure being the cause of elevated PA pressure. Tissue Doppler imaging provides important information on left atrial pressure, but lateral mitral annular velocities should be used since septal velocities are affected by right ventricular dysfunction or electrical delay, which are common in congenital heart disease.[9]

- Pulsed-wave Doppler flow velocity of the right ventricular outflow tract is an excellent indicator of the pulmonary impedance. Several variables may be measured including acceleration time, velocity-time integral (VTI), and qualitative notching. Shorter acceleration time (the time from the initiation of flow to the peak velocity) correlates with higher pulmonary artery pressure and PVR (Figure 9-4).

- Mid-systolic notching of the flow velocity envelope represents systolic flow deceleration in the setting of reflected pressure waves and strongly suggests elevated PVR and increased pulmonary artery stiffness (Figure 9-5).[10] Notching is the Doppler correlate of the historically reported finding of a "flying W" pattern of pulmonary valve motion on M-mode imaging (Figure 9-6).

INVASIVE (CARDIAC CATHETERIZATION) EVALUATION OF SUSPECTED PULMONARY HYPERTENSION

- All patients with suspected pulmonary arterial hypertension (ie, high PVR) in the setting of CHD, without unusual extenuating issues, should undergo diagnostic catheterization.

Table 9-1 Hemodynamic Definitions and Equations

RAP = right atrial pressure (mm Hg)

MAP = mean systemic arterial pressure (mm Hg)

DPAP = diastolic pulmonary artery pressure (mm Hg)

SPAP = systolic pulmonary artery pressure (mm Hg)

MPAP = mean pulmonary artery pressure (mm Hg)

PAWP = pulmonary artery wedge pressure

(PA occlusion pressure and PA capillary wedge pressure are clinically equivalent terms) (mm Hg)

HR = heart rate (bpm)

CO = Qs = cardiac output (l/min)

SV = stroke volume (mL/beat) = (CO × 1000)/HR

BSA = body surface area (m^2)

CI = Qsi = cardiac index (l/min/m^2) = CO/BSA

SVI = stroke volume index (mL/beat/m^2) = SV/BSA

PVR = pulmonary vascular resistance (WU/m^2 or dyne × second × s^{-5}/m^2)

PVRI = pulmonary vascular resistance indexed to BSA = PVR × BSA)

SVR = systemic vascular resistance (either WU or dyne × second × s^{-5})

WU = Wood unit (mm Hg/l/min)

1 WU = 80 dynes × seconds × cm^{-5}

CaO_2 = oxygen content of blood (mL/L)

PaO_2 = partial pressure of oxygen

VO_2 = O_2 consumption (mL/min/m^2)

MPAP ≈ 0.67 × DPAP + 0.33 × SPAP

Transpulmonary gradient (TPG) = MPAP − PAWP

cO_2 (mL/L) = (1.34 × [Hg] [g/dL] × SO_2 × x 10) + (PaO_2 × 0.003)

cO_2 (mL/L) ≈ (1.34 × [Hg] [g/dL] × SO_2 × x 10)

CO (Fick) = (VO_2)/(systemic arterial cO_2 − mixed venous cO_2)

PVR = TPG/CO

SVR = (MAP − RAP)/CO

CI = CO/BSA

PVRI = TPG/CI

SVRI = (MAP − RAP)/CI

For the cO_2 calculation, O_2 saturation is entered as a decimal (eg, 0.99 instead of 99%). To convert units from g/dL to g/L, the x10 term is included [Hg] = hemoglobin concentration.

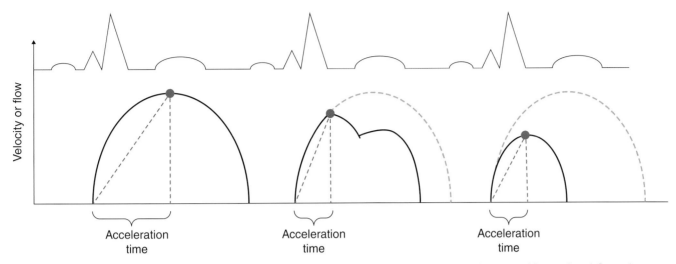

FIGURE 9-4 Measurement of right ventricular outflow tract (RVOT) acceleration time, the time between the onset of flow and peak flow velocity. Acceleration time is usually greater than 100 ms, and values less than that (especially <80 ms) are suggestive of elevated pulmonary vascular resistance.

- The vast majority of pulmonary hypertension (ie, elevated mean PA pressure) in the general population is due to left heart disease and this is also true for a sizable subset of adults with CHD.

- Discussion of the mechanics of catheterization and catheterization techniques in the presence of intracardiac shunting or complex defects is beyond the scope of this chapter, but it is important to review the fundamental hemodynamic evaluation of elevated PA pressure.

- As such, a standard right heart catheterization (RHC) will be discussed.

TECHNIQUE FOR RIGHT HEART CARDIAC CATHETERIZATION

- For adults, right heart catheterization is usually performed with a single or double-lumen balloon-tipped radiopaque catheter with distance markings every 10 cm, with or without a near-the-catheter

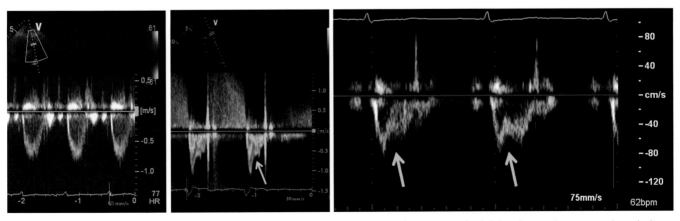

FIGURE 9-5 Three examples of right ventricular outflow tract (RVOT) pulse-wave Doppler tracings. The left-hand example is a normal parabolic shape. The middle and right-hand examples demonstrate short acceleration time and systolic notching (flow deceleration).

tip thermistor (for thermodilution output measurements). When 2 fluid-filled lumens are present the proximal lumen opens approximately 30 cm from the catheter tip and the distal lumen opens at the tip beyond the balloon. A third lumen is used to transmit gas or fluid from a syringe to the balloon, which usually has a capacity of 1.5 mL.

- Intracardiac pressures should be measured with neutral intrathoracic pressure, most closely approximated at end expiration for spontaneously breathing patients. Mean pressures should generally not be substituted for end-expiratory pressure.

- In the presence of marked shifts in intrathoracic pressure with breathing, often seen in patients with labored breathing, digitally averaged pressure over the entirely respiratory cycle may variably over- or underestimate true chamber; steps should be taken to limit respiratory variation such as encouraging an end-expiratory maneuver. The ability of patients to comply with such requests is critical, and support performance of catheterization with limited, if any, sedation to the extent possible.

- Intrathoracic pressure can be estimated using esophageal manometry, but this is very rarely employed in clinical practice and has limitations.

- It is important to confirm a PA "wedge" pressure. It can be difficult to completely obstruct antegrade flow in patients with PH; CHD patient with systemic-pulmonary arterial collateral flow also poses challenges to optimal wedge positioning.

- With care not to dissect the occluded branch vessel or to extravasate, a small amount of contrast (see discussion of wedge angiography later) may be slowly injected to similarly confirm wedge position.

MEASUREMENT OF CARDIAC OUTPUT

There are 2 methods to estimate cardiac output commonly used in clinical practice, indicator dilution and Fick.

Indicator Dilution Method

- Indicator dilution involves injecting an indicator, usually room temperature or cold saline, through a proximal catheter port. In the case of thermodilation there is a thermistor near the distal end of the catheter which measures temperature change after injection of a specified volume of saline of known temperature.

- Using these data, cardiac output is estimated using the Stewart-Hamilton equation. Dilution techniques are inaccurate in the setting of intracardiac shunts, and the accuracy is questionable with severe tricuspid regurgitation or cardiogenic shock.

- Measurement should be repeated at least 3 times (or more if measurements are not consistent) to ensure an accurate estimate. Dilution techniques do not require an estimate of oxygen consumption, which avoids an important source of error in the use of the Fick principle when this variable is assumed based on population data.

The Fick Principle

- The quantity of O_2 extracted from the blood is equivalent, during aerobic metabolism, to the amount of O_2 used by the tissues. Whatever volume of blood the heart is able to deliver (cardiac output), the

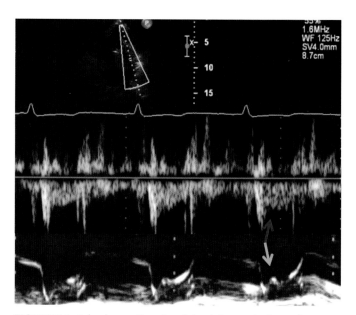

FIGURE 9-6 Pulsed-wave Doppler of the right ventricular outflow tract (RVOT) (top) and M-mode of the pulmonary valve (bottom) in a patient with pulmonary arterial hypertension. Red arrow identifies mid-systolic flow deceleration while the blue arrow identifies transient movement of the pulmonary valve toward the closed position ("flying W") as a consequence, both related to reflected waves in the pulmonary circulation.

tissues must extract some absolute amount of oxygen to support a given level of aerobic metabolism.

- If the cardiac output doubles, half as much oxygen per unit of blood will need to be extracted to support a given degree of oxygen consumption.

- The Fick equation uses this relationship to estimate the cardiac output using oxygen consumption (measured or assumed/estimated) and the arteriovenous difference in oxygen content.

- Cardiac output (l/min) = [oxygen consumption (mL/min)]/ (arterial O_2 content − venous O_2 content). See Table 9-1.

- The blood's oxygen content is mostly composed of oxygen molecules bound to hemoglobin, with a small contribution by oxygen molecules in solution.

- Catheterization should be performed with the patient using their baseline supplemental oxygen, and there is a negligible absolute amount of dissolved oxygen. Therefore, the estimate of oxygen content usually ignores dissolved oxygen. Only when a patient is on high concentrations of supplemental oxygen with high PaO_2 does this importantly impact cardiac output estimates (see Table 9-1).

- Oxygen consumption can be directly measured during catheterization. In clinical practice, however, O_2 consumption is usually estimated using normative equations derived from population averages.

- Many clinicians use a standard value of 125 mL/min/m^2, though empiric normative values by age, sex, body size, and heart rate are available. At the extremes of body size and age, these estimates are of questionable validity even on a population scale.

- On an individual basis, the inaccuracy of assumed $\dot{V}O_2$ constitutes one of the most important limitations of the accuracy of Fick of cardiac output estimates.[11-13]

HEMODYNAMIC DATA FROM CARDIAC CATHETERIZATION

PVR usually refers to the prevenous component of resistance. Resistance describes the relationship between pressure and flow, in this case between mean pulmonary artery pressure (MPAP) and pulmonary blood flow which approximates systemic cardiac output in the absence of intracardiac shunting.

The main hemodynamic parameters of interest in the evaluation of PH are as follows:

- Mean PA pressure: The presence of elevated mean PA pressure is integral to the definition of PH, but the degree of pressure elevation itself has limited diagnostic and prognostic value.

- PVR: Elevated PVR is the primary hemodynamic feature of PAH. The hemodynamic criteria for PAH are as follows:
  a. MPAP greater than 25 mm Hg
  b. PVR greater than 3 WU
  c. Pulmonary artery occlusion pressure (PAOP) less than or equal to 15 mm Hg

- Some patients with left-sided heart failure or pulmonary vein stenosis develop high PVR. The PVR is usually mildly elevated, but can occasionally be greater than 4.5 WU.[14] While such patients are not classified as having PAH (group I PH), elevated PVR is correlated with impaired functional capacity and may sometimes be a reasonable target for therapy.

- Cardiac output/index: The capacity to perform work is directly related to the ability to increase the systemic cardiac output.

- Right atrial and right ventricular end-diastolic pressure (RVEDP): Elevated RAP and RVEDP reflect right ventricular failure and are markers of poor prognosis.

LIMITATIONS OF CARDIAC CATHETERIZATION

- While catheterization is the clinical "gold standard" for evaluating the hemodynamics of PH, there are several important limitations. RHC provides data about hemodynamics at a single moment in an unnatural setting, sometimes with positive pressure ventilation or sedation. Symptoms tend to be exertional while catheterization is performed at rest.

- Further, catheterization is almost always limited to assessment of supine values, even when "exercise" is performed. The cardiovascular response to exercise is dramatically different in the supine and upright positions. The definition, diagnosis, and management of "exercise-induced pulmonary arterial hypertension" is controversial.

- There is value in pursuing invasive hemodynamic evaluation during exercise in a subset of ACHD patients with unexplained dyspnea or other symptoms suggestive of PH or heart failure, as this provides a better understanding of what is truly limiting the patient. The results are often surprising, and can identify noncardiac limits such as pulmonary mechanical limits to effort. PVR, used clinically as a marker of overall impedance to RV output, does not provide data on the pulsatile characteristics of the pulmonary circulation. Perhaps most important, the quality of data and interpretation are variable and operator dependent.

- Catheterization for the evaluation of PH in CHD, especially in the presence of shunting or complex disease, should be performed by experienced clinicians.

ANGIOGRAPHY

Wedge, Pulmonary Arterial

- Pulmonary wedge angiography involves hand injection of a small amount (usually ~5 cc) of radiopaque contrast material distal though a "wedged" pulmonary arterial catheter in order to opacify the distal pulmonary vasculature. The balloon is deflated, and the contrast flows through the pulmonary vasculature, providing a dynamic impression of flow and outlining the pulmonary venous drainage.

- Wedge angiography confirms catheter placement, and also provides data on the physical appearance of the branch pulmonary arteries and perfusion, with the ability to diagnose chronic thromboembolic disease, pulmonary arteriovenous malformations, and pulmonary venous obstruction. Rapid branch pulmonary arterial tapering, longer pulmonary circulation time, and decrease in background "haze" correlate with increased PVR and more severe lung biopsy findings among patients with congenital heart disease.[15]

- The angiographic appearance of the pulmonary vasculature may reflect long-term pathologic changes. That being said, the clinical application of this information is less straightforward.

Pulmonary Arterial Angiography

- Nonselective pulmonary artery angiography is indicated in a subset of adults with congenital heart disease, to allow further definition of branch pulmonary artery stenosis or thromboembolic disease prior to surgical or interventional therapy.

- This chapter will not provide a detailed review of this technique, but the role of purely diagnostic invasive pulmonary angiography is in flux given impressive advances in noninvasive anatomic and physiologic imaging, including V/Q scanning, CT angiography, and magnetic resonance angiography.

CLINICAL SITUATIONS

Pulmonary Hypertension Due to Elevated Distal Pressures

PATIENT STORY 1: HIGH LEFT ATRIAL PRESSURE

A 68-year-old woman presented with mild dyspnea and was noted on examination to have a grade 2 holosystolic murmur. She was referred for a transthoracic echocardiogram which revealed moderate mitral regurgitation, severe left atrial dilation, and a markedly dilated vascular structure posterior to the left ventricle and left atrium (Figure 9-7). MR angiography demonstrated a fistula between left circumflex coronary artery and the coronary sinus. Catheterization revealed pulmonary hypertension with PA pressure of 47/20 with a mean of 32 mm Hg and pulmonary artery wedge pressure (PAWP) of 24 mm Hg with Qp:Qs of 1.2:1 and pulmonary flow of 4.1 l/min, with a calculated PVR of just under 2 WU.

CASE EXPLANATION

- This case describes a common clinical scenario of a patient with pulmonary hypertension but with normal pulmonary flow and resistance. It should be highlighted that while this patient had mildly elevated PA pressure, even severely elevated PA pressure can be caused by elevated PAWP, especially in the setting of high-normal PVR and pulmonary flow.

- For this reason, echocardiographic estimation of PA systolic pressure is a fatally flawed surrogate for pulmonary vascular disease. Even if echocardiographic estimates of PA systolic pressure are accurate, they provide very little information on why and therefore cannot be used in isolation to guide therapy or diagnosis.[8]

PATHOPHYSIOLOGY OF PULMONARY HYPERTENSION DUE TO ELEVATED DISTAL PRESSURE

- We tend to focus on aspects of PH that are particular to patients with CHD, such as increased flow due to shunts or pulmonary vascular remodeling related to long-standing shunt, and we tend to pay less thought to the third physiologic underpinning of elevated PA pressure.

- The most common cause of elevated pulmonary artery pressure in the general population is elevated pulmonary venous and left atrial

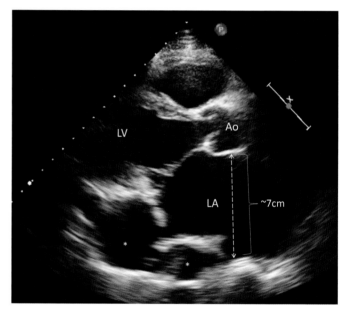

FIGURE 9-7 A parasternal long-axis image demonstrating severe left atrial dilation in this patient with long-standing mitral regurgitation in the setting of a coronary artery fistula (*). Ao, aorta; LA, left atrium; LV, left ventricle.

pressure, often with normal PVR and flow. While precise figures are not available for ACHD, elevated pulmonary venous pressure is a common cause of PH in this population also. This applies to left-sided obstructive lesions such as congenital mitral stenosis, obstructive cor triatriatum, aortic stenosis, or coarctation with a consequently stiff left ventricle. Aortic or mitral regurgitation can have a similar effect.

- Elevated left heart filling pressure, however, can also play a role in causing pulmonary hypertension to varying degrees to right-sided lesions and more complex lesions. Left ventricular systolic and diastolic dysfunction and elevated left ventricular end-diastolic pressure (LVEDP) are not rare in patients with repaired tetralogy of Fallot, for example, and these findings are associated with adverse outcomes.[16-18]

Pulmonary Hypertension Due to Elevated Flow

PATIENT STORY 2: AN INTRACARDIAC SHUNT WITH ELEVATED PULMONARY FLOW

A 64-year-old woman presented for evaluation of an atrial septal defect with pulmonary hypertension. She carried a diagnosis of chronic atrial fibrillation for several years, but was incidentally found to have a secundum ASD on imaging obtained during an admission for nausea and vomiting.

An electrocardiogram showed atrial fibrillation with right ventricular hypertrophy (Figure 9-8). Transthoracic echocardiogram showed a large secundum atrial septal defect (~2.8 × 2.3 cm) with severe RV and RA dilation and moderate-severe tricuspid regurgitation (Figures 9-9 through 9-11). Pulmonary artery systolic pressure was estimated at 69 mm Hg plus right atrial pressure (Figure 9-12). The patient was referred for catheterization, with hemodynamic and oximetric data provided in Table 9-2.

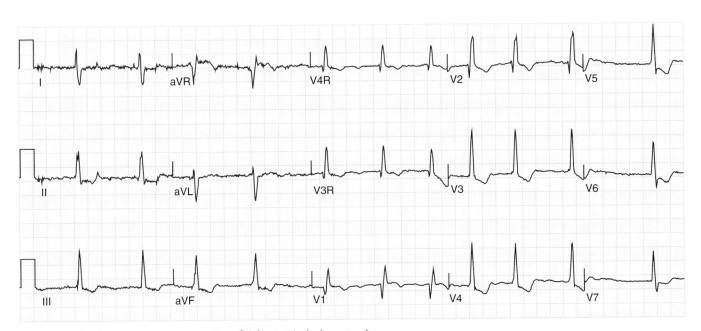

FIGURE 9-8 An electrocardiogram suggestive of right ventricular hypertrophy.

The estimated systemic cardiac index (Qsi) using the Fick principle with an assumption of $\text{vo}_2 = 125$ cc/min/m^2 was 3.1 l/min/m^2, while the Qp:Qs was approximately 3:1 with a pulmonary blood flow of approximately 9.2 l/min/m^2. While the patient had elevated PA pressure, in the setting of such high pulmonary flow the calculated pulmonary vascular resistance was normal (2.7 WU/m^2 or 1.6 WU). The defect was closed percutaneously and the patient continues to do well 2 years later.

CASE EXPLANATION

- This presentation is not uncommon and highlights that even in the presence of markedly elevated PA systolic pressure the pulmonary vascular resistance and distal filling pressures may be normal or nearly so.

- In some cases, there may even be exertional cyanosis unrelated to elevated PVR, but rather due to streaming, eccentric tricuspid regurgitation, or other causes of decreased right heart compliance such as pulmonary valve stenosis or regurgitation.[19]

PATHOPHYSIOLOGY OF PULMONARY HYPERTENSION DUE TO ELEVATED FLOW

- High pulmonary arterial flow can result in elevated pressure with increased pulse pressure. In the absence of structural heart disease this can be seen in patients with severe anemia, cirrhosis, hyperthyroidism, or other high output states.

- This is a specific concern for patients with a congenital heart defect that permits large volume of left-to-right shunting (eg, atrial septal defect). Severe pulmonary regurgitation also causes high PA pulse pressure, akin to what is seen in the systemic circulation with aortic regurgitation.

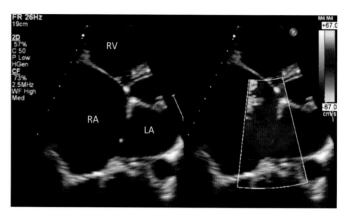

FIGURE 9-9 A transthoracic echocardiogram showing a secundum atrial septal defect (*) with left-to-right shunting. Ao, aorta; LA, left atrium; RA, right atrium; RV, right ventricle.

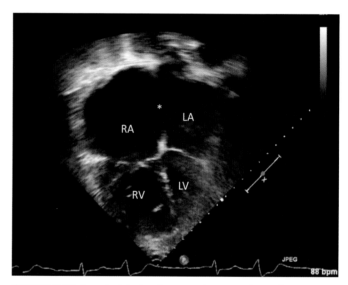

FIGURE 9-10 An apical 4-chamber transthoracic echocardiogram image showing a secundum atrial septal defect (*) with right atrial and right ventricular enlargement. LA, left atrium; LV, left ventricle; RA, right atrium; RV, right ventricle.

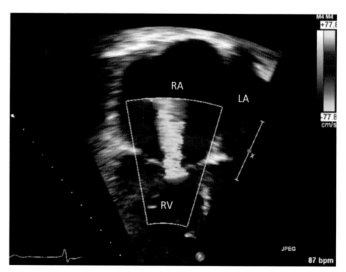

FIGURE 9-11 An apical 4-chamber transthoracic echocardiogram image with color Doppler showing moderate tricuspid regurgitation. LA, left atrium; RA, right atrium; RV, right ventricle.

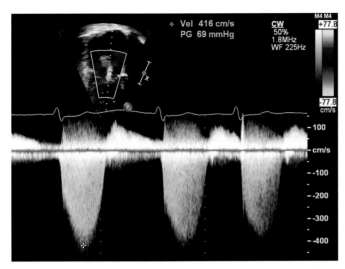

FIGURE 9-12 Transtricuspid continuous-wave Doppler imaging demonstrating increased systolic velocity between the right ventricle and right atrium, consistent with elevated right ventricular systolic pressure.

Table 9-2 Case Hemodynamic Data, Patient Story 2.

	Pressure(s), mm Hg	O$_2$ Saturation, %
SVC	16	71
RA	16	86
PA	73/20, mean 40	87
PAWP/pulmonary veins	16	95
Ao	102	95

Pulmonary Hypertension Due to Elevated Pulmonary Vascular Resistance

PATIENT STORY 3a: AN ADULT WITH EISENMENGER SYNDROME

A 35-year-old woman from Thailand presented with increasing cough with blood-tinged sputum, occasional episodes of her fingers turning a blush tint with exertion. She also noted progressive exertional dyspnea over the prior several years. She was found to have a periph eral noninvasive O$_2$ saturation of approximately 75% which did not improve with administration of supplemental oxygen. On examination there was a widely split S2 with a loud pulmonic component as well as a right-sided S3. PA and lateral chest radiography showed an enlarged proximal pulmonary artery and right ventricular hypertrophy (Figures 9-13A and 9-13B). An echocardiogram was performed which suggested the presence of a secundum ASD with bidirectional shunting, right ventricular hypertrophy, dilation and dysfunction (Figure 9-14), and an estimated right ventricular systolic pressure of approximately 100 mm Hg + right atrial pressure. There was moderate tricuspid regurgitation by color Doppler (Figure 9-15), and marked systolic ventricular septal flattening suggestive of elevated pulmonary arterial impedance (Figures 9-16 and 9-17). The echocardiogram also demonstrated dilated proximal pulmonary arteries with thrombus (Figure 9-18), which was confirmed by CT angiography.

Catheterization revealed RA pressure of 1 to 2 mm Hg, with PA pressure of 100/50, mean 68 mm Hg and equivalent aortic pressure with PAWP of approximately 3 to 4 mm Hg. Estimated pulmonary

blood flow was 2.1 l/min/m^2 and PVR was calculated at greater than 30 WU/m^2. Oximetry suggested a bidirectional shunt at atrial level. Saturations in the superior vena cava (SVC), RA, RV, and PA were 63%, 71%, 73%, and 72%, respectively. The left upper pulmonary vein saturation was 99% breathing room air, with LV and aortic saturations of 89%. There was severe distal pruning of the pulmonary vasculature on right lower lobe selective wedge angiography (Figure 9-19).

The patient was started on bosentan, an endothelin receptor blocker, and warfarin. Given the apparent lack of intrinsic pulmonary parenchymal disease (no improvement in so$_2$ with supplemental oxygen), she was not prescribed supplemental oxygen.

CASE EXPLANATION 3a: AN ADULT WITH EISENMENGER SYNDROME

• Eisenmenger syndrome, as defined by Paul Wood, refers to "pulmonary hypertension due to a high pulmonary vascular resistance with reversed or bidirectional shunt at aortopulmonary, ventricular, or atrial level."[20,21] That is, Eisenmenger syndrome refers to a combination of a congenital heart defect allowing left-to-right shunting (eg, ASD, VSD, or patent ductus arteriosus [PDA]) with subsequent pulmonary vascular remodeling resulting in elevated PVR.

• Eventually, the forces driving shunting (eg, relative right and left heart compliance in the case of ASD) will no longer strongly favor

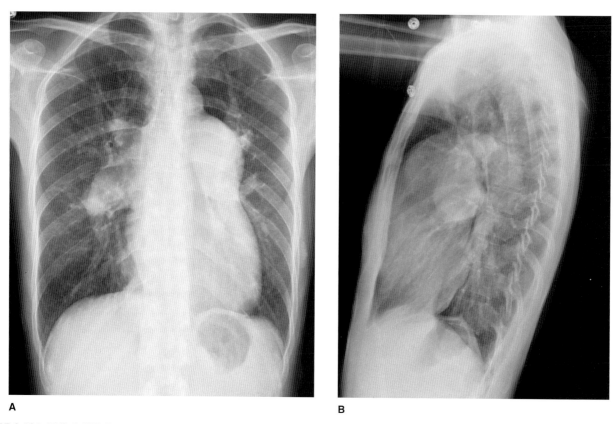

A

B

FIGURE 9-13A AND 9-13B Posterior-anterior and lateral chest radiographs of a patient with Eisenmenger syndrome demonstrating proximal PA dilation and right ventricular enlargement, suggested by loss of the retrosternal air space.

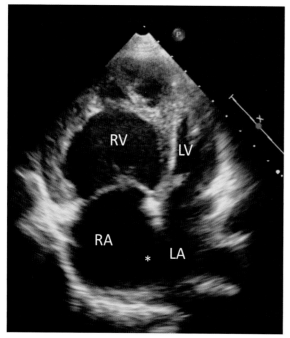

FIGURE 9-14 An apical 4-chamber transthoracic echocardiogram image showing right ventricular enlargement and severe right ventricular hypertrophy in a patient with Eisenmenger syndrome. The atrial septal defect is marked by an asterisk (∗). LA, left atrium; LV, left ventricle; RA, right atrium; RV, right ventricle.

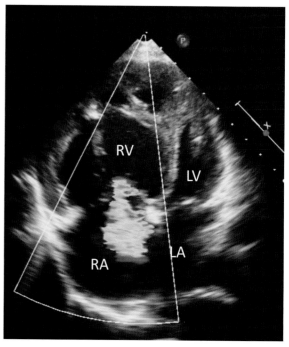

FIGURE 9-15 An apical 4-chamber transthoracic echocardiogram image with color Doppler showing tricuspid regurgitation. LA, left atrium; LV, left ventricle; RA, right atrium; RV, right ventricle.

left-to-right shunting. The histopathology of the pulmonary vasculature in Eisenmenger syndrome is equivalent to that observed in other forms of pulmonary arterial hypertension.

- Even with the development of several classes of pulmonary vasodilator medications, however, these changes are essentially irreversible. Paul Wood, in 1958, described that surgical repair was the proximate cause of patient death for many patients,[20,21] and the high risk of surgical intervention in these patients has not changed.

- Surgical or percutaneous repair is not recommended for patients with severely elevated PVR, and as described in the next section, it is unclear whether those with more than mildly elevated PVR but without Eisenmenger syndrome or even cyanosis truly benefit from repair.

- Despite the similar pathology, there are several distinctions in the natural history, complications, and management of patients with Eisenmenger syndrome compared with other forms of PAH. A few of the notable differences include the following:

  - The prognosis for a patient with Eisenmenger syndrome is generally more favorable. This may be due to the extended period of time during which the right ventricle can remodel before sustaining very high pulmonary arterial impedance, or the earlier age of onset. Other potential mechanisms include beneficial right-left ventricular interaction or the presence of a "pop-off" valve for the struggling right ventricle, a concept which provides the foundation for specific interventions of PAH without a patent shunt.[22,23]

  - The most obvious clinical feature of patients with Eisenmenger syndrome is hypoxemia with consequent secondary erythrocytosis and cyanosis.

  - Eisenmenger syndrome is associated with increased risk of bleeding and thrombosis.

  - Thrombosis of the large- and medium-sized pulmonary arteries is more common in Eisenmenger syndrome than in other forms of PAH.[24] This is due to in situ thrombosis and not venous thromboembolism. While the presence of pulmonary thrombus is a poor prognostic sign, it is unclear if the benefits of anticoagulation outweigh the risks of bleeding.

  - The presence of a patent shunt lesion may provide benefit (as earlier), but it can also be a mechanism for specific complications. Peripheral embolism is one concern, as is the potential that acute drops in peripheral vascular tone (eg, systemic vasodilation after jumping in a hot tub) may result in clinically significant hypoxemia due to a decrease in pulmonary blood flow.

PATIENT STORY 3b: PROGRESSIVE PULMONARY VASCULAR REMODELLING AFTER REPAIR OF CONGENITAL HEART DISEASE WITH LEFT-TO-RIGHT SHUNT

The patient is a 33-year-old woman born with a primum ASD and cleft mitral valve status post (s/p) surgical repair at age 18 with a fenestrated ASD closure in the setting of left-to-right shunting and mildly elevated PVR. Initially after closure, pulmonary artery pressures improved to less than one-half systemic, but over the following

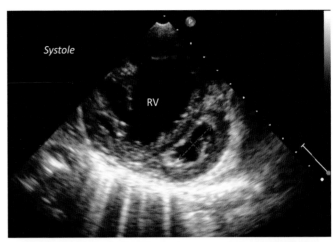
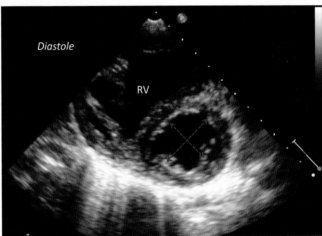

FIGURES 9-16 AND 9-17 Parasternal short-axis images in systole (Figure 9-16) and diastole (Figure 9-17) at the papillary muscle level showing marked systolic ventricular septal bowing into the left ventricle, with more preserved, relatively normal septal configuration in diastole. RV, right ventricle.

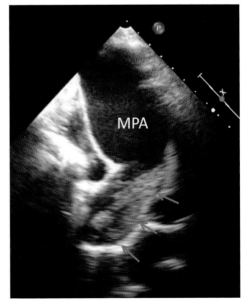

FIGURE 9-18 An off-axis parasternal view demonstrating thrombus in the branch pulmonary artery (orange arrows). MPA, main pulmonary artery.

5 to 7 years there was progressive increase in pressures and eventually she was determined to have progressive pulmonary vascular remodeling despite no residual shunt by echocardiography or catheterization (ie, $Qp = Qs$).

Despite therapy with an oral endothelin receptor blockade and phosphodiesterase inhibitor, catheterization demonstrated right atrial pressure (RAP) = 13, right ventricular pressure (RVP) = 122/16, PA 123/62, mean 84 with PAWP = LVEDP = 9 mm Hg in the setting of a cardiac index of 2 L/min/m^2 (pulmonary vascular resistance index [PVRI] = 38 WU/m^2). With nitric oxide there was little change in pulmonary or cardiac pressures but there was an increase in cardiac index to 4.3 L/min/m^2

(PVRI = 17 WU/m^2). Selective wedge pulmonary angiography showed tortuous branch pulmonary arteries with distal pruning (Figure 9-20). CT angiography of the pulmonary arteries demonstrated proximal chronic pulmonary artery thrombus (Figure 9-21A through C).

CASE EXPLANATION 3b: PROGRESSIVE PULMONARY VASCULAR REMODELLING AFTER REPAIR OF CONGENITAL HEART DISEASE WITH LEFT-TO-RIGHT SHUNT

- The development of surgical and percutaneous approaches to repair various forms of simple shunt lesions has made Eisenmenger syndrome a rare finding, at least in parts of the world with extensive access to health care. There are 3 more common scenarios currently seen in clinical practice, with defects shown in patients as below:
  1. Closed early in life
  2. Closed later in life
  3. Diagnosed late in life, usually of a simple shunt lesion, a secundum ASD, or sinus venosus defect

- There are data suggesting that early repair is associated with excellent long-term outcomes and little risk of progressive pulmonary vascular disease. Even for atrial shunt lesions identified late in life, prevention of PAH is not a major player in recommending closure; improving effort intolerance, preventing heart failure, and possible preventing arrhythmia are more salient goals.

- One reason is that for patients with small ventricular septal defect (VSD) or moderate-large atrial shunt lesions, the development of PAH is not inevitable and occurs in a minority (~10%-20% in the case of ASD) of patients. Another issue is that in some cases, especially when there is mildly or moderately elevated PVR prior to closure, there is progressive development of pulmonary vascular disease despite elimination of any ongoing shunting. That is, chronic shunting seems to initiate a process of pulmonary vascular remodeling but may not be, in all cases, necessary to maintaining that process. While this phenomenon is well known, there is much less certainty on what criteria confidently identify those patients who would benefit from repair and those who may be harmed (for the reasons outlined earlier describing the various ways patients with Eisenmenger syndrome may have better prognosis than PAH in the absence of a patent shunt).

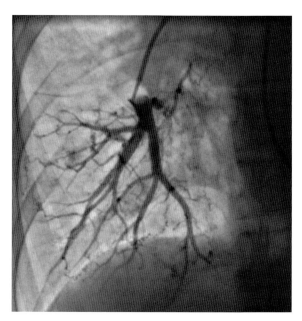

FIGURE 9-19 Wedge pulmonary angiography of a right lower lobe segment demonstrating severe pruning of the distal pulmonary vasculature.

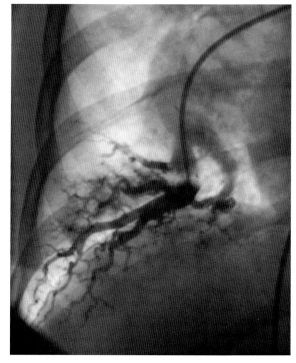

FIGURE 9-20 Wedge pulmonary angiography of a right lower lobe segment showing tortuous branch pulmonary arteries with milder pruning of the distal pulmonary vasculature.

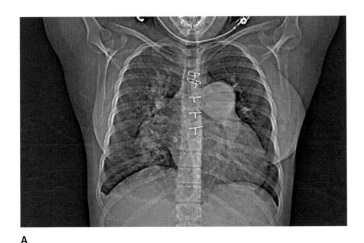

A

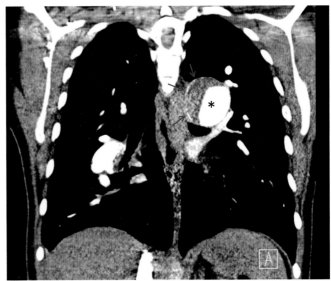

B

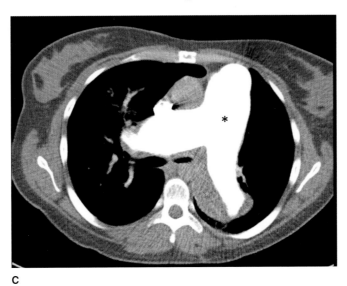

C

FIGURE 9-21 Computed tomography (CT) angiography of a patient with progressive pulmonary vascular disease and chronic thrombosis 15 years after fenestrated closure of a primum atrial septal defect with no residual shunt. Panel A shows the scout film, while panels B and C provide coronal and axial images, respectively. Red arrows identify calcification of pulmonary artery wall, with the **blue star** signifying thrombus and the black asterisk identifying the vessel lumen.

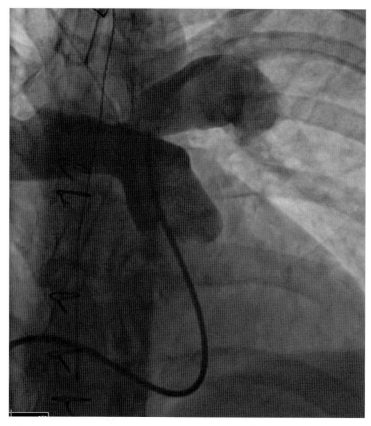

FIGURE 9-22 Pulmonary angiogram in an asymptomatic patient with tetralogy of Fallot surgically repaired with a transannular patch approach in childhood, without previous palliative shunt. There is stenosis of the proximal left pulmonary artery. Nuclear perfusion imaging confirmed that only 27% of pulmonary blood flow was directed to the left lung.

- It is difficult to define the degree of intrinsic pulmonary vascular disease in a given, with a sizable, left-to-right shunt, as high flow is associated with maximal pulmonary arterial recruitment and dilation (Figure 9-2). Balloon occlusion during catheterization provides very short-term data on what may happen with closure, but that provides limited insight into medium- and long-term consequences.

- These patients often do very well for a number of years after closure before deterioration due to pulmonary vascular remodeling, providing a false impression that the approach was safe and beneficial.

MISCELLANEOUS PULMONARY VASCULAR DISEASE

- Patients with congenital heart disease without small vessel pulmonary arteriolar remodeling may have additional reasons for elevated pulmonary vascular impedance. Gross abnormalities in the proximal and branch pulmonary arteries are relatively common among patients with moderately or severely complex disease after repair, such as those with tetralogy of Fallot (Figure 9-22). This can be due to developmental abnormalities or prior palliative or reparative surgery (Figure 9-23).

- Less appreciated in clinical practice, abnormal pulmonary distensibility and stiffness are almost ubiquitous in patients with right ventricular outflow tract and large pulmonary artery defects, or those who have undergone prior pulmonary artery surgical or percutaneous repair.

- Pulmonary vascular resistance only captures mean pulmonary vascular impedance (ie, the ratio of mean pressure drop to mean flow) but the pulmonary circulation is pulsatile. Data suggest that low pulmonary artery compliance is an independent predictor of impaired exercise capacity in various populations,[25,26] though there are few data in patients with congenital heart disease.

- Pulmonary vein stenosis is relatively uncommon, but when present can cause severe pulmonary hypertension. This can be due to pulmonary venous hypertension, but over time it may cause irreversible pulmonary arteriolar remodeling similar to that seen in pulmonary arterial hypertension or Eisenmenger syndrome. The segments affected by a stenotic vein, however, tend to have low flow and there may be little or no evidence of pulmonary vascular remodeling despite long-standing pulmonary vein stenosis (Figures 9-24 and 9-25).

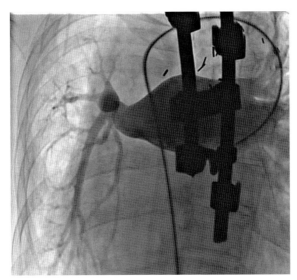

FIGURE 9-23 A pulmonary angiogram in a patient with complex congenital heart disease and a left Blalock-Taussig shunt demonstrating a severely dilated proximal artery and diminutive distal vessels with little flow to the right upper lobe. The patient also had a restrictive ventilatory defect related partly to severe scoliosis s/p Harrington rod placement. This is a common comorbidity in patients with cyanotic heart disease.

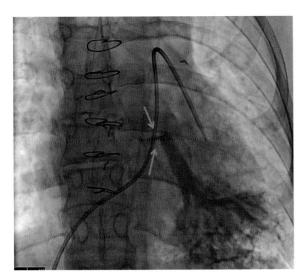

FIGURE 9-24 Delayed phase of a selective left lower lobe pulmonary angiogram in a 26-year-old woman with left upper pulmonary vein atresia demonstrating severe left lower pulmonary vein stenosis (orange arrows).

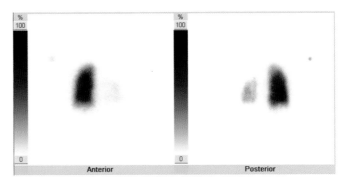

FIGURE 9-25 Nuclear perfusion imaging from the same patient described in Figure 9-24 demonstrates that only 9% of pulmonary blood flow was directed to the left lung, with an absence of any flow to the left upper lobe. Invasively measured pulmonary artery pressure and resistance were normal. Nevertheless, cardiopulmonary exercise testing demonstrated normal peak vo_2 (>100% predicted), normal ventilator response to exercise, normal end-tidal CO_2 and normal $Ve:Vco_2$ slope.

REFERENCES

1. Dexter L, Dow JW, Haynes FW, et al. Studies of the pulmonary circulation in man at rest; normal variations and the interrelations between increased pulmonary blood flow, elevated pulmonary arterial pressure, and high pulmonary "capillary" pressures. *J Clin Invest*. 1950;29:602-613.

2. McLaughlin VV, Archer SL, Badesch DB, et al. ACCF/AHA 2009 expert consensus document on pulmonary hypertension: a report of the American College of Cardiology Foundation Task Force on Expert Consensus Documents and the American Heart Association: developed in collaboration with the American College of Chest Physicians, American Thoracic Society, Inc., and the Pulmonary Hypertension Association. *Circulation*. 2009;119:2250-2294.

3. Fisher MR, Forfia PR, Chamera E, et al. Accuracy of Doppler echocardiography in the hemodynamic assessment of pulmonary hypertension. *Am J Respir Crit Care Med*. 2009;179:615-621.

4. Ryan T, Petrovic O, Dillon JC, Feigenbaum H, Conley MJ, Armstrong WF. An echocardiographic index for separation of right ventricular volume and pressure overload. *J Am Coll Cardiol*. 1985;5:918-927.

5. Ghio S, Constantin C, Klersy C, et al. Interventricular and intraventricular dyssynchrony are common in heart failure patients, regardless of QRS duration. *Eur Heart J*. 2004;25:571-578.

6. Marcus JT, Gan CT, Zwanenburg JJ, et al. Interventricular mechanical asynchrony in pulmonary arterial hypertension: left-to-right delay in peak shortening is related to right ventricular overload and left ventricular underfilling. *J Am Coll Cardiol*. 2008;51:750-757.

7. Walker RE, Moran AM, Gauvreau K, Colan SD. Evidence of adverse ventricular interdependence in patients with atrial septal defects. *Am J Cardiol*. 2004;93:1374-1377, A6.

8. Opotowsky AR, Ojeda J, Rogers F, et al. A simple echocardiographic prediction rule for hemodynamics in pulmonary hypertension. *Circ Cardiovasc Imaging*. 2012;5:765-775.

9. Ruan Q, Nagueh SF. Clinical application of tissue Doppler imaging in patients with idiopathic pulmonary hypertension. *Chest*. 2007;131:395-401.

10. Arkles JS, Opotowsky AR, Ojeda, J et al. Shape of the right ventricular Doppler envelope predicts hemodynamics and right heart function in pulmonary hypertension. *Am J Respir Crit Care Med*. 2011;183:268-276.

11. Kendrick AH, West J, Papouchado M, Rozkovec A. Direct Fick cardiac output: are assumed values of oxygen consumption acceptable? *Eur Heart J*. 1988;9:337-342.

12. Shanahan CL, Wilson NJ, Gentles TL, Skinner JR. The influence of measured versus assumed uptake of oxygen in assessing pulmonary vascular resistance in patients with a bidirectional Glenn anastomosis. *Cardiol Young*. 2003;13:137-142.

13. Fakler U, Pauli C, Hennig M, Sebening W, Hess J. Assumed oxygen consumption frequently results in large errors in the determination of cardiac output. *J Thorac Cardiovasc Surg*. 2005;130:272-276.

14. Butler J, Chomsky DB, Wilson JR. Pulmonary hypertension and exercise intolerance in patients with heart failure. *J Am Coll Cardiol*. 1999;34:1802-1806.

15. Rabinovitch M, Keane JF, Fellows KE, Castaneda AR, Reid L. Quantitative analysis of the pulmonary wedge angiogram in congenital heart defects. Correlation with hemodynamic data and morphometric findings in lung biopsy tissue. *Circulation*. 1981;63:152-164.

16. Khairy P, Harris L, Landzberg MJ, et al. Implantable cardioverter-defibrillators in tetralogy of Fallot. *Circulation*. 2008;117:363-370.

17. Aboulhosn JA, Lluri G, Gurvitz MZ, et al. Left and right ventricular diastolic function in adults with surgically repaired tetralogy of Fallot: a multiinstitutional study. *Can J Cardiol*. 2013;29:866-872.

18. Broberg CS, Aboulhosn J, Mongeon FP, et al. Prevalence of left ventricular systolic dysfunction in adults with repaired tetralogy of fallot. *Am J Cardiol*. 2011;107:1215-1220.

19. Dexter L. Atrial septal defect. *Br Heart J*. 1956;18:209-225.

20. Wood P. The Eisenmenger syndrome or pulmonary hypertension with reversed central shunt. *Br Med J*. 1958;2:755-762.

21. Wood P. The Eisenmenger syndrome or pulmonary hypertension with reversed central shunt. I. *Br Med J*. 1958;2:701-709.

22. Kurzyna M, Dabrowski M, Bielecki D, et al. Atrial septostomy in treatment of end-stage right heart failure in patients with pulmonary hypertension. *Chest*. 2007;131:977-983.

23. Esch JJ, Shah PB, Cockrill BA, et al. Transcatheter Potts shunt creation in patients with severe pulmonary arterial hypertension: initial clinical experience. *J Heart Lung Transplant*. 2013;32:381-387.

24. Silversides CK, Granton JT, Konen E, Hart MA, Webb GD, Therrien J. Pulmonary thrombosis in adults with Eisenmenger syndrome. *J Am Coll Cardiol*. 2003;42:1982-1987.

25. Saggar R, Lewis GD, Systrom DM, Champion HC, Naeije R. Pulmonary vascular responses to exercise: a haemodynamic observation. *Eur Respir J*. 2012;39:231-234.

26. Lewis GD, Murphy RM, Shah RV, et al. Pulmonary vascular response patterns during exercise in left ventricular systolic dysfunction predict exercise capacity and outcomes. *Circ Heart Fail*. 2011;4:276-285.

10 EISENMENGER SYNDROME IN THE ADULT WITH CONGENITAL HEART DISEASE

W. Aaron Kay, MD
Curt J. Daniels, MD
Ali N. Zaidi, MD

PATIENT STORY

A 35-year-old-young man from Guatemala presented with chronic cough and progressive fatigue. He was told that he had a "hole in his heart" when he was a child but never underwent surgical repair. His oxygen saturations at rest were 84%, heart rate of 106 bpm, and a BP of 118/78 mm Hg. He had equal saturations in all 4 extremities. He had a loud second heart sound, and a III/VI holosystolic murmur at the left sternal border (LSB) with a mild right parasternal heave on palpation and clear lungs. He had only trivial edema around his ankles. On echo-cardiography he was found to have a large perimembranous ventricular septal defect (VSD) with predominantly right-to-left shunting with color flow Doppler assessment (Figures 10-1A, 10-1B, and 10-2). There was no evidence of any right ventricular outflow tract obstruction. He underwent a cardiac catheterization and was found to have irreversible pulmonary vascular disease with a pulmonary vascular resistance of 14 Wood units (WU) and no reversibility with a vasodilator challenge (Figure 10-3). He was not a candidate for late surgical closure of the defect. He was treated with pulmonary vasodilators for symptomatic relief. His symptoms of chronic cough did improve. He also had sig-nificant erythrocytosis and an elevated hematocrit. He did not manifest any symptoms of hyperviscosity and therefore did not undergo any phlebotomy.

CASE EXPLANATION

- The triad of systemic-to-pulmonary cardiovascular communica-tion, pulmonary arterial disease, and cyanosis is called Eisenmenger syndrome. The diagnosis of Eisenmenger syndrome implies that the development of pulmonary arterial disease is a consequence of increased pulmonary blood flow, and requires exclusion of other causes of pulmonary arterial hypertension (PAH).

- Eisenmenger syndrome (ES) is a multisystem disease and affects nearly all organs of the body, including the lungs, brain, hemato-logic, endocrine, and reproductive system.

- This case vividly outlines the epidemiologic pattern of ES in devel-oping countries where ES is common sequelae of unrepaired intra-cardiac shunt lesions.

- These patients often develop markedly elevated pulmonary vascular resistance (PVR) and are more likely to be inoperable secondary to Eisenmenger physiology.

EPIDEMIOLOGY

- ES usually develops before puberty but may develop in adolescence and early adulthood.

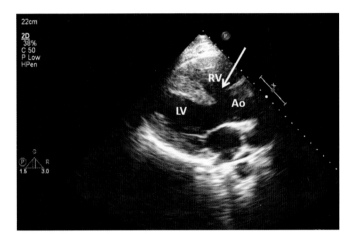

A

FIGURE 10-1A Parasternal long image on a 2D transthoracic echocar-diographic image showing a large-sized perimembranous ventricular septal defect (arrow). Ao, aorta; LV, left ventricle; RV, right ventricle.

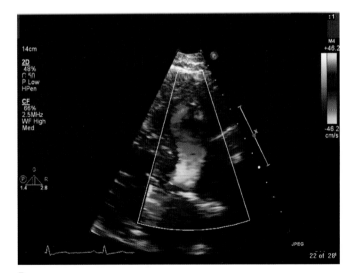

B

FIGURE 10-1B Parasternal long-axis image of a large perimembranous ventricular septal defect (VSD) with color flow Doppler with predomi-nantly right-to-left shunting across the defect.

- Overall prevalence of ES is unknown, but is rare in developed countries.

- In developing nations, ES is common sequelae of unrepaired intracardiac shunt lesions. These patients may have markedly elevated PVR and are more likely to be inoperable secondary to Eisenmenger physiology.

- Rarely, ES is first diagnosed in adulthood, after the development of symptoms of pulmonary hypertension (PH), heart failure, or arrhythmias or after symptomatic presentation of the multiorgan effects of ES.

ETIOLOGY AND PATHOPHYSIOLOGY

- Eisenmenger syndrome can occur in patients with large, congenital cardiac, or surgically created extracardiac left-to-right shunts. These shunts cause increased pulmonary blood flow. If left uncorrected this will lead to remodeling of the pulmonary

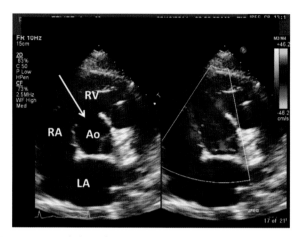

FIGURE 10-2 Side-by-side parasternal short-axis echocardiographic images showing the perimembranous ventricular septal defect (VSD) (arrow) in 2D and with color flow across the defect. Ao, aorta; LA, left atrium; RA, right atrium; RV, right ventricle.

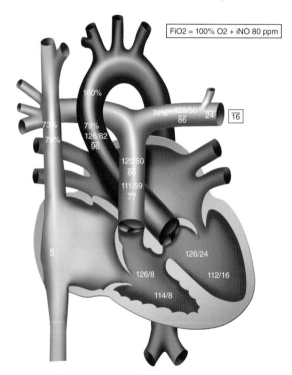

FIGURE 10-3 Hemodynamic cardiac catheterization data in a 35-year-old patient with an unrepaired ventricular septal defect (VSD). The hemodynamic data shown in the image is after vasoreactive testing using iNO and 100% FiO₂.

(1) There were systemic RV and PA pressures in all phases.
(2) Baseline hemodynamic measurements on room air are as follows:
- Qp/Qs = 0.25:1, PVR = 30.2 WU
- Saturations: SVC 73%, LPA 74%, aAo 79%
- Pressures: RA 3 mm Hg, RV 126/8 mm Hg, PA 120/50/86 mm Hg, LPA 120/50/86 mm Hg, LPCW 24 mm Hg
- LV 126/24 mm Hg, dAo 126/82/96 mm Hg

(3) Hemodynamic measurements after 100% oxygen are as follows:
- Qp/Qs = 1.24:1 PVR 30.9 WU
- Saturations: SVC 71%, LPA 85%, aAo 96%
- Pressures: RA 4 mm Hg, RV 111/8 mm Hg, PA 116/60/80 mm Hg, LPCW 16 mm Hg, dAo 116/79/92 mm Hg

(4) Hemodynamic measurements with 100% oxygen and iNO 80 ppm are as follows:
- Qp/Qs = 1.8:1, PVR 17.8 WU
- Saturations: SVC 79%, LPA 90%, LV 100%, aAo 100%
- Pressures: RA 3 mm Hg, RV 114/8 mm Hg, PA 111/59 mm Hg, LPA 111/59/77 mm Hg, LPCW 16 mm Hg
- dAo 118/80/93

aAo, ascending aorta; dAo, descending aorta; iNO, inhaled nitric oxide; LPA, left pulmonary artery; LPCW, left pulmonary capillary wedge pressure; LV, left ventricle; PA, pulmonary artery; PVR, pulmonary vascular resistance; RA, right atrium; RV, right ventricle; SVC, superior vena cava; VSD, ventricular septal defect.

microvasculature, with subsequent obstruction to pulmonary blood flow. This is commonly referred to as pulmonary vascular obstructive disease (PVOD).

- Eventually, the pulmonary vascular resistance exceeds systemic vascular resistance, leading to PAH, reversal of the shunt (now right to left), and resultant cyanosis.[1,2]

- The incidence of PAH and development of reversed shunting depends on the specific heart defect as well as any interventions performed. The risk of developing ES is determined by the size of the initial left-to-right shunt as well as the volume of pulmonary blood flow. The volume of pulmonary blood flow is determined by the PVR, which is normally high in the neonatal period, and gradually drops over a period of about 2 months. Larger shunts have an increased risk of progressing to ES.

- The progression to Eisenmenger syndrome is represented by a spectrum of morphologic changes in the capillary bed that progress from reversible lesions to irreversible ones. Endothelial dysfunction and smooth muscle proliferation result from the changes in flow and pressure, increasing the PVR.[3]

- Unrepaired atrial septal defects (ASD) are less likely to lead to pulmonary hypertension (Figures 10-4A and 10-4B). Only 10% of unrepaired ASDs progress to PH, and PH typically develops after the third decade of life.

- Approximately 50% of infants with a large, nonrestrictive VSD (Figures 10-1A, 10-1B, and 10-2) or patent ductus arteriosus (PDA) (Figure 10-5) develop pulmonary hypertension within the first year of life, if the shunt is not surgically closed. Almost 40% of patients develop pulmonary hypertension within the first year of life if they have unrepaired VSD or PDA and transposition of the great arteries. Virtually all patients with truncus arteriosus (with unrestricted pulmonary blood flow) and patients with common atrioventricular (AV) canal defect, if unrepaired in infancy, will develop irreversible pulmonary vascular disease by the second year of life.[4] Rarely an unrepaired aortopulmonary (AP) window is found in adults who have developed ES (Figure 10-6).

- Iatrogenic ES can occur after placement of a surgical systemic-to-pulmonary artery shunt, such as a Blalock-Taussig-Thomas shunt. The risk of PAH depends on the diameter and length of the shunt as well as the anatomic location. Ten percent of patients with a classic Blalock-Taussig-Thomas shunt (subclavian artery–to–pulmonary artery anastomosis) have been found to develop PAH. Waterston (ascending aorta to pulmonary artery) and Potts (descending aorta to pulmonary artery) shunts, which are no longer performed, had a much higher incidence of PAH. Newer modifications to shunt procedures have significantly decreased the risk of acquired PAH.

- The extent of intracardiac shunting is assessed as the ratio of measured pulmonary blood flow (Qp) to systemic blood flow (Qs). In a normal heart, where no shunting exists, the Qp:Qs ratio is 1:1. A net left-to-right shunt (acyanotic physiology) results in a Qp:Qs greater than 1, whereas a net right-to-left shunt (cyanotic physiology) results in a Qp:Qs less than 1. The Qp:Qs can be calculated based on differential oxygen saturations in the catheterization laboratory (Fick equation) or estimated by a variety of noninvasive imaging techniques which are beyond the scope of this chapter.

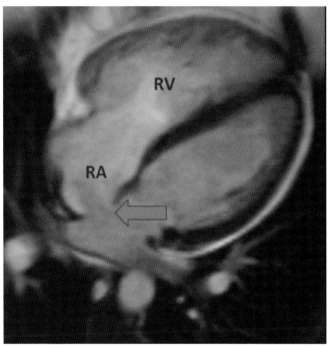

A

FIGURE 10-4A A 4-chamber view of the heart using steady-state free precession (SSFP) cine imaging showing a large atrial secundum atrial septal defect (ASD) with right atrium (RA) and, right ventricle (RV) enlargement (blue arrow).

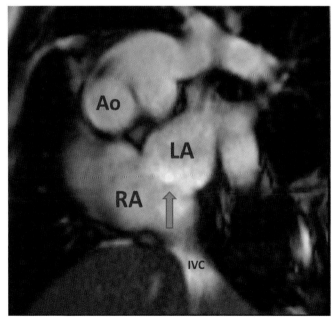

B

FIGURE 10-4B Biatrial short-axis view using steady-state free precession (SSFP) cine imaging showing the atrial septal defect (ASD) (blue arrow); Ao, aorta; IVC, inferior vena cava; LA, left atrium; RA, right atrium.

DIAGNOSIS

Cardiac/Pulmonary Historical Features

- If a patient has known congenital heart disease (CHD) with suspected PAH, it is important to obtain records of all prior surgical and catheter-based interventions.[5]

- Patients who develop Eisenmenger syndrome may be asymptomatic for long periods of time. The elevated PVR prevents pulmonary overcirculation and the symptoms of heart failure. This can result in a delay in diagnosis.

- Patients with ES may present with a multitude of symptoms including dyspnea, fatigue, severely reduced exercise tolerance with a prolonged recovery phase, presyncope, and syncope. Patients may also have symptoms suggestive of heart failure including exertional dyspnea, orthopnea, paroxysmal nocturnal dyspnea, edema, and ascites.

Historical Features From Extracardiac Organ Involvement

Other symptoms are caused by various multisystem complications associated with cyanotic congenital heart disease as listed below:

- Hematologic symptoms secondary to erythrocytosis that may include myalgia, muscle weakness, paresthesias of the digits and lip, visual changes due to retinal involvement including episodes of transient visual loss and spontaneous hyphemas, headaches, and dizziness.

- Hyperviscosity may lead to thromboembolic events, cerebrovascular complications, gout, chest pain from pulmonary infarction, and hemoptysis. Most of the symptoms are nonspecific and are confirmed if they are relieved by phlebotomy.

- Symptoms of a tendency toward bleeding include mild mucocutaneous bleeding, epistaxis, hemoptysis, and rarely pulmonary hemorrhage.

- Vascular symptoms of presyncope or syncope can arise from systemic vasodilation.

- Symptoms of cholelithiasis include abdominal or right upper quadrant pain, biliary colic, pale stool and jaundice.

- Patients can also suffer from nephrolithiasis giving rise to renal colic, secondary gout and joint pain and swelling.

- Joint symptoms that can arise include long bone pain and tenderness.

Physical Examination

Cardiovascular findings include the following:

- Central cyanosis (differential cyanosis in the case of a patient with a PDA).

- Digital clubbing can often be pronounced.

- Elevated jugular venous pulse wave suggestive of prominent central venous pressures. There may be a dominant A-wave. In the presence of a significant tricuspid regurgitation, the V-wave may be prominent.

- Precordial palpation reveals a right ventricular heave and, frequently, a palpable S2.

- A pulmonary ejection click with a loud P2, can be heard.

- High-pitched early diastolic murmur of pulmonic insufficiency.

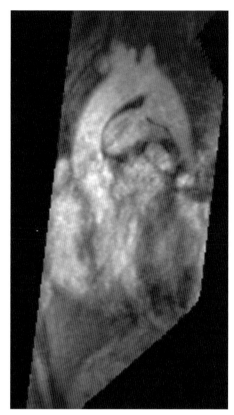

FIGURE 10-5 Left anterior oblique cine magnetic resonance angiogram. The image shows a large patent ductus arteriosus (PDA) connecting the aorta (Ao) and the pulmonary artery (PA).

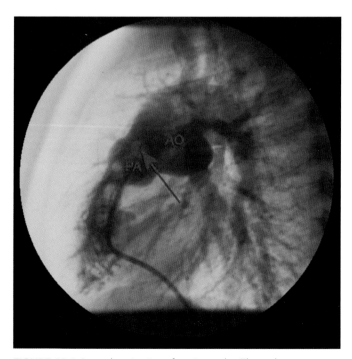

FIGURE 10-6 Lateral projection of angiography. The catheter courses through the right ventricle and pulmonary artery. Contrast is seen passing directly through the aortopulmonary window (red arrow) from the pulmonary artery (PA) into the aorta (Ao). Note the opacification of head and neck vessels.

- Peripheral edema is common in advanced stages of right heart failure due to ES.
- Ascites and hepatomegaly are common.

Noncardiac examination findings include the following:

- Respiratory findings of cyanosis and tachypnea.
- Hematologic findings may include bruising and bleeding.
- Ocular examination can reveal conjunctival injection and rubeosis iridis. Changes from retinal hyperviscosity on funduscopic examination reveal engorged vessels, papilledema, microaneurysms, and blot hemorrhages secondary to erythrocytosis.
- Abdominal signs include jaundice, right upper quadrant tenderness, and positive Murphy sign that may signify acute cholecystitis.
- Rarely there can be vascular findings of postural hypotension and focal ischemia from paradoxical embolus.
- Findings of hypertrophic osteoarthropathy include clubbing, small joint tenderness, and joint effusions.
- A hallmark of the transition to Eisenmenger physiology can be a seemingly improving clinical condition, despite the absence of change in therapy for congestive heart failure. It represents a physiologically normalized condition caused by the progressively worsening pulmonary vascular obstructive disease (PVOD), with resolution of pulmonary over circulation and heart failure.

Electrocardiogram

- Frontal plane QRS right-axis deviation (Figure 10-7).
- Right or biventricular hypertrophy with associated ST-T wave changes.

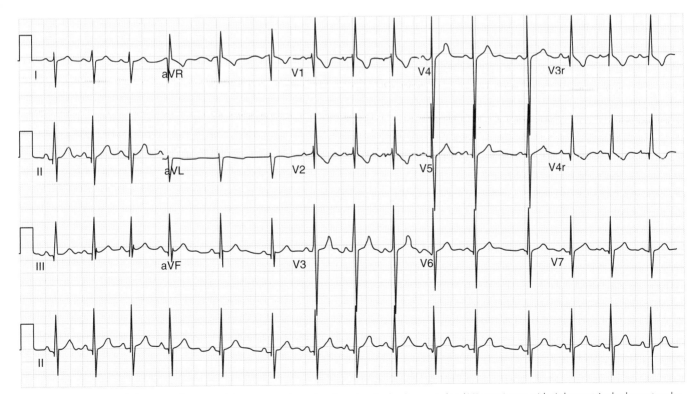

FIGURE 10-7 A 15-lead electrocardiogram of the same patient showing elevated voltages in lead V1 consistent with right ventricular hypertrophy. Note also the net negative voltages in leads I and aVL consistent with right-axis deviation, commonly found in right ventricular hypertrophy secondary to pulmonary hypertension.

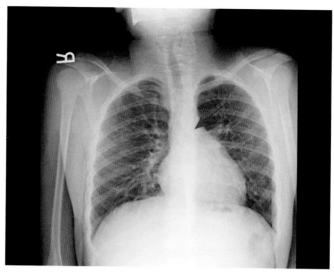

FIGURE 10-8 Anteroposterior chest radiograph demonstrates increased pulmonary vascular markings. The silhouette of the pulmonary artery trunk is also enlarged (red arrow).

- Right atrial abnormality (tall, narrow P-wave—also called P-pulmonale).

- Left-axis deviation is seen in patients with an atrioventricular septal defect.

Chest Radiography

- In the early stages, chest radiography reveals a typical appearance of increased pulmonary flow with right ventricular or biventricular enlargement, right atrial or biatrial enlargement, pulmonary vascular plethora, and an enlarged main pulmonary artery (Figure 10-8).

- With ES, often there is significant dilation of central pulmonary arteries.

- Peripheral artery "pruning" (abrupt attenuation and/or termination of peripheral pulmonary artery branches) can be visualized.

- Cardiomegaly with right heart enlargement can be seen.

Echocardiography

- Two-dimensional (2D) transthoracic imaging can reveal the particular features of the structural cardiac defect responsible for the shunt (Figures 10-1A and 10-1B). Color flow Doppler is useful for demonstrating the direction of intracardiac blood flow (Figure 10-2). It may be difficult to detect shunting across the defect due to equalization of pressures within the left and right heart.

- Pulsed- and continuous-wave Doppler measurements permit quantification of the intracardiac shunt, right ventricular pressures, and estimation of pulmonary artery systolic/diastolic and mean pressures by means of the modified Bernoulli equation.

- With chronic right ventricular pressure overload and right ventricular hypertrophy, there is often flattening of the interventricular septum into the left ventricle during systole (Figure 10-9).

- In advanced right heart failure, right ventricular dilation and hypokinesis may also occur.

- The intraventricular septum may show abnormal systolic flattening.

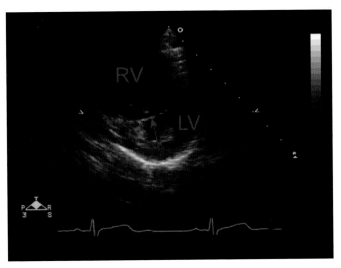

FIGURE 10-9 Echocardiogram showing evidence of right ventricular pressure overload. The left ventricle (LV) is D-shaped rather than round due to flattening of the interventricular septum (red arrow).

- The right atrium dilates, and tricuspid and pulmonary regurgitation are commonly seen secondary to dilation of the valve annuli.

Cardiac Magnetic Resonance Imaging

- Cardiac magnetic resonance imaging (MRI) can give further anatomic definition when echocardiographic images are suboptimal (Figures 10-4A and 10-4B). It can provide accurate and volumetric definition of the size and function of the right (and left) ventricular chambers. Like echocardiography, chronic right ventricular pressure overload can give rise to flattening of the interventricular septum into the left ventricle during systole.

- Using phase-contrast velocity-encoded imaging, cardiac MRI can be used to measure the magnitude of the right-to-left shunt by providing accurate Qp/Qs quantification (Figure 10-10). Phase-contrast imaging can also be utilized to quantify the degree of blood flow in each lung across the right and left pulmonary arteries.

Computed Tomography

- Computed tomography (CT) pulmonary artery angiography—may show dilation, aneurysm, thrombosis, and mural calcification of the pulmonary trunk and proximal branches.[6,7]

- When needed, CT of the lung parenchyma can identify embolic infarction, hemorrhage, neovascularity, lobular ground glass opacification, and hilar and intercostal collaterals in patients with ES.[8]

Cardiac Catheterization

Cardiac catheterization can be of value, after collecting clinical and noninvasive data, to confirm and/or demonstrate the following:

- Cardiac catheterization permits the examination of the intracardiac structure and exclusion of potentially reversible causes of pulmonary hypertension, as well as assessment of ventricular function (systolic and diastolic), examination of the intracardiac shunt, determination of pulmonary artery pressure and flow, and calculation of PVR.

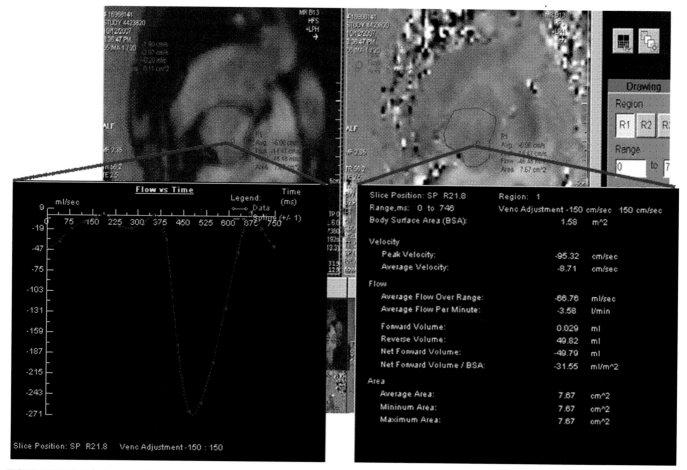

FIGURE 10-10 Velocity-encoded phase-contrast (PC) imaging is often used to measure flow and calculate Qp:Qs. Magnitude (left) and phase (right) images of a phase-contrast magnetic resonance imaging study is shown. An imaging plane is placed perpendicular to the aorta such that cross-section of the vessel and through-plane velocity of blood are measured. Total flow (Qs) is calculated by summing velocity across the luminal cross-section across the aorta. The same principle is applied to the pulmonary artery (PA) to get the total flow (Qp) across the PA. The resultant flow measurements across the aorta and the PA can then be used to calculated the Qp:Qs ratio.

- Cardiac catheterization in suspected ES should be performed at a center with expertise in hemodynamic catheterization, PAH, and management of CHD-related PAH. If the pulmonary artery pressures do not fall with inhalation of 100% oxygen or nitric oxide, the pulmonary hypertension is considered irreversible, and the patient is not a candidate for surgical repair.[9]

- The reactivity of the pulmonary vascular bed can be determined by a trial of inhaled 100% oxygen and nitric oxide. After 5 minutes of inhalational therapy, the hemodynamics are repeated. Responsiveness to these agents is associated with longer midterm survival.[10]

- Pulmonary angiography can reveal structural alterations in the pulmonary vascular bed. Irreversible changes (consistent with Heath-Edwards III severity) can be visualized and may include loss of normal arborization, as well as tortuosity, narrowing, or cutoff of small pulmonary arteries.

Exercise Testing

- The 6-minute walk test (6MWT), which requires minimal equipment and subspecialty experience, is simpler than the more formal and involved traditional cardiopulmonary exercise test (CPET) and is better tolerated in young children.

- The 6MWT may be effective in patients with a walk distance of less than 300 m. In patients above the 300-m threshold, however, a CPET should be considered.[11]

Laboratory Studies

- Laboratory studies used in the diagnosis of Eisenmenger syndrome include complete blood count (CBC), biochemical profiles, and iron studies, in addition to blood gas assessments.
- Hemoglobin and hematocrit levels should be followed due to erythrocytosis secondary to chronic cyanosis. The red cell mass increases with chronic erythrocytosis.
- Ferritin and iron studies need to be followed in patients with ES, since despite the elevated red blood cell mass, iron deficiency is common and can adversely affect the oxygen carrying capacity. There is reduced serum ferritin due to phlebotomy-related iron store reduction with increased total iron-binding capacity.
- Biochemical profile should be documented including conjugated bilirubin, uric acid, urea, creatinine which are often elevated.
- Urinary biochemical analysis reveals proteinuria.
- Arterial blood gas (ABG) reflects reduced resting partial pressure of carbon dioxide ($PaCO_2$) due to resting tachypnea and reduced partial pressure of oxygen (PaO_2) due to right-to-left shunting, mixed respiratory and metabolic acidosis.
- Recent data suggests that brain natriuretic peptide (BNP) may be a marker for prognosis in PAH and ES.[12,13]

MANAGEMENT

The medical treatment of Eisenmenger syndrome is directed toward the improvement of symptoms related to heart failure and pulmonary hypertension and the prevention and management of complications related to cyanotic congenital heart disease.

The treatment of Eisenmenger syndrome varies widely and depends on the patient's age, degree of cyanosis, and subsequent polycythemia. Asymptomatic patients require periodic evaluation, with anticipation of potential needs. Much of the therapy currently used for Eisenmenger syndrome has been studied in the treatment of idiopathic pulmonary arterial hypertension (IPAH). Because of the similarities between these entities, therapies found useful in patients with IPAH are very attractive for use in Eisenmenger physiology.

MEDICAL MANAGEMENT

Oxygen Therapy

- The use of oxygen supplementation in patients with Eisenmenger syndrome is controversial. It has been shown to have no impact on exercise capacity and survival in adult patients with this condition. Some patients, however, may benefit from nocturnal supplementation, although oxygen therapy is most useful as a bridge to heart-lung transplant.[14,15]

Pulmonary Vasodilator Therapy

- Studies of patients with IPAH have shown an imbalance between vasoconstrictors (endothelin, thromboxane) and vasodilators (prostacyclin, nitric oxide) in the pulmonary vasculature, and current therapy is directed at correcting this imbalance.[16]

- Vasodilator studies for IPAH (most of which have been performed in adults) have revealed a significant improvement in exercise tolerance, 6-minute walk distance, or New York Heart Association (NYHA) class. Subgroups, as well as smaller studies, have shown improvement in pulmonary hypertension caused by congenital heart disease.

Prostacyclins

- Long-term prostacyclin therapy was shown to improve hemodynamics (decrease in mean pulmonary artery pressure, improvement in cardiac index, decrease in PVR) and the quality of life in patients with congenital heart disease and PAH.[17]
- Epoprostenol requires a continuous intravenous infusion via a central catheter because of its short half-life (5 minutes). Patients must carry a portable pump in a waist pack and must maintain the drug at a cool temperature during the infusion. This therapy is extremely expensive but has been shown to improve pulmonary pressure, 6MWT distance, oxygenation, and quality of life in patients.[18]
- Treprostinil is a prostacyclin analogue that is administered by continuous subcutaneous infusion.
- Iloprost is an inhaled prostacyclin administered intermittently 6 to 9 times daily via nebulizer and is approved for adults with IPAH.

Endothelin Receptor Antagonists

- Bosentan, an endothelin receptor antagonist that has been approved for patients with IPAH.
- A multicenter, prospective, double-blind, placebo-controlled study (the Bosentan Randomized Trial of Endothelin Antagonist Therapy-5 [BREATH-5] study) found that bosentan reduced the mean pulmonary arterial pressure and improved exercise capacity and World Health Organization (WHO) class. The study tested the effect of bosentan titrated to 125 mg bid in 54 patients with Eisenmenger syndrome.[19]
- A longer follow up study in the BREATH-5 population (up to 40 weeks) showed that bosentan remained safe and had a positive impact on patients with Eisenmenger syndrome.[20]

Phosphodiesterase Inhibitors

- Sildenafil, another vasodilatory agent, was originally used for erectile dysfunction but has since been approved by the US Food and Drug Administration (FDA) for IPAH. It acts as an inhibitor of phosphodiesterase 5, resulting in an increase in cyclic guanosine monophosphate (cGMP) and vascular relaxation.[21]
- Studies suggest that sildenafil is safe and effective in patients with Eisenmenger syndrome. In a randomized, placebo-controlled study of 20 patients with PAH (10 patients with Eisenmenger syndrome and 10 with IPAH), sildenafil improved the patient's NYHA class, 6MWT distance, and exercise duration. Furthermore, sildenafil therapy resulted in a decrease in systolic pulmonary arterial pressure from 98 to 78 mm Hg. The effects of the drug were similar for the 2 patient populations in this study.[22]

Erythrocytosis and Iron Deficiency

- Erythrocytosis is almost always present in patients with Eisenmenger syndrome. This can result in symptoms of hyperviscosity, including visual disturbances, fatigue, headache, dizziness, and paresthesias. Routine phlebotomy is not usually recommended for this condition, except in the presence of hyperviscosity symptoms. Before initiating phlebotomy, dehydration must be ruled out, since it can falsely increase the hematocrit level. Phlebotomy should always be performed with concomitant fluid replacement.

- As for other patients with cyanotic heart disease, iron deficiency should be avoided in Eisenmenger patients.

Prevention of Thrombosis, Stroke, and Systemic Vascular Events

Patients with Eisenmenger syndrome are prone to thrombotic events as part of their hyperviscosity. At the same time, they are susceptible to bleeding because their platelets are dysfunctional. Therefore, patients who have a hematocrit level greater than 65% and are undergoing noncardiac surgery could be considered for phlebotomy and concomitant fluid replacement in order to decrease the risk of thrombotic and bleeding events.[23]

Role of Anticoagulation

- Although an increased risk of thrombosis is observed in patients with Eisenmenger syndrome, an increased risk of bleeding and pulmonary hemorrhage is also recognized. Thus, anticoagulation is still not routinely recommended and often has to be individualized for patient care.

SURGICAL MANAGEMENT

- Heart and lung transplantation or lung transplantation with intracardiac repair are treatment options in Eisenmenger patients. Transplantation should be reserved for severely symptomatic patients, since overall survival with medical management is usually quite good even in patients with severe pulmonary arterial disease.[24]

- Repair of the primary defect is contraindicated in the context of established severe PAH. However, corrective surgery may be possible in certain cases if a significant degree of left-to-right shunting remains and if responsiveness of the pulmonary circulation to vasodilator therapy can be demonstrated.

- Heart-lung transplantation is the procedure of choice if repair of the underlying cardiac defect is not possible in Eisenmenger syndrome. This procedure was performed successfully for the first time in 1981.

- Patients can undergo lung transplantation only if they have pulmonary hypertension and Eisenmenger syndrome with surgically correctable congenital anomalies and maintained right ventricular function. Patients may undergo heart-lung transplantation with complex congenital heart defects and those with severe right ventricular failure along with ES.

- Excellent results can be obtained with transplantation, with return to normal pulmonary function.

WOMEN WITH EISENMENGER SYNDROME

Contraception in Women With ES

- Women with severe CHD-PAH, especially those with Eisenmenger syndrome, and their partners should be counseled about the absolute avoidance of pregnancy in view of the high risk of maternal death, and should be educated regarding safe and appropriate methods of contraception. Given the risks associated with pregnancy, women with Eisenmenger syndrome should use a nonreversible method of contraception, such as hysteroscopic sterilization/tubal ligation.[25]

- Other options include progestin-only contraception, such as depot medroxyprogesterone acetate (DMPA) injections or the etonogestrel implant (Implanon), which are highly effective reversible methods of contraception.

- Estrogen-containing oral contraceptives should be avoided when possible given the increased risk of thrombosis and stroke in ES.

- An intrauterine device (IUD) is an option for acyanotic or mildly cyanotic women who want a reversible method of contraception and are at low risk of acquiring a sexually transmitted infection. However, due to the approximately 5% risk of vasovagal reaction at the time of implantation, an IUD is an option only if other alternatives are unacceptable and the device should be implanted in a monitored setting.[26]

Reproductive Concerns in Women With ES

- Miscarriage is common in cyanotic women. Intrauterine growth restriction is seen in 30% of pregnancies as a result of maternal hypoxemia. Premature labor is found in 50% to 60% of instances and the high perinatal mortality rate (28%) is due mostly to prematurity. In one study of women with Eisenmenger syndrome, 47% delivered at term, 33% between 32 and 36 weeks, and 20% before 31 weeks of gestation.[27]

- Pregnancy is a cause of significant mortality in most published series of women with Eisenmenger syndrome. A systematic review of published studies from 1978 to 1996 examined maternal mortality rates in women with Eisenmenger syndrome and demonstrated mortality rates of 56%.[2] A more recent review suggested that mortality remains high.[3] Most complications occur near-term and early (first week) postpartum, and therefore extended postpartum hospital observation is suggested. Mortality is typically from heart failure, sudden death presumably due to arrhythmias, or thromboembolic events.[28]

- Women with ES of childbearing age should be strongly advised to avoid pregnancy.[29]

- Bleeding as well as thrombotic complications in the postpartum period cause a significant morbidity and mortality. Although the maternal mortality rate in Eisenmenger syndrome ranges from 23% to 52% in different series, it is estimated that the mortality rate is in excess of 50%. The most critical time is postpartum, and the majority of deaths occur in the first week after delivery.

- The fetal mortality rate ranges from 7.8% to 28%, and only 15% of babies are born at term.

- Women with CHD and ES who become pregnant should receive individualized counseling from cardiovascular and obstetric caregivers with expertise in the management of CHD-PAH and should undergo the earliest possible pregnancy termination after such counseling.

LONG TERM OUTCOMES

Long-Term Morbidity

Patients with ES have multiple complications that often result from multiorgan systems include, but not limited to, the following

- Hematologic complications including hyperviscosity syndromes related to secondary erythrocytosis and bleeding diatheses.

- Nervous system complications which include brain abscess, transient cerebral ischemia, thrombotic stroke, and intracerebral hemorrhage.

- Patients can have significant hyperbilirubinemia increasing the risk of gallstones.

- Hyperuricemia can cause nephrolithiasis and secondary gout.

- Hypertrophic osteoarthropathy can cause bone pain and tenderness.

- Vision loss has been reported with transient vision loss related to peripheral retinal microvascular abnormalities.

- Cardiovascular complications include congestive heart failure, arrhythmias, risk of infective endocarditis, and syncope since the systemic vascular bed is prone to vasodilation and subsequent systemic arterial hypotension, which can cause syncope.

- Pulmonary infarction and hemorrhage with infective endocarditis has also been described.

Long-Term Mortality

- Patients with ES usually do not survive beyond the second or third decade without any forms of treatment. The mean age of death is 37 years, although survival into the 60s has been reported.[30-32]

- Long-term survival depends on the patient's age at the onset of pulmonary hypertension and the coexistence of additional adverse features, such as Down syndrome.

- Life expectancy is generally more severely reduced in Eisenmenger patients with complex congenital heart disease than in Eisenmenger patients with simple lesions.

- A double-blind, randomized multicenter study (BREATHE-5) showed improved outcomes in patients with ES using bosentan therapy. The pulmonary vascular resistance decreased, pulmonary artery pressure decreased, and exercise capacity increased over a 16-week study period.[33]

- Eisenmenger patients have a better life expectancy than patients with primary pulmonary hypertension (PPH) who have similar hemodynamics.[34,35] This was illustrated in a report of patients with severe PAH (37 Eisenmenger, 57 PPH).[34] Actuarial survival at 1 and 3 years of those not receiving transplants was higher in those with Eisenmenger syndrome (97% vs 77% and 77% vs 35%, respectively). The reason for this is unknown, but may be because both ventricles, rather than just the right ventricle, share the increased hemodynamic load of increased PVR.[36]

- The mortality rate in pregnant patients with Eisenmenger syndrome is reported to be approximately 50%, although it may be higher.[30-32]

- Most patients are thought to die from worsening heart failure, arrhythmias, sudden death, or thromboembolism or intrapulmonary hemorrhage due to rupture of a major vessel.[9-10,16,30,31,37]

- ES is a chronic disease and requires lifelong specialty care. Patients with ES should follow at least yearly in a dedicated Adult Congenital Heart Disease (ACHD) program with capabilities of providing care for patients with pulmonary hypertension.

CONCLUSION

- Patients with congenital heart disease (CHD) and ES should be seen by a CHD-PAH trained provider at least yearly. All planned interventions should be discussed with the provider.

- The following evaluation is recommended at least yearly:
  - Comprehensive evaluation of functional capacity and assessment of secondary complications.
  - Hemoglobin, platelet count, iron studies, creatinine, and uric acid.
  - Digital oximetry, both with and without supplemental oxygen therapy. Oxygen-responsive hypoxemia should be investigated.

- All medication changes should be rigorously reviewed for potential impact on the systemic blood pressure, loading conditions, intravascular shunting, and renal or hepatic perfusion or function.

- Patients with Eisenmenger syndrome should seek prompt attention for arrhythmias and infections.

REFERENCES

1. Wood P. The Eisenmenger syndrome or pulmonary hypertension with reversed central shunt. I. *Br Med J*. 1958;2:701.

2. Vongpatanasin W, Brickner ME, Hillis LD, Lange RA. The Eisenmenger syndrome in adults. *Ann Intern Med*. 1998;128:745.

3. Humbert M, Sitbon O, Simonneau G. Treatment of pulmonary arterial hypertension. *N Engl J Med*. 2004;351:1425-1436.

4. Granton JT, Rabinovitch M. Pulmonary arterial hypertension in congenital heart disease. *Cardiol Clin*. 2002;20:441.

5. Warnes CA, Williams RG, Bashore TM, et al. ACC/AHA 2008 Guidelines for the Management of Adults with Congenital Heart Disease: a report of the American College of Cardiology/American Heart Association Task Force on Practice Guidelines (writing committee to develop guidelines on the management of adults with congenital heart disease). *Circulation*. 2008;118:e714.

6. Perloff JK, Hart EM, Greaves SM, et al. Proximal pulmonary arterial and intrapulmonary radiologic features of Eisenmenger syndrome and primary pulmonary hypertension. *Am J Cardiol*. 2003;92:182.

7. Silversides CK, Granton JT, Konen E, et al. Pulmonary thrombosis in adults with Eisenmenger syndrome. *J Am Coll Cardiol*. 2003;42:1982.

8. Sheehan R, Perloff JK, Fishbein MC, et al. Pulmonary neovascularity: a distinctive radiographic finding in Eisenmenger syndrome. *Circulation*. 2005;112:2778.

9. Balzer DT, Kort HW, Day RW, et al. Inhaled Nitric Oxide as a Preoperative Test (INOP Test I): the INOP Test Study Group. *Circulation*. 2002;106(12 suppl 1):176-181.

10. Post MC, Janssens S, Van de Werf F, Budts W. Responsiveness to inhaled nitric oxide is a predictor for mid-term survival in adult patients with congenital heart defects and pulmonary arterial hypertension. *Eur Heart J*. 2004;25:1651-1656.

11. Lammers AE, Diller GP, Odendaal D, Tailor S, Derrick G, Haworth SG. Comparison of 6-min walk test distance and

cardiopulmonary exercise test performance in children with pulmonary hypertension. *Arch Dis Child.* 2011;96:141-147.

12. Bernus A, Wagner BD, Accurso F, Doran A, Kaess H, Ivy DD. Brain natriuretic peptide levels in managing pediatric patients with pulmonary arterial hypertension. *Chest.* 2009;135:745-751.

13. Diller GP, Alonso-Gonzalez R, Kempny A, et al. B-type natriuretic peptide concentrations in contemporary Eisenmenger syndrome patients: predictive value and response to disease targeting therapy. *Heart.* 2012;98:736-742.

14. Bowyer JJ, Busst CM, Denison DM, Shinebourne EA. Effect of long term oxygen treatment at home in children with pulmonary vascular disease. *Br Heart J.* 1986;55:385-390.

15. Sandoval J, Aguirre JS, Pulido T, et al. Nocturnal oxygen therapy in patients with the Eisenmenger syndrome. *Am J Respir Crit Care Med.* 2001;164:1682-1687.

16. Humbert M, Sitbon O, Simonneau G. Treatment of pulmonary arterial hypertension. *N Engl J Med.* 2004;351:1425-1436.

17. Rosenzweig EB, Kerstein D, Barst RJ. Long-term prostacyclin for pulmonary hypertension with associated congenital heart defects. *Circulation.* 1999;99:1858-1865.

18. Ivy DD, Doran A, Claussen L, Bingaman D, Yetman A. Weaning and discontinuation of epoprostenol in children with idiopathic pulmonary arterial hypertension receiving concomitant bosentan. *Am J Cardiol.* 2004;93:943-946.

19. Galiè N, Beghetti M, Gatzoulis MA, et al. Bosentan therapy in patients with Eisenmenger syndrome: a multicenter, double-blind, randomized, placebo-controlled study. *Circulation.* 2006;114:48-54.

20. Gatzoulis MA, Beghetti M, Galiè N, et al. Longer-term bosentan therapy improves functional capacity in Eisenmenger syndrome: results of the BREATHE-5 open-label extension study. *Int J Cardiol.* 2008;127:27-32.

21. Chau EM, Fan KY, Chow WH. Effects of chronic sildenafil in patients with Eisenmenger syndrome versus idiopathic pulmonary arterial hypertension. *Int J Cardiol.* 2007;120:301-305.

22. Singh TP, Rohit M, Grover A, Malhotra S, Vijayvergiya R. A randomized, placebo-controlled, double-blind, crossover study to evaluate the efficacy of oral sildenafil therapy in severe pulmonary artery hypertension. *Am Heart J.* 2006;151:851.e1-e5.

23. Brickner ME, Hillis LD, Lange RA. Congenital heart disease in adults. Second of two parts. *N Engl J Med.* 2000;342:334-342.

24. Hopkins WE, Ochoa LL, Richardson GW, Trulock EP. Comparison of the hemodynamics and survival of adults with severe primary pulmonary hypertension or Eisenmenger syndrome. *J Heart Lung Transplant.* 1996;15(1 pt 1):100-105.

25. Miño M, Arjona JE, Cordón J, Pelegrin B, Povedano B, Chacon E. Success rate and patient satisfaction with the Essure sterilisation in an outpatient setting: a prospective study of 857 women. *BJOG.* 2007;114:763-766.

26. European Society of Gynecology (ESG), Association for European Paediatric Cardiology (AEPC), German Society for Gender Medicine (DGesGM), Regitz-Zagrosek V, Blomstrom Lundqvist C, Borghi C, et al. ESC Committee for Practice Guidelines on the management of cardiovascular diseases during pregnancy: the Task Force on the Management of Cardiovascular Diseases during Pregnancy of the European Society of Cardiology (ESC). *Eur Heart J.* 2011;32:3147-3197.

27. Weiss BM, Zemp L, Seifert B, Hess OM. Outcome of pulmonary vascular disease in pregnancy: a systematic overview from 1978 through 1996. *J Am Coll Cardiol.* 1998;31:1650-1657.

28. Weiss BM, Zemp L, Seifert B, Hess OM. Outcome of pulmonary vascular disease in pregnancy: a systematic overview from 1978 through 1996. *J Am Coll Cardiol.* 1998;31:1650-1657.

29. Bédard E, Dimopoulos K, Gatzoulis MA. Has there been any progress made on pregnancy outcomes among women with pulmonary arterial hypertension? *Eur Heart J.* 2009;30(3):256-265.

30. Niwa K, Perloff JK, Kaplan S, et al. Eisenmenger syndrome in adults: ventricular septal defect, truncus arteriosus, univentricular heart. *J Am Coll Cardiol.* 1999;34:223.

31. Daliento L, Somerville J, Presbitero P, et al. Eisenmenger syndrome. Factors relating to deterioration and death. *Eur Heart J.* 1998;19:1845.

32. Warnes CA, Boger JE, Roberts WC. Eisenmenger ventricular septal defect with prolonged survival. *Am J Cardiol.* 1984;54:460.

33. Galiè N, Beghetti M, Gatzoulis MA, et al. *Circulation.* Bosentan therapy in patients with Eisenmenger syndrome: a multicenter, double-blind, randomized, placebo-controlled study. 2006;114:48-54.

34. Hopkins WE, Ochoa LL, Richardson GW, Trulock EP. Comparison of the hemodynamics and survival of adults with severe primary pulmonary hypertension or Eisenmenger syndrome. *J Heart Lung Transplant.* 1996;15:100.

35. Hayden AM, Robert RC, Kriett JM, et al. Primary diagnosis predicts prognosis of lung transplant candidates. *Transplantation.* 1993; 55:1048.

36. Hopkins WE, Waggoner AD. Severe pulmonary hypertension without right ventricular failure: the unique hearts of patients with Eisenmenger syndrome. *Am J Cardiol.* 2002;89:34.

37. Saha A, Balakrishnan KG, Jaiswal PK, et al. Prognosis for patients with Eisenmenger syndrome of various aetiology. *Int J Cardiol.* 1994;45:199.

11 PREGNANCY AND CONGENITAL HEART DISEASE

Sara L. Partington, MD
Anne Marie Valente, MD

Congestive Heart Failure in a Pregnant Woman with Transposition of the Great Arteries S/P Atrial Switch Surgery

A 29-year-old woman with complete transposition of the great arteries (TGA) repaired with a Mustard atrial switch surgery presented with heart failure symptoms 7 days postpartum. TGA is a form of cyanotic congenital heart disease (CHD) in which the aorta originates from the right ventricle (RV) pumping deoxygenated blood to the body and the pulmonary artery (PA) originates from the left ventricle (LV) pumping oxygenated blood to the lungs. This lesion is often incompatible with life and many adults currently living with TGA have undergone atrial switch surgeries as infants to direct deoxygenated blood to the LV to be pumped to the lungs and oxygenated blood to the RV to be pumped to the body (Figure 11-1A). The RV in patients who have undergone the atrial switch procedure is the systemic ventricle and becomes hypertrophied, dilated, and often dysfunctional.

This woman had an uncomplicated pregnancy and underwent a cesarean section for obstetrical reasons during which time she received several liters of intravenous fluids. On presentation, one week postpartum, she presented with dyspnea and edema. She underwent an echocardiogram that did not reveal any changes in systemic ventricular function and tricuspid valve regurgitation (Figure 11-1B). She was treated with intravenous furosemide and her symptoms dramatically improved. The increased volume load of pregnancy is not tolerated well in some women with CHD, particularly those with underlying ventricular dysfunction. Symptoms may be exacerbated in the postpartum period when afterload increases and dramatic changes in volume loading may occur.

CASE EXPLANATION

- The presence of cardiovascular disease in pregnant women poses a difficult clinical scenario in which the responsibility of the treating physician extends not only to the mother but also to the unborn fetus.
- Pregnancy has a profound effect on the circulatory system. Most of these hemodynamic changes start in the first trimester, peak during the second trimester, and plateau during the third trimester.
- The delivery and immediate postpartum period is associated with further profound and rapid changes in the circulatory system. During delivery, cardiac output, heart rate, blood pressure, and systemic vascular resistance increase with each uterine contraction.[1]
- Immediately postpartum, the delivery of the placenta increases afterload by removing the low-resistance circulation and increases the preload by returning placental blood to the maternal circulation. This increase in preload is accentuated by the elimination of the mechanical compression of the inferior vena cava (IVC). Blood loss is typically 300 to 400 mL during vaginal delivery and 500 to 800 mL during cesarean delivery. These changes can place an intolerable strain on an abnormal heart necessitating aggressive medical management, such as in the case of this patient, and very occasionally, invasive hemodynamic monitoring.[2]

DIAGNOSIS

- In the United States, CHD is now the most common form of heart disease complicating pregnancy.
- Women with complete transposition of the great arteries are reaching reproductive age because of operative interventions, which in the earlier days of surgical repair involved atrial switch repairs, such as the Mustard or Senning procedures.
- Gestational risks after Mustard or Senning repairs are related chiefly to the functional status of the subaortic morphologic right ventricle, the presence of pulmonary hypertension, and to conduction and rhythm abnormalities.
- Patients with known or suspected systemic ventricular dysfunction should have an echocardiogram before conception, or as soon as possible after pregnancy is confirmed, to determine baseline ventricular function. Pregnancy should be discouraged if there is a significant reduction in ventricular function (ejection fraction <40%).[3]
- There are several modalities that may be utilized to follow women with CHD throughout pregnancy and the postpartum period at risk of congestive heart failure. These include laboratory testing including B-type natriuretic peptide (BNP), exercise testing, and imaging studies.

- Vaginal delivery is preferred because it causes smaller shifts in blood volume, less hemorrhage, fewer clots, and fewer infections. Cesarean delivery is generally indicated only for obstetric reasons.[4]

B-Type Natriuretic Peptide

- Plasma brain natriuretic peptide (BNP) and N-terminal pro-brain natriuretic peptide (NT-pro-BNP) levels are well-recognized markers of heart failure and these markers may also be helpful in monitoring women with cardiovascular disease during pregnancy.

- The BNP increases in response to increased volume loading and predicts adverse outcomes in women with congenital heart disease during pregnancy.

- Tanous et al reported that a BNP value of less than or equal to 100 pg/mL during pregnancy had a negative predictive value of 100% for identifying cardiac events in women with CHD[5] (Figure 11-2).

- In patients with repaired tetralogy of Fallot, Kamiya reported that the peak BNP after the second trimester was most useful in predicting adverse maternal cardiac events in women with repaired tetralogy of Fallot.[6]

Exercise Testing

- Another useful tool in risk stratification is objective exercise testing.

- Cardiopulmonary exercise testing is often used to evaluate exercise capacity in adults with congenital heart disease including women who are considering pregnancy. A multicenter study including 89 pregnancies in 83 women with CHD identified a low chronotropic index as a risk factor for an adverse maternal cardiac outcome.[7]

Echocardiography

- Echocardiography may be used to assess cardiac function in the setting of the hemodynamic burden of pregnancy, though the frequency of echocardiographic screening in woman with various forms of congenital heart disease is not well established.

- There are normal echocardiographic changes during pregnancy that should not be considered pathologic (Table 11-1).[8,9]

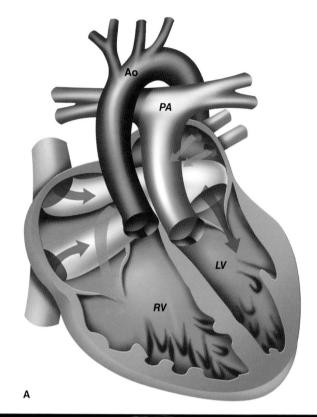

A

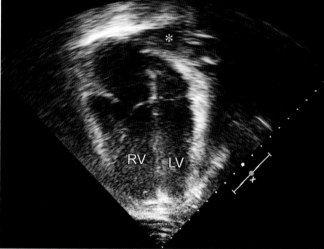

B

FIGURE 11-1 A. D-transposition Transposition of the great arteries with an atrial switch procedure. **B.** Postpartum echocardiogram in a woman with d-transposition of the great arteries and an atrial switch procedure demonstrating a dilated, hypertrophied systemic right ventricle who presented with heart failure in the postpartum period. Ao, aorta; LV, left ventricle; PA, pulmonary artery; RV, right ventricle. *Pulmonary vein entering the pulmonary venous atrium.

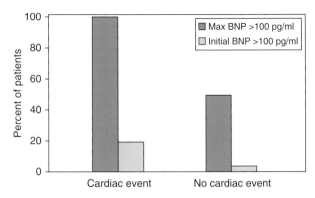

FIGURE 11-2 Elevated B-type natriuretic peptide (BNP) predicts cardiac events in pregnant women with congenital heart disease. (*Adapted from Tanous D, Siu SC, Mason J, Greutmann M, Wald RM, Parker JD, Sermer M, Colman JM, Silversides CK. B-type natriuretic peptide in pregnant women with heart disease. J Am Coll Cardiol. 2010;56:1247-1253.*)

Table 11-1 Normal Echocardiographic Changes During Pregnancy

Left atrium	Slight ↑ in size (3-4 mm)
Left ventricular end-diastolic volume	↑
Left ventricular mass	↑
Left ventricular ejection fraction	Slight ↓ or no change*
Aortic root	↑ in diameter (2-3 mm)
Left ventricular outflow tract velocity	↑ ~0.3 m/s
Pericardial effusion, small	Present in ~25% of women

*May be affected by positional changes.

Fetal Diagnosis of CHD in a Pregnant Woman with Truncus Arteriosus

PATIENT STORY 2

A 28-year-old woman with truncus arteriosus (Figure 11-3A), born with a single arterial trunk containing the aorta and the pulmonary artery was surgically repaired by removing the pulmonary arteries from the common arterial trunk and attaching them to a conduit from the right ventricle. She had a routine screening fetal echocardiogram given her history of CHD and the fetus was also found to have truncus arteriosus (Figures 11-3B and 11-3C) and a plan to have neonatology present at time of delivery with initiation of intravenous prostaglandins was arranged.

CASE EXPLANATION

• Women who were born with complex congenital cardiac lesions such as transposition of the great vessels, tricuspid atresia, single ventricle physiology, and truncus arteriosus are now reaching reproductive age due to the success of surgical procedures.

• This case outlines the close collaboration between both cardiac and obstetric teams that is needed for optimal care for both women and fetuses with congenital heart disease.

DISCUSSION

• Current guidelines recommend screening all fetuses of parents with CHD with fetal echocardiography to assess risk to the fetus and to ensure that the parents are properly counseled and post-delivery plans are appropriate.[32]

• Women with moderate- or high-risk lesions, especially cyanotic lesions, have an increased risk of fetal growth restriction and should be followed with monthly ultrasounds for fetal growth.

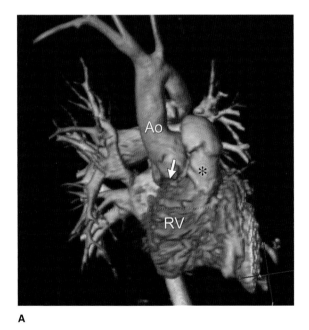

A

FIGURE 11-3A A cardiovascular magnetic resonance (CMR) of a woman with truncus arteriosus. Ao, aorta; RV, right ventricle; arrow, single truncal valve; *, RV-PA conduit

- Decisions about timing and mode of delivery must be made well in advance of labor.

- Continuous electronic fetal heart rate monitoring is recommended to assess fetal well-being during labor and allow timely intervention if non-reassuring fetal heart rate patterns occur.

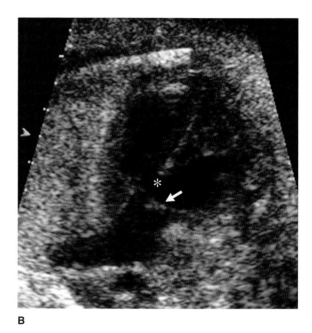

B

FIGURE 11-3B At 20 weeks' gestation, she underwent a screening fetal echocardiogram that detected truncus arteriosus in the fetus. Arrow, single truncal valve; ∗, ventricular septal defect.

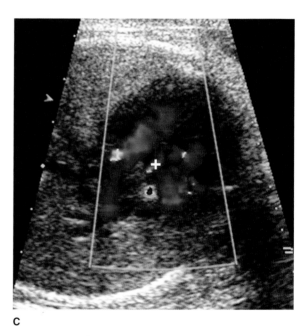

C

FIGURE 11-3C The fetal echocardiographic Doppler demonstrates truncal valve regurgitation in the fetus. +, truncal valve regurgitation.

Infective Endocarditis in a Pregnant Woman with CHD

PATIENT STORY 3

A 38-year-old woman with a bicuspid aortic valve (BAV) with no prior cardiac interventions and only minimal valvar regurgitation presented at 23 weeks' gestation with myalgias, fevers, chills, and a worsening murmur of aortic regurgitation. She was found to have *Streptococcus bacteremia*, a vegetation on her aortic valve (Figure 11-4A) and severe aortic regurgitation on echocardiogram (Figure 11-4B). She was treated with intravenous antibiotics with clinical stability; however, at 29 weeks' gestation she presented with premature labor and signs of heart failure. She underwent an emergent cesarean section, followed by aortic valve and aortic root replacements 1 week later.

CASE EXPLANATION

- Aortic stenosis (AS) in women of childbearing age is primarily due to a congenital bicuspid aortic valve.

- Mild bicuspid aortic stenosis or insufficiency generally is well tolerated during pregnancy because left ventricular ejection fraction (LVEF) is usually above normal.[10]

- Even though this patient did develop infective endocarditis, a BAV is not a lesion requiring endocarditis prophylaxis unless it has been subjected to valve replacement.

DISCUSSION

- Common valvular lesions for which antimicrobial prophylaxis is no longer recommended in the 2007 AHA guidelines include bicuspid aortic valve, acquired aortic or mitral valve disease (including mitral valve prolapse with regurgitation), and hypertrophic cardiomyopathy with latent or resting obstruction.[11]

- In addition, uncomplicated vaginal or cesarean delivery is not considered an indication for antibiotic prophylaxis.

- Infectious endocarditis (IE) is very rare in pregnancy, with an incidence reported to be 1.7 to 5.5/100,000.

- However, the maternal mortality rate is high, with reported rates between 22% and 33%, with the most deaths related to heart failure or an embolic event.

- The rate of fetal mortality is equally high and ranges between 15% and 33%.[12,13]

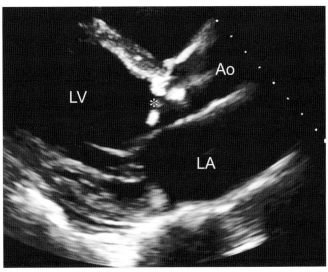

A

FIGURE 11-4A A 2D echocardiogram of a woman presenting with endocarditis of her bicuspid aortic valve at 25 weeks' gestation. She has ascending aorta dilation associated with her bicuspid valve disease. Ao, aorta; LA, left atrium; LV, left ventricle; *, large vegetation on aortic valve.

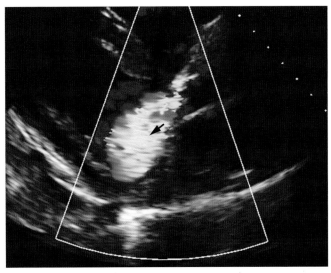

B

FIGURE 11-4B Doppler echocardiogram demonstrates severe aortic regurgitation. (see arrow)

The Pregnant Woman With Connective Tissue Disease With Aortopathy

A 40-year-old woman with Marfan syndrome (MFS) and a dilated aortic root measuring 4.1 cm was treated with atenolol during her pregnancy. She underwent an uncomplicated cesarean section delivery of twins and 6 days later developed neck and back pain. An echocardiogram demonstrated a type 1 aortic dissection (Figure 11-5A) and moderate-to-severe aortic regurgitation (Figure 11-5B). She underwent emergent surgery involving mechanical aortic valve replacement, ascending aortic graft and saphenous vein bypass graft from the aortic graft to the right coronary artery.

CASE EXPLANATION

- This case highlights that pregnant women with MFS with aortic root dilatation are at increased risk for aortic dissection and/or rupture, although a normal dimension or a mildly dilated aorta does not exclude the possibility of dissection.

- The diagnosis and management of aortic dissection that occurs during pregnancy are similar to that for aortic dissection in general.

- Given the lethal nature of aortic dissection, prompt diagnosis and intervention are critical.

- Complications can occur at any time during pregnancy or postpartum, but are most often seen after the second trimester or during the postpartum period. There is general agreement that risk increases at larger aortic root diameters.

DISCUSSION

- The Marfan syndrome is an autosomal dominant condition with a reported incidence of 1 in 3000 to 5000 individuals.

- Women with connective tissue disorders have an increased risk of aortic root dilation and dissection during the peripartum period.[14]

- Accelerated aortic growth rates result in increased aortic dimensions during pregnancy that may not return to baseline levels following delivery in women with Marfan syndrome.[15]

- If pregnancy is contemplated in a woman with Marfan syndrome, she should be advised to consider aortic root and ascending aortic replacement if the diameter of the aorta exceeds 4 cm (class IIa guideline, level of evidence C).[16]

- Serial clinical assessment should include echocardiographic monitoring in all pregnant women with MFS, even among women with baseline aortic root diameter less than or equal to 40 mm.

- Transthoracic echocardiography is not a sensitive enough technique to rule out dissection and frequently an alternative technique such as transesophageal echocardiography, computed tomography (CT), or magnetic resonance imaging (MRI) may be required.[17]

- The frequency of clinical and imaging follow-up should be individualized depending on patient and aorta characteristics.

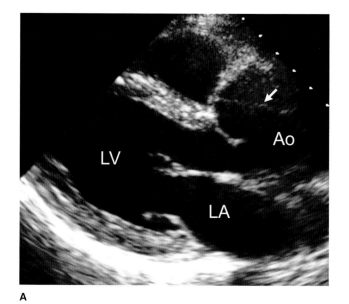

A

FIGURE 11-5A A postpartum 2D echocardiogram of a woman with Marfan syndrome and a dilated aortic root presenting with a type 1 aortic dissection. Ao, aorta; LA, left atrium; LV, left ventricle; arrow, dissection flap.

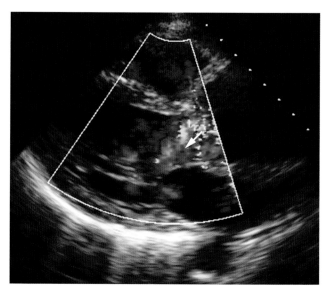

B

FIGURE 11-5B Doppler echocardiogram demonstrates severe aortic regurgitation. (see arrow)

- The 2011 European Society of Cardiology (ESC) guidelines suggest repeat echocardiographic imaging every 4 to 8 weeks during pregnancy in patients with ascending aorta dilatation (aortic diameter >40 mm).[18]

- Similarly, the 2010 American College of Cardiology/American Heart Association/American Association of Thoracic Surgeons (ACC/AHA/AATS) guidelines recommend monthly or bimonthly echocardiographic measurement of the ascending aortic dimensions in this setting.[16,19]

- Beta-blocker, preferably labetalol or metoprolol, along with strict blood pressure control is recommended for all pregnant women with MFS in an attempt to minimize aortic dilation and the risk of aortic dissection.[20] All women with Marfan syndrome should be counseled on the genetic risk to their offspring, as this is an autosomal dominant condition.

The Pregnant Woman with Repaired Tetralogy of Fallot S/P Bioprosthetic Pulmonary Valve Replacement

PATIENT STORY 5

A 30-year-old woman with a history of rheumatic heart disease underwent mechanical mitral and aortic valve replacements at the age of 20 years. She was diagnosed with a desired but unplanned pregnancy at 8 weeks gestation. Prior to pregnancy, she was taking warfarin 5 mg/day to maintain an INR of 2.5–3.5 and she had well-functioning mechanical aortic and mitral valve prostheses with stable gradients. The peak gradient across the aortic valve was 44 mmHg and the peak gradient across the mitral valve was 6 mmHg with normal biventricular size and function. At her cardiology visit in the first trimester of pregnancy, she was asymptomatic and had no change in her mechanical valve function or gradients. There was a discussion regarding the risks of valve thrombosis and her anticoagulation options during pregnancy and the patient opted to switch her warfarin to enoxaparin for the remainder of the pregnancy.

She presented at 14 weeks gestation with left facial droop and slurred speech that completely resolved within 1 hour of symptoms onset. A MRI of the head demonstrated a left cerebellar infarct (image 1). Her anti-Xa level 3 days prior to her cerebral vascular accident was therapeutic (1.2 U/mL). A transesophageal echocardiogram demonstrated normal mobility of her mechanical aortic and mitral valves, no valve thrombosis (images 2a, b) and stable gradients across the valves. She was diagnosed with a transient ischemic attack most likely secondary to mechanical valve thrombosis without a large, visible thrombosis on either valve. Her enoxaparin was changed to warfarin with a target INR of 2.5–3.5 with a plan to convert to IV heparin closer to term and a daily aspirin was added.

At 32 weeks gestation, she presented with elevated blood pressures. She was admitted to hospital, her warfarin was stopped and intravenous (IV) heparin was started when her INR was < 2.5. She underwent a semi-urgent Cesarean section 3 days later when she developed evidence of preeclampsia. Heparin was restarted 4 hours after Cesarean section and warfarin was restarted the next day. She developed a large abdominal wall hematoma on post-operative day 5 requiring cessation of warfarin and bridging with IV heparin. She was eventually restarted back on her warfarin when the hematoma began to resolve. (Figures 11-6A through 11-6C).

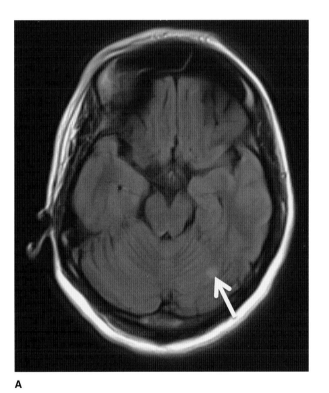

A

FIGURE 11-6A MRI of the head in a pregnant woman with mechanical aortic and mitral valves demonstrating a left cerebellar infarct. Arrow shows area of cerebellar infarct. (*Copyright © McGraw-Hill Education, Photographer: Dr. Sara L. Partington.*)

CASE EXPLANATION

- Management of women with bioprosthetic heart valves may be particularly challenging during pregnancy.

- Mechanical valves require intense attention to anticoagulation during pregnancy. Tissue valves may have an accelerated rate of degeneration with pregnancy; however, the evidence for this is controversial.[21,22]

DISCUSSION

- Managing pregnant women who require ongoing anticoagulation for the prophylaxis or treatment of thrombotic complications is a challenging dilemma.

- Therapeutic anticoagulation is recommended in all pregnant women with mechanical prosthetic heart valves to prevent valve thrombosis and thromboembolic events.[20]

- There are different modalities for anticoagulation that can be used during pregnancy including warfarin, intravenous unfractionated heparin [UFH]), and low-molecular-weight heparin (LMWH).

- For patients with mechanical valves, Warfarin is the long-term anticoagulant of choice in nonpregnant patients, but freely crosses the placental barrier in pregnant women because of its low molecular weight and can cause fetal embryopathy. The exact risk of warfarin embryopathy is difficult to predict with the best overall estimate of the risk for fetal embryopathy being less than 10%. A dose-dependent effect of warfarin on fetal embryopathy has also been reported, with warfarin less than or equal to 5 mg having lower rates of fetal complications than warfarin greater than 5 mg per day.[23-25]

- UFH does not cross the placenta in pregnant women due to its large molecular size and therefore does not carry the same risk of embryopathy as warfarin. There is limited data on the use of UFH throughout pregnancy in women with mechanical valves, though some have advocated for the use of UFH in the first trimester, followed by oral anticoagulants during the remainder of pregnancy till closer to delivery.

- LMWH can be considered during pregnancy and has several advantages over UFH including more predictable therapeutic levels for anticoagulation, less effect on bone, less bleeding and thrombocytopenia, and like UFH does not cross the placenta.

- The 2008 ACC/AHA guidelines emphasize that anticoagulation should be uninterrupted once pregnancy is achieved with frequent monitoring. Women can elect to stop warfarin between 6 and 12 weeks of gestation especially if the warfarin dose is > 5 mg/day, but should be treated with dose-adjusted continuous intravenous UFH, subcutaneous UFH, or LMWH. Between 12 and 36 weeks, the patient can be treated with warfarin, dose-adjusted continuous intravenous UFH, subcutaneous UFH, or LMWH. With warfarin compared to the different heparin regimens, the fetal risk is higher but the maternal risk appears to be *lower* for prosthetic valve thrombosis and risk for systemic embolization. Strict monitoring is essentially with dose-adjusted LMWH which should be given subcutaneously twice daily to maintain the anti-Xa level between 0.7 and 1.2 U/mL at 4 hours and 0.8-1.2 U/mL at 4-6 hours after dosing. LMWH should not be given if such monitoring cannot be performed. With dose-adjusted UFH, the activated partial

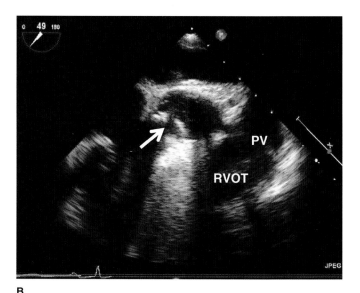

B

FIGURE 11-6B A transesophageal echocardiogram demonstrating a short axis view of the aortic mechanical valve leaflets. The aortic valve leaflets have normal mobility with no evidence of thrombus. RVOT, right ventricular outflow tract; PV, pulmonary valve; arrow shows mechanical aortic valve. (*Copyright © McGraw-Hill Education, Photographer: Dr. Sara L. Partington.*)

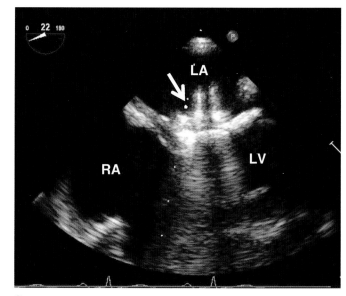

C

FIGURE 11-6C A transesophageal echocardiogram demonstrating the mechanical mitral valve. The mitral valve leaflets have normal mobility with no evidence of thrombus. RA, right atrium; LA, left atrium, LV, left ventricle; arrow, mechanical mitral valve. (*Copyright © McGraw-Hill Education, Photographer: Dr. Sara L. Partington.*)

thromboplastin time (aPTT) should be at least twice controlled. Beginning 2 to 3 weeks prior to delivery, warfarin should be discontinued and continuous intravenous UFH should be started. After delivery, UFH should be resumed 4 to 6 hours after delivery and warfarin should be restarted, in the absence of significant bleeding.[20]

Cardiac Catheterization in Pregnant Woman With CHD

PATIENT STORY 6

A 24-year-old woman with Alagille syndrome (AGS) with hypoplastic branch pulmonary arteries presented at 24 weeks' gestation with dyspnea on exertion and severely elevated right ventricular (RV) pressure on Doppler echocardiography. She underwent fluoroscopic angiography for dilation and stenting to the proximal left pulmonary artery (Figure 11-7) with abdominal shielding that resulted in a good angiographic and symptomatic improvement.

CASE EXPLANATION

- Rarely patients may need to undergo cardiac catheterization with directed intervention to optimize hemodynamics during the course of pregnancy.

- This is a rare case of a patient with Alagille syndrome who needed to undergo cardiac catheterization and a directed intervention during the course of her pregnancy, with successful outcomes for both the mother and the fetus.

DISCUSSION

- The AGS is a multisystem autosomal dominant condition with hepatic, cardiac, ophthalmic, skeletal, renal, and craniofacial anomalies with a prevalence of 1 in 100,000 live births.

- Patients may become pregnant prior to optimization of hemodynamics and in order to improve outcomes for the mother and fetus, interventions are occasionally required during pregnancy.

- Radiation doses greater than100 mGy are likely to cause dose-dependent developmental effects.

- Catheterization should be avoided in the first trimester if possible. At the time of catheterization of any pregnant woman, abdominal shielding should be performed.[26]

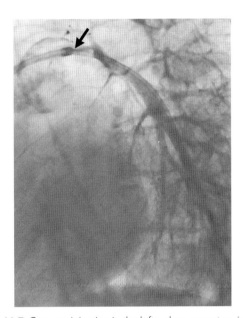

FIGURE 11-7 Contrast injection in the left pulmonary artery in a woman with Alagille syndrome and hypoplastic branch pulmonary arteries who presents with an unplanned pregnancy at 24 weeks' gestation with symptomatic left pulmonary artery stenosis. Directed dilation and stenting to the proximal left pulmonary artery (arrow) with abdominal shielding with a good angiographic result.

Pregnancy and Congenital Heart Disease

EPIDEMIOLOGY

- Improved medical and surgical management of patients with CHD have resulted in more women with CHD surviving to childbearing age.[27]

- CHD has become the most common form of heart disease complicating pregnancy in the United States. With improved medical, surgical, and transcatheter therapies, more than 85% of children born with CHD are expected to reach adulthood.

- It naturally follows that more adult women with underlying CHD are therefore surviving and becoming pregnant.[28]

- The majority of women with CHD tolerate pregnancy well; however, cardiac disease accounts for 15% of pregnancy-related mortality in the United States.[29]

- Fetal outcomes are also worse in women with complex CHD with more frequent premature delivery and small for gestational age infants.[30]

- Women with CHD of childbearing age should be counseled[4] on the importance of planning pregnancy to ensure that hemodynamics are optimized prior to conception and discuss possible risks of pregnancy to the mother and fetus.[31]

- A team of cardiologists, obstetricians, and anesthesiologists should create pregnancy and delivery care plans to help prevent and manage any complications that occur throughout the peripartum period in these higher risk patients.[32]

- The European Society of Cardiology has published risk stratification guidelines for women with heart disease (Table 11-2).[18]

ETIOLOGY/PHYSIOLOGIC CHANGES OF PREGNANCY

- Pregnancy results in dramatic hemodynamic changes (Figure 11-8).

- Understanding the normal hemodynamic changes of pregnancy in the context of residual cardiac lesions helps to properly counsel women regarding risks of pregnancy.

- Changes such as increased blood volume and cardiac output can act as a circulatory burden in patients with impaired systolic function or left-sided obstructive lesions, while other changes such as decreased afterload can temporarily decrease the severity of regurgitant lesions.[33]

- Pregnancy is also associated with a hypercoagulable state due to relative increases in fibrinogen, plasminogen activator inhibitors, clotting factors VII, VIII, X, von Willebrand factor, and platelet adhesion molecules; as well as relative decreases in protein S activity.[34]

- Normal alterations in circulatory and respiratory physiology during pregnancy can have deleterious effects on the mother with congenital heart disease and on her developing fetus.

- Blood pressure typically falls early in gestation and is usually 10 mm Hg below baseline in the second trimester, declining to a mean of 105/60 mm Hg. This response reflects a reduction in systemic vascular resistance which serves to increase flow across right-to-left shunts.

- A 30% to 50% increase in intravascular volume and cardiac output occurs in normal pregnancy by the early to mid-third trimester. In patients whose cardiac output is limited by myocardial dysfunction or valvular lesions, volume overload is poorly tolerated and may result in congestive heart failure. Pregnancy may also result in ascending aortic aneurysm or dissection in patients with an anatomic predisposition (eg, Marfan syndrome, coarctation of the aorta, or bicuspid aortic valve).

ROLE OF CARDIAC SURGERY DURING PREGNANCY

- Maternal survival is good and similar to nonpregnant women of similar age.

- Fetal loss remains high with retrospective studies suggesting fetal loss rates of 14% in a contemporary cohort of women undergoing cardiothoracic surgery during pregnancy.[35]

- Cesarean section prior to cardiac surgery is generally recommended for a fetus greater than 28 weeks.

- If an emergency occurs before 28 weeks' gestation, it is advisable to wait until beyond the first trimester for maternal cardiac surgery to allow for organogenesis and to employ high flow, high pressure, normothermic cardiopulmonary bypass for as brief an episode as possible to enhance placental blood flow.[36]

COMPLICATIONS

Maternal Outcomes

- Maternal cardiac risks of pregnancy in congenital heart disease include heart failure, arrhythmia, stroke or cardiac death, and complicate 13% to 20% of pregnancies.[3,37]

- Risk factors for cardiac events during pregnancy (Table 11-3) include a cardiac event or arrhythmia prior to pregnancy, poor functional class, cyanosis (oxygen saturation <90%), systemic ventricular systolic dysfunction (ejection fraction <40%), and left heart obstruction (mitral valve area <2 cm^2, aortic valve area <1.5 cm^2, left ventricular outflow tract gradient of >30 mm Hg)[3] (Figures 11-9A and 11-9B).

- Risk of a cardiac event is less than 5% if the patient has no risk factors, however the event rate increases to 75% if there are 2 or more risk factors.[3]

- One study demonstrated that decreased subpulmonary ejection fraction and/or severe pulmonary regurgitation independently predict maternal events.[37]

- Recent data suggests that women with a cardiac event during pregnancy have a greater risk of long-term cardiac complications.[38]

Table 11-2 Modified WHO Classification of Maternal Cardiovascular Risk. (*From Regitz-Zagrosek (2011). Esc guidelines on the management of cardiovascular diseases during pregnancy: The task force on the management of cardiovascular diseases during pregnancy of the european society of cardiology (esc). Eur Heart J. 2011;32:3147-3197 by permission of Oxford University Press.*)

WHO class 1: No increased risk maternal mortality and no/mild risk of morbidity

Uncomplicated, small or mild
 –Pulmonary stenosis
 –Patent ductus arteriosus
 –Mitral valve prolapse

Successfully repaired simple shunt lesions
 –Atrial septal defect
 –Ventricular septal defect
 –Patent ductus arteriosus
 –Anomalous pulmonary venous drainage

WHO class 2: Small increased risk of maternal mortality or moderate increase in morbidity

Unrepaired
 –Atrial septal defect
 –Ventricular septal defect

Repaired tetralogy of Fallot

WHO class 2-3: Depending on individual patient

Mild left ventricular dysfunction

Hypertrophic cardiomyopathy

Native or bioprosthetic valve heart disease (not considered WHO class 1 or 4)

Marfan syndrome without aortic dilation

Aorta <4 mm in aortic disease associated with bicuspid aortic valve

Repaired aortic coarctation

WHO class 3: Significantly increased risk of maternal mortality or severe morbidity[a]

Mechanical valve

Systemic right ventricle

Fontan circulation

Cyanotic heart disease (unrepaired)

Other complex congenital heart disease

Marfan syndrome with aortic dilation 40-45 mm

Aorta 45-50 mm in aortic disease with bicuspid aortic valve

WHO class 4: Extremely high risk of maternal mortality or severe morbidity (pregnancy contraindicated)[b]

Pulmonary arterial hypertension of any cause

Severe systemic ventricular dysfunction (ejection fraction <30%, NYHA III-IV)

Previous peripartum cardiomyopathy with any residual impairment of left ventricular function

Severe left-sided obstructive lesions
 –Severe mitral stenosis
 –Severe symptomatic aortic stenosis

Marfan syndrome with dilated aorta >45 mm

Aorta >50 mm in aortic disease associated with bicuspid aortic valve

Native severe aortic coarctation

---

[a]Expert counselling required. If pregnancy is decided upon, intensive specialist cardiac and obstetric monitoring needed throughout pregnancy, childbirth and the puerperium.
[b]If pregnancy occurs, termination should be discussed. If pregnancy continues, care as for Class 3.

Fetal Outcomes in Pregnant Women With CHD

Women with CHD have an increased risk of having children with CHD. The incidence of CHD in children with a parent with nonsyndromic CHD is approximately 4% compared to a risk of approximately 1% in the general population.[39]

- Fetal echocardiography frequently detects major forms of CHD but may miss less severe lesions that can often be detected on pediatric cardiac examination following delivery.[40]

- Current guidelines recommend screening all fetuses of parents with CHD with fetal echocardiography to assess risk to the fetus and to ensure that the parents are properly counseled and postdelivery plans are appropriate.[32]

CONCLUSION

- The majority of women with CHD tolerate pregnancy well but CHD results in increased maternal mortality, morbidity, and worse fetal outcomes.

- Given the heterogeneity of diseases, individual assessment and appropriate counseling by an adult congenital heart disease specialist is recommended for women with congenital heart disease who are contemplating pregnancy.

- Reparative surgery has substantially increased the number of females with congenital heart disease who reach childbearing age. Cardiac optimization, which may include surgical repair, before gestation is pivotal in reducing maternal and fetal risks. The risks of pregnancy after surgery are determined chiefly by the presence, type, and degree of cardiac and vascular residua and sequelae.

- Although cardiac disease complicates a small percentage of all pregnancies in developed countries (1%-4% in the United States), cardiac disease is a major cause of nonobstetric maternal morbidity and mortality. As a result, care of these high-risk patients often requires a team approach including specialists in maternal-fetal medicine, cardiology, and obstetrical anesthesiology.

- There are several diagnostic tests that may aid in risk stratification and identify cardiac complications in pregnant women with CHD.

- Percutaneous cardiac interventions and cardiac surgery can be done during pregnancy but are best avoided, if possible.

- Women with biologic prosthetic heart valves who are hemodynamically stable and do not require anticoagulation generally tolerate pregnancy well. The risk of pregnancy is high for both the mother and fetus when a mechanical valve is present, mainly due to the increased risk of thrombosis and the complications related to anticoagulation.

- There are different modalities for anticoagulation that can be used during pregnancy including warfarin, intravenous unfractionated heparin [UFH]) and low-molecular-weight heparin (LMWH).

- Virtually all pregnant women with cardiac disease can expect to attempt vaginal delivery because it poses less cardiac risk than cesarean delivery. Cardiac indications for cesarean delivery largely involve aortic disease including aortopathy with a dilated root greater than 4-4.5 cm, progressive aortic enlargement, or aortic dissection or hemodynamic instability. In general, cesarean delivery is most commonly reserved for obstetric indications.

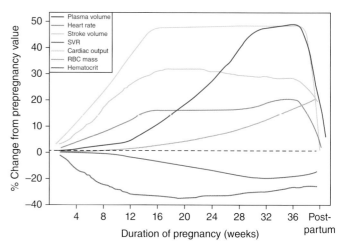

FIGURE 11-8 Normal hemodynamic changes with pregnancy. (*Textbook of Perinatal Medicine, 2nd edition, A. Kurjak and FA Chervenak, Copyright © 2006, Taylor & Francis Group, LLC, reproduced by permission of Taylor & Francis Books UK.*)

Table 11-3 Predictors of Maternal Cardiac Events During Pregnancy (*From Siu SC, Sermer M, Colman JM, Alvarez AN, Mercier LA, Morton BC, et al. Prospective multicenter study of pregnancy outcomes in women with heart disease. Circulation. 2001;104:515-21.*)

Cardiac event prior to pregnancy
- –TIA or CVA
- –Congestive Heart Failure
- –Arrhythmia

Decreased baseline functional capacity or cyanosis
- –NYHA class > II OR
- –Resting oxygen saturation <90%

Left heart obstruction
- –Peak left ventricular outflow tract gradient >30 mm Hg (echocardiography)
- –Mitral valve area <2 cm²
- –Aortic valve area <1.5 cm²

Reduced systemic ventricular systolic function
- –Ejection fraction <40%

TIA: transient ischemic attack. CVA: cerebral vascular accident. CARPREG risk score: for each CARPREG predictor that is present, a point is assigned.
Risk estimation for cardiovascular maternal complications:
0 point = 5%
1 point = 27%
>1 point = 75%
NYHA: New York Heart Association.

- Pregnant patients with complex CHD should be followed by a multidisciplinary team including cardiologists and obstetricians skilled in the care of women with heart disease to decrease the risks of pregnancy and to improve outcomes for both mother and fetus.

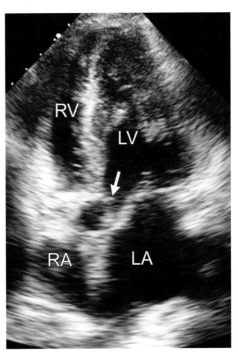

FIGURE 11-9A A 2D echocardiogram of a pregnant woman with a bicuspid aortic valve with combined aortic stenosis and aortic regurgitation. LA, left atrium; LV, left ventricle; RA, right atrium; RV, right ventricle; arrow, thickened aortic valve.

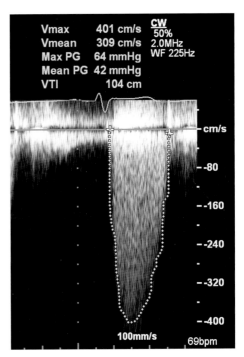

FIGURE 11-9B Doppler echocardiogram demonstrates severe aortic regurgitation. Spectral Doppler demonstrates aortic stenosis with a peak gradient across the aortic valve of 64 mm Hg which is a known risk factor for an adverse maternal cardiovascular event during pregnancy.

REFERENCES

1. Shime J, Mocarski EJ, Hastings D, et al. Congenital heart disease in pregnancy: short- and long-term implications. *Am J Obstet Gynecol.* 1987;156:313-322.

2. Stout KK, Otto CM. Pregnancy in women with valvular heart disease. *Heart.* 2007;93:552-558.

3. Siu SC, Sermer M, Colman JM, Alvarez AN, Mercier LA, Morton BC, et al. Prospective multicenter study of pregnancy outcomes in women with heart disease. *Circulation.* 2001;104:515-521.

4. Steer PJ. Pregnancy and contraception. In: Gatzoulis MA, Swan L, Therrien J, Pantely GA, eds. *Adult Congenital Heart Disease: A Practical Guide.* Oxford, UK: BMJ Publishing, Blackwell Publishing; 2005:16-35.

5. Tanous D, Siu SC, Mason J, et al. B-type natriuretic peptide in pregnant women with heart disease. *J Am Coll Cardiol.* 2010;56:1247-1253.

6. Kamiya CA, Iwamiya T, Neki R, et al. Outcome of pregnancy and effects on the right heart in women with repaired tetralogy of fallot. *Circ J.* 2012;76:957-963.

7. Lui GK, Silversides CK, Khairy P, et al. Heart rate response during exercise and pregnancy outcome in women with congenital heart disease. *Circulation.* 2011;123:242-248.

8. Geva T, Mauer MB, Striker L, Kirshon B, Pivarnik JM. Effects of physiologic load of pregnancy on left ventricular contractility and remodeling. *Am Heart J.* 1997;133:53-59.

9. Rossi A, Cornette J, Johnson MR, et al. Quantitative cardiovascular magnetic resonance in pregnant women: cross-sectional analysis of physiological parameters throughout pregnancy and the impact of the supine position. *J Cardiovasc Magn Reson.* 2011;13:31.

10. Lao TT, Sermer M, MaGee L, Farine D, Colman J. Congenital aortic stenosis and pregnancy—a reappraisal. *Am J Obstet Gynecol.* 1993;169:540-545.

11. Wilson W, Taubert KA, Gewitz M, et al. Prevention of infective endocarditis: guidelines from the American Heart Association: a guideline from the American Heart Association Rheumatic Fever, Endocarditis, and Kawasaki Disease Committee, Council on Cardiovascular Disease in the Young, and the Council on Clinical Cardiology, Council on Cardiovascular Surgery and Anesthesia, and the Quality of Care and Outcomes Research Interdisciplinary Working Group. American Heart Association Rheumatic Fever, Endocarditis, and Kawasaki Disease Committee, American Heart Association Council on Cardiovascular Disease in the Young, American Heart Association Council on Clinical Cardiology, American Heart Association Council on Cardiovascular Surgery and Anesthesia, Quality of Care and Outcomes Research Interdisciplinary Working Group. *Circulation.* 2007;116:1736-1754.

12. Montoya ME, Karnath BM, Ahmad M. Endocarditis during pregnancy. *South Med J.* 2003;96:1156-1157.

13. Campuzano K, Roque H, Bolnick A, Leo MV, Campbell WA. Bacterial endocarditis complicating pregnancy: case report and systematic review of the literature. *Arch Gynecol Obstet.* 2003;268:251-255.

14. Lipscomb KJ, Smith JC, Clarke B, Donnai P, Harris R. Outcome of pregnancy in women with Marfan's syndrome. *Br J Obstet Gynaecol.* 1997;104:201-206.

15. Donnelly RT, Pinto NM, Kocolas I, Yetman AT. The immediate and long-term impact of pregnancy on aortic growth rate and mortality in women with Marfan syndrome. *J Am Coll Cardiol.* 2012;60:224-229.

16. Hiratzka LF, Bakris GL, Beckman JA, et al. 2010 ACCF/AHA/AATS/ACR/ASA/SCA/SCAI/SIR/STS/SVM guidelines for the diagnosis and management of patients with thoracic aortic disease: A report of the American College of Cardiology Foundation/American Heart Association Task Force on Practice Guidelines, American Association for Thoracic Surgery, American College of Radiology, American Stroke Association, Society of Cardiovascular Anesthesiologists, Society for Cardiovascular Angiography and Interventions, Society of Interventional Radiology, Society of Thoracic Surgeons, and Society for Vascular Medicine. *Circulation.* 2010;121:e266-e369.

17. Simpson IA, de Belder MA, Treasure T, Camm AJ, Pumphrey CW. Cardiovascular manifestations of Marfan's syndrome: improved evaluation by transoesophageal echocardiography. *Br Heart J.* 1993;69:104-108.

18. Regitz-Zagrosek V, Blomstrom Lundqvist C, Borghi C, et al. ESC guidelines on the management of cardiovascular diseases during pregnancy: the task force on the management of cardiovascular diseases during pregnancy of the European Society of Cardiology (ESC). *Eur Heart J.* 2011;32:3147-3197.

19. Hiratzka LF, Bakris GL, Beckman JA, et al. 2010 ACCF/AHA/AATS/ACR/ASA/SCA/SCAI/SIR/STS/SVM guidelines for the diagnosis and management of patients with Thoracic Aortic Disease: a report of the American College of Cardiology Foundation/American Heart Association Task Force on Practice Guidelines, American Association for Thoracic Surgery, American College of Radiology, American Stroke Association, Society of Cardiovascular Anesthesiologists, Society for Cardiovascular Angiography and Interventions, Society of Interventional Radiology, Society of Thoracic Surgeons, and Society for Vascular Medicine. *Circulation.* 2010;121:e266.

20. Nishimura R et al. *Circulation.* 2014.

21. Cleuziou J, Horer J, Kaemmerer H, et al. Pregnancy does not accelerate biological valve degeneration. *Int J Cardiol.* 2010;145:418-421.

22. Avila WS, Rossi EG, Grinberg M, Ramires JA. Influence of pregnancy after bioprosthetic valve replacement in young women: a prospective five-year study. *J Heart Valve Dis.* 2002;11:864-869.

23. Wagoner LE, Taylor DO, Olsen SL, et al. Immunosuppressive therapy, management, and outcome of heart transplant recipients during pregnancy. *J Heart Lung Transplant.* 1993;12:993-999; discussion 1000.

24. Silversides CK, Harris L, Haberer K, Sermer M, Colman JM, Siu SC. Recurrence rates of arrhythmias during pregnancy in women with previous tachyarrhythmia and impact on fetal and neonatal outcomes. *Am J Cardiol.* 2006;97:1206-1212.

25. Howie PW. Anticoagulants in pregnancy. *Clin Obstet Gynaecol.* 1986;13:349-363.

26. Chambers CE, Fetterly KA, Holzer R, et al. Radiation safety program for the cardiac catheterization laboratory. *Catheter Cardiovasc Interv.* 2011;77:546-556.

27. Marelli AJ, Mackie AS, Ionescu-Ittu R, Rahme E, Pilote L. Congenital heart disease in the general population: changing prevalence and age distribution. *Circulation.* 2007;115:163-172.

28. Balint OH, Siu SC, Mason J, et al. Cardiac outcomes after pregnancy in women with congenital heart disease. *Heart.* 2010;96:1656-1661.

29. Berg CJ, Mackay AP, Qin C, Callaghan WM. Overview of maternal morbidity during hospitalization for labor and delivery in the United States: 1993–1997 and 2001–2005. *Obstet Gynecol.* 2009;113:1075-1081.

30. Drenthen W, Pieper PG, Roos-Hesselink JW, et al. Outcome of pregnancy in women with congenital heart disease: a literature review. *J Am Coll Cardiol.* 2007;49:2303-2311.

31. Kovacs AH, Harrison JL, Colman JM, Sermer M, Siu SC, Silversides CK. Pregnancy and contraception in congenital heart disease: what women are not told. *J Am Coll Cardiol.* 2008;52:577-578.

32. Warnes CA, Williams RG, Bashore TM, et al. ACC/AHA 2008 guidelines for the management of adults with congenital heart disease: a report of the American College of Cardiology/American Heart Association Task Force on Practice Guidelines (writing committee to develop guidelines on the management of adults with congenital heart disease). *Circulation.* 2008;118:e714-833.

33. Traill TA. Valvular heart disease and pregnancy. *Cardiol Clin.* 2012;30:369-381.

34. Brenner B, Grabowski EF, Hellgren M, et al. Thrombophilia and pregnancy complications. *Thromb Haemost.* 2004;92:678-681.

35. John AS, Gurley F, Schaff HV, et al. Cardiopulmonary bypass during pregnancy. *Ann Thorac Surg.* 2011;91:1191-1196.

36. Chandrasekhar S, Cook CR, Collard CD. Cardiac surgery in the parturient. *Anesth Analg.* 2009;108:777-785.

37. Khairy P, Ouyang DW, Fernandes SM, Lee-Parritz A, Economy KE, Landzberg MJ. Pregnancy outcomes in women with congenital heart disease. *Circulation.* 2006;113:517-524.

38. Balint OH, Siu SC, Mason J, et al. Cardiac outcomes after pregnancy in women with congenital heart disease. *Heart.* 2010;96:1656-1661.

39. Burn J, Brennan P, Little J, et al. Recurrence risks in offspring of adults with major heart defects: results from first cohort of British collaborative study. *Lancet.* 1998;351:311-316.

40. Thangaroopan M, Wald RM, Silversides CK, et al. Incremental diagnostic yield of pediatric cardiac assessment after fetal echocardiography in the offspring of women with congenital heart disease: a prospective study. *Pediatrics.* 2008;121:e660-e665.

12 AORTOPATHIES IN THE ADULT WITH CONGENITAL HEART DISEASE

Mary Hunt Martin, MD
Angela T. Yetman, MD

PATIENT STORY

A 28-year-old woman presented to her local rural hospital with acute-onset severe chest pain which came on at rest. There was no inciting physical or emotional stressor. She had a known diagnosis of Turner syndrome (XO) with prior documentation of a normal functioning bicuspid aortic valve. Her diagnosis of bicuspid aortic valve was based on a cardiac catheterization performed in early childhood and subsequent clinical examinations. She had no murmur to suggest aortic insufficiency or stenosis and had no prior cardiac imaging evaluations. She was seen routinely by a pediatric cardiologist every 2 years until the age of 18 years. She was subsequently lost to follow up.

At the time of her last routine pediatric cardiology visit 10 years ago she had been provided with instructions regarding the need for routine care and the possible need for cardiovascular surgery in the future but had not been instructed on where to seek care now that she had reached adult age. She assumed she could no longer be seen at a pediatric institution and did not successfully transition to an adult facility.

At the time of her presentation to the emergency room, she had a blood pressure (BP) in both arms of 160/80 mm Hg. A chest x-ray was performed which showed a widened mediastinum thus prompting a computed tomography (CT) angiogram which demonstrated a dilated ascending aorta measuring 3.6 cm yielding an indexed score of 2.4 cm/m^2 (with a normal value for this patient population defined as <2.2 cm/m^2).[1] There was no dissection of the ascending aorta. She had a bovine arch wherein the first head and neck vessel gave rise to both carotid arteries.[2] There was focal aneurysmal dilation of the distal aortic arch extending to the proximal portion of the left subclavian artery and proximal descending thoracic aorta. There was a focal dissection beginning in the distal aortic arch with propagation into the proximal left subclavian artery and into the descending thoracic aorta. The right subclavian artery was aberrant in origin arising from the descending thoracic aorta just distal to the left subclavian artery.

The patient was started on a labetalol infusion with an achieved goal systolic BP of 100 mm Hg. Attempts were made to transfer the patient to an appropriate medical facility for further management. In light of the limited nature of the dissection, the lack of ascending aortic involvement, and a maximal aortic diameter less than established surgical criteria, an attempt at conservative management was attempted.[3] Despite optimal blood pressure control, serial scans over a period of 4 days demonstrated progressive dilation of the involved aortic segment and thus the decision was made to proceed with intervention. A hybrid procedure approach was undertaken. Bilateral carotid artery to subclavian artery bypass grafts were first placed to establish flow to both subclavian vessels. This was then followed by placement of a covered stent in the distal arch at the site of the dissection. The patient was discharged on pravastatin, aspirin, and lisinopril.

CASE EXPLANATION

- Aortic dilation, aneurysms, and dissections can be seen in a wide variety of connective tissue diseases, patients with known syndromes (like Turner). It is now being increasingly reported in adult patients with congenital heart disease. Aortic dilatation has been described in adult women with Turners syndrome, where aortic valve morphology, age, and blood pressure can be major determinants of the aortic diameter.

- Such patients may face a significant risk of premature cardiovascular death due to aortic dissection, ischemic heart disease, and stroke. Careful and continuous monitoring of the aorta in this patient group is therefore of vital importance.

- This case also highlights the importance of timely transition of care for adults with congenital heart disease, so patients are not lost to follow up and continue to receive appropriate lifelong care.

EPIDEMIOLOGY

- Frequency of aortic dilation varies according to the underlying syndrome, mutation, or congenital cardiac defect.

- Aortic dilation was historically underdiagnosed in patients with all of these entities for the following reasons:
  - Failure to image affected portion of the aorta which is often in the mid-to-high ascending aorta
  - Lack of consideration of body size and age in determining whether an aortic diameter was normal
  - Lack of appreciation of aortic dilation as pathologic in contrast to a normal part of the underlying structural disease entity (ie post stenotic dilation)[4]
  - Lack of routine screening of high-risk patients, namely family members of patients with a bicuspid aortic valve,[5] and family members of older patients with aortic dissection

- Patients with bicuspid aortic valve may have an isolated cardiac defect which is often familial, or the valvular abnormality may be indicative of an underlying syndrome or well characterized familial aortopathy (Figure 12-1 and Tables 12-1 and 12-2).

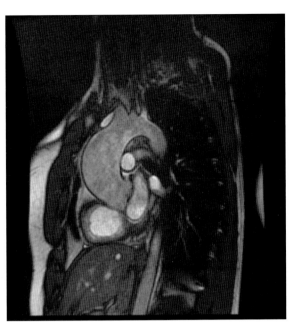

FIGURE 12-1 A 20-year-old man with history of bicuspid aortic valve, status post surgical valvotomy for stenosis, now with dilation of the ascending aorta, maximum diameter 44 mm.

Table 12-1 Syndromes With Aortopathies

Syndrome	Incidence	Aneurysm/Dissection Frequency	Dissection Site
Turner syndrome	1/2000 liveborn	50%, rare	Asc Ao, arch, IC
Marfan syndrome	1/5000-1/10000	>80%, common	Asc Ao, Dao, arch, IC
Loeys-Dietz syndrome		Unknown, very common	Asc Ao, arch, Dao, IC, P
Type IV EDS	1/100000-1/200000	NA,[a] universal	Asc Ao, arch, Dao, IC, P
Neurofibromatosis-1	1/3000	10%, rare	Dao, IC, Asc Ao, P
ADPKD	1/1000	8%, rare	Asc Ao, Dao, IC

ADPKD, autosomal dominant polycystic kidney disease; Asc Ao, ascending aorta; Dao, descending thoracoabdominal aorta; EDS, Ehlers-Danlos syndrome; IC, intracranial arteries; P, peripheral branches of the aorta including coronary arteries; TA, transverse arch; [a] NA, not applicable as these patients often experience dissection in the absence of aneurysms. Dissection is considered an eventual consequence of all survivors as many patients die from organ rupture.

Table 12-2 Familiar Thoracic Aortic Aneurysms due to the Genetic Mutations

Genetic Mutation	Other Cardiac Features	Craniofacial Features	Other Features
MYH11[47]	PDA, premature CAD	None	None
ACTA2[48]	BAV, premature CAD Arterial occlusions	Moyamoya, stroke	Livedo reticularis, iris floccule
TGFBRI/II[21]	BAV, aneurysmal PDA	Hypertelorism, bifid uvula Abnormal palate	Translucent skin
SMAD3[49]	Vessel tortuosity, MVP, BAV	Hypertelorism, bifid uvula Abnormal palate	Early-onset OA Scoliosis Velvety skin

BAV, bicuspid aortic valve; CAD, coronary artery disease; MVP, mitral valve prolapse; OA, osteoarthritis; PDA, patent ductus arteriosus.

- Within a population of children and young adults, moderate or severe ascending aortic dilation was present in 5% and 16%, respectively.[6] Aortic dissection or rupture has been documented to occur in 8% of those with dilation.[7]

- In patients with tetralogy of Fallot the aorta is typically larger than normal since birth.[8] A subset of these patients will have ongoing pathologic aortic dilation placing them at risk for aortic insufficiency[9] and aortic dissection.[10] Within this population, male gender, pulmonary atresia type tetralogy of Fallot, and persistent ventricular septal defects (Figures 12-2, 12-3A, and 12-3B) have been identified as risk factors for aortic complications.[9]

- The incidence of progressive aortic dilation in patients with conotruncal abnormalities like those with d-transposition of the great arteries (D-TGA) (Figure 12-4) and patients with single ventricles s/p Fontan palliation (Figure 12-5) are not yet fully appreciated given that this adult patient population remains in its infancy. Rare cases of patients with D-TGA with aortic dilation causing coronary compression and dissection have been reported.[11]

ETIOLOGY

- Progressive aortic dilation and aortic dissection are seen in the following categories:

  A. The following are the names of certain genetic syndromes:
    - Turner syndrome[1]
    - Marfan syndrome[12]
    - Loeys-Dietz syndrome[13]
    - Type IV Ehlers-Danlos syndrome (EDS)[14]
    - Others (neurofibromatosis,[15] Shprintzen-Goldberg syndrome,[16] autosomal dominant polycystic kidney disease, etc)[4] with the incidence of the syndrome and aortic dilation noted in Table 12-1.

  B. Patients with the following congenital cardiac conditions:
    - Bicuspid aortic valve[7]
    - Coarctation or interruption of the aorta[7] (Figure 12-6)
    - Conotruncal defects including D-TGA (Figure 12-4),[17] tetralogy of Fallot,[18] pulmonary atresia/ventricular septal defect (VSD) (s/p Fontan palliation)[9]
    - Others including aberrant subclavian artery[19] and bovine aortic arch[2]
    - Postoperative patients following the Ross procedure[20]

  A. Familiar thoracic aortic aneurysms[21] due to the genetic mutations identified in Table 12-2:
    - There continues to be some controversy as to whether the aortic dilation seen in association with congenital cardiac defects represents an intrinsic aortopathy or whether the dilation occurs secondary to abnormal flow dynamics.

- Evidence that it stems from an intrinsic aortopathy includes the following:
  - The degree of aortic stenosis does not relate to the degree of aortic dilation.[22]
  - Patients with a normal functioning bicuspid aortic valve (BAV) often have significant dilation.[22]

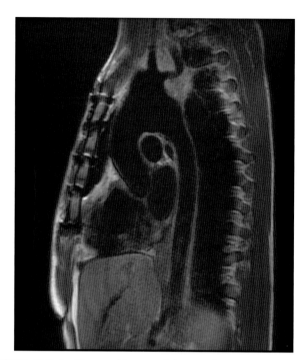

FIGURE 12-2 An 18-year-old man with history of ventricular septal defect (VSD) and aortic arch interruption type B, who initially underwent pulmonary artery band and arch repair with 8-mm conduit from ascending to descending aorta in infancy. One year later he underwent VSD repair, and 6 years later repeat arch repair with end-to-end anastomosis. He now has progressive dilation of the transverse arch shown by magnetic resonance imaging (MRI), currently measuring 58 mm.

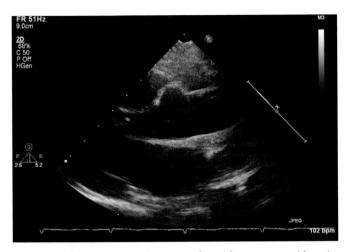

FIGURE 12-3A A 32-year-old woman referred for murmur and found to have an incidental finding of aneurysm of the right sinus of Valsalva on echocardiogram.

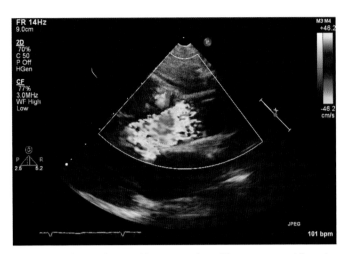

FIGURE 12-3B A 32-year-old woman referred for murmur and found to have an incidental finding of aneurysm of the right sinus of Valsalva on echocardiogram (Color flow Doppler image showing severe aortic regurgitation).

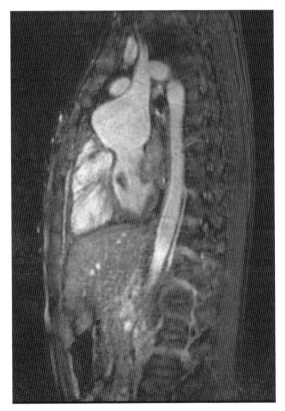

FIGURE 12-4 A 10-year-old boy with d-transposition of the great arteries (D-TGA) with ventricular septal defect (VSD) and coarctation of the aorta, status post arterial switch operation with VSD closure and coarctation repair in infancy, now with progressive dilation of the aortic root measuring 39 × 44 mm by MRI.

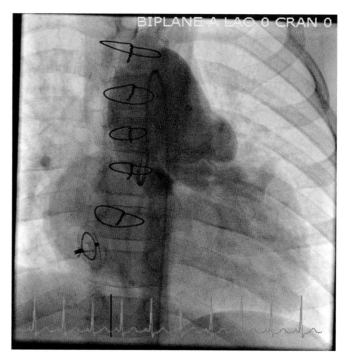

FIGURE 12-5 An 8-year-old girl with a history of hypoplastic left heart syndrome, status post Norwood palliation with Damus-Kaye-Stansel anastomosis in infancy, followed by Glenn and Fontan, now with progressive dilation of ascending neoaortic root and ascending aorta showed by angiography with pigtail catheter in the native aortic root. There is moderate and progressive neoaortic insufficiency.

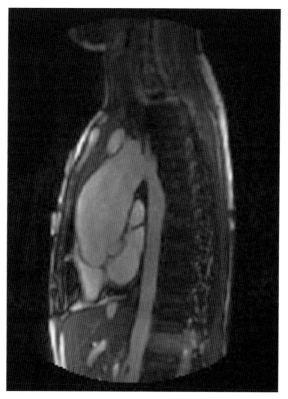

FIGURE 12-6 A 24-year-old woman with a history of moyamoya disease and coarctation of the aorta that was repaired in infancy with end-to-side anastomosis. Currently, with progressive dilation of the ascending aorta is shown by MRI, maximum diameter 44 mm.

- Dilation is present from early childhood and the rate of aortic growth is abnormal.[6,22]
- First-degree family members of probands with BAV have increased incidence of aortic aneurysm and dissection even in the presence of a tri-leaflet valve.[5]
- Decreased fibrillin content has been documented in the aorta of patients with BAV.[23]

- Evidence that aortic dilation occurs secondary to abnormal flow dynamics includes data documented as follows:
  - The angle between the systolic ejection jet and the ascending aorta correlates aortic diameter in both patients with BAV as well as normal controls.[24]
  - Ascending aortic curvature has been shown to be more important than aortic size in predicting aortic dissection in a mathematical model.[25]

- It is most probable that a combination of a genetic predisposition yielding to abnormal aortic wall architecture exists which then results in abnormal aortic stiffness and distensibility[7,26] thereby predisposing to progressive aortic dilation which may be accentuated by abnormal flow jets.
  - Aortic dissection, irrespective of the underlying cause of aortic dilation, is often preceded by an inciting factor[27] namely a physical or emotional stressor,[28] and occurs more commonly in those with the following comorbidities: hypertension,[29] smoking,[30] obesity,[31] and hyperlipidemia.[31]

PATHOPHYSIOLOGY

- Irrespective of the underlying cause of aortopathy, common physiologic processes exist and lead to maladaptive arterial remodeling. Features common to aneurysm formation include the following:
  - An increase in proteolytic enzymes known as matrix metalloproteinases (MMPs) at the site of aneurysm formation[7]
  - An imbalance of the degradative enzymes (MMPs) and their endogenous tissue inhibitors (tissue inhibitors of metalloproteinases [TIMPs])[7]
  - An increase in angiotensin-mediated transforming growth factor (TGF) beta signaling[7]
  - Even prior to the development of aneurysm formation, aortic function is abnormal with documentation of increased arterial wall stiffness and decreased distensibility. These alterations in flow mechanics likely play a key role in aneurysm development and have been shown to be present in patients with bicuspid aortic valve (Figure 12-1), first-degree family members of patients with bicuspid aortic valve, conotruncal defects, Marfan syndrome, and the familial aortopathies.

DIAGNOSIS

- A detailed multigeneration pedigree and careful physical examination are often imperative in establishing the etiology of the aortic dilation.
- Genetic testing plays a valuable role in confirming the diagnosis in many patients and is helpful in determining frequency and type of follow-up surveillance and in establishing whether first-degree family members require cardiac evaluation. Aortopathy panels are now

commercially available which allow for testing of the most common genetic alterations.[26]

- In patients without an obvious source of aortic dilation, clinical examination should focus on the presence or absence of the clinical features noted in Table 12-2 in order to hone in on the underlying diagnosis.
- Diagnosis of aortic dilation requires a maximal diameter of the native aorta that is outside of the range of normal for age and body size.[3]
- Normal datasets have been established for age and body size.[32,33]
- Appropriate nomograms[6,34] must be used to determine the presence of aortic dilation.

MEDICAL MANAGEMENT

- Patients with dilated aortas should avoid extreme isometrics, weight lifting,[35] and smoking.
- Recommendation of routine aerobic exercise to avoid hypertension, obesity, and hyperlipidemia.
- Importance of blood pressure control at less than 130/85 mm Hg in adults with aortic dilation without prior dissection and less than 120/80 mm Hg for those with prior dissection should be stressed.
- Medications are used to attain BP goals but also in attempts to alter the disease process.
- Beta-blockers play an essential role in the hypertensive patient but their impact in the normotensive young patient is unclear.[36] Their impact on the pathophysiologic processes involved in aneurysm formation is thought to be minimal.
- In addition to being effective antihypertensive agents, angiotensin-converting enzyme (ACE) inhibitors have been shown to lower the risk of dissection, decrease aortic growth rate, decrease aortic stiffness, and decrease MMP levels in patients with aneurysms of diverse cause.[37-39]
- Angiotensin receptor blockers have been shown to have a beneficial effect on aortic growth in a Marfan mouse model.[40] Several trials are ongoing in order to assess the impact of this class of medication in humans with aortic dilation.[41]
- Doxycycline, through its inhibition of MMPs, has been shown to decrease aneurysm progression in adults with abdominal aortic aneurysms and to have a beneficial effect on the aortic aneurysms in Marfan and Ehlers-Danlos mouse models.[42-44]
- Celiprolol, a β_1 antagonist with β_2 agonist properties, has been shown in a randomized trial to significantly decrease the rate of arterial complications in patients with the vascular form of Ehlers-Danlos syndrome.[45] Unfortunately, the medication is not available in the United States.

SURGICAL MANAGEMENT

- The indications for surgical intervention vary between lesions due to the varying risk of aortic dissection and are outlined in Table 12-3.

Table 12-3 Surgical Criteria

Underlying Diagnosis	Surgical Size Criteria
BAV	50 cm or aortic CSA/height (m) >10, whichever is less[3]
Conotruncal defects	55 cm[50]
Marfan syndrome	45-50 cm or Ao CSA/height (m) >10, whichever is less[3]
Loeys-Dietz syndrome	40 cm (adults) Z-score >3 (child)[5]
Turner syndrome	Asc Ao >2.5 cm/m^2 or Ao CSA/height (m) >10, whichever is less[51,3]

Ao, aorta; Asc Ao, ascending aorta; CSA, cross-sectional area (diameter/2 × 3.1415); m, meters.

- In order to account for body size, the American Heart Association (AHA) guidelines have recommended the following criteria for surgical intervention for all "at risk" patients with their native aorta: maximal cross-sectional aortic area/height (meters) greater than 10[3].

FOLLOW-UP

- Serial imaging is required for all patients with aortic aneurysms.
- Frequency of imaging is dictated by the underlying disease, the degree of dilation, and the rate of change and is outlined in Table 12-4.
- For routine follow-up, adequate imaging of the ascending aorta can be obtained in the majority of patients with transthoracic echo, magnetic resonance imaging (MRI), or computed tomography (CT).
- Evaluation of the descending aorta should be performed periodically in patients at risk for distal dissection (Table 12-1) and requires MRI or CT (Figure 12-6).

Long-Term Complications

- Progressive aortic dilation leading to aortic insufficiency.
- Dissection of the native ascending aorta with a high risk of mortality often due to coronary involvement or pericardial tamponade.

Table 12-4 Imaging Frequency

Underlying Diagnosis	Imaging Modality	Imaging Frequency
Turner syndrome	TTE; MR/CT if >18 y or other lesions present (CoA, aberrant SCA, bovine Ao)	Children: q3-5y Adults or any patient with dilation q1-2y[46]
Marfan syndrome	TTE; MR/CT if >18 y or postop	TTE annually; MR/CT q3-5y
Loeys-Dietz syndrome	TTE and MR/CT	TTE annually, MR/CT annually
BAV w dilation	TTE	q1-2y
BAV w/o dilation	TTE	q5y
Conotruncal abnormalities	TTE	Dictated by other cardiac lesions

Ao, aorta; BAV, bicuspid aortic valve; CoA, coarctation; MR/CT = MRA or CTA; SCA, subclavian artery; TTE, transthoracic echo; w, with; w/o, without.

- While anastomotic suture lines prevent the extension of a dissection in patients with a Ross procedure, aortic rupture can occur albeit rarely.

- Peripheral and distal aortic aneurysms occur in a subset of these patients.

CONCLUSION

- Aortopathy is common in several forms of CHD (Figures 12-3A, 12-3B, 12-4, and 12-7).

- Aortic disease can have overwhelming effects on affected individuals, resulting in severe morbidities including aneurysms (Figure 12-7), tears, dissections, and aortic valve regurgitation secondary to annular dilatation. Progressive aortic dilation and dissection are often the most worrying complications.

- Patients with syndromes (like Turner syndrome) or congenital heart defects including those with bicuspid aortic valves and conotruncal defects have been associated with dilated aortas, dissections and aneurysm formation.

- Care should be individualized to each patient, with detailed assessment of the patient's underlying CHD, associated comorbidities, and need for medical or surgical therapies.

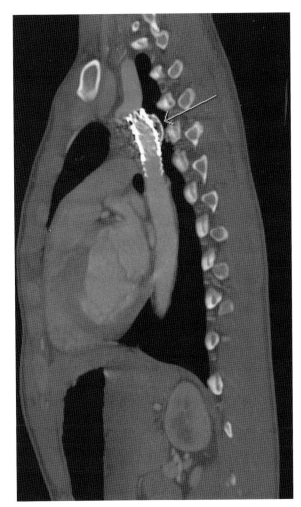

FIGURE 12-7 A 26-year-old man with a history of coarctation of the aorta, discovered at age 18, status post balloon dilation and stenting, which was complicated by late aneurysm formation at the proximal end of the stent. This was treated with placement of a covered stent. This computed tomography (CT) image shows the isolated aneurysm posterior to the covered stent (see arrow).

REFERENCES

1. Matura LA, Ho VB, Rosing DR, Bondy CA. Aortic dilatation and dissection in Turner syndrome. *Circulation*. 2007;116:1663-1670.

2. Wanamaker KM, Amadi CC, Mueller JS, Moraca RJ. Incidence of aortic arch anomalies in patients with thoracic aortic dissections. *J Card Surg*. 2013;28:151-154.

3. Hiratzka LF, Bakris GL, Beckman JA, et al. 2010 ACCF/AHA/AATS/ACR/ASA/SCA/SCAI/SIR/STS/SVM guidelines for the diagnosis and management of patients with thoracic aortic disease. *Circulation*. 2010;121:e266-2369.

4. Drummond IA. Polycystins, focal adhesions and extracellular matrix interactions. *Biochem Biophys Acta*. 2011;1812:1322-1326.

5. Biner S, Rafique AM, Ray I, Cuk O, Siegel RJ, Tolstrup K. Aortopathy is prevalent in relatives of bicuspid aortic valve patients. *J Am Coll Cardiol*. 2009;53:2288-2295.

6. Fernandes S, Khairy P, Graham DA, et al. Bicuspid aortic valve and associated aortic dilation in the young. *Heart*. 2012;98:1014-1019.

7. Yetman AT, Graham T. State-of-the-Art Paper. Aortopathies in congenital heart disease. *J Am Coll Cardiol*. 2009;53: 461-467.

8. Seki M, Kurishima C, Kawasaki H, Masutani S, Senzaki H. Aortic stiffness and aortic dilation in infants and children with tetralogy of Fallot before corrective surgery: evidence for intrinsically abnormal aortic mechanical property. *Eur J Cardiothorac Surg*. 2012;41:277-282.

9. Nagy CD, Alejo DE, Corretti MC, et al. Tetralogy of Fallot and aortic root dilation: a long-term outlook. *Pediatr Cardiol*. 2013;34:809-816.

10. Konstantinov IE, Fricke TA, d'Udekem Y, Robertson T. Aortic dissection and rupture in adolescents after tetralogy of Fallot repair. *J Torac Cardiovasc Surg*. 2010;140:71-73.

11. McMahon CJ, Nihill MR, Denfield S. Neoartic root dilation associated with left coronary stenosis following arterial switch procedure. *Pediatr Cardiol*. 2003;24:43-46.

12. Schoenhoff FS, Jungi S, Czerny M, et al. Acute aortic dissection determines the fate of initially untreated aortic segments in Marfan syndrome. *Circulation*. 2013;127:1569-1575.

13. Williams JA, Loeys BL, Nwakanma LU, et al. Early surgical experience with Loeys-Dietz: a new syndrome of aggressive thoracic aortic aneurysm disease. *Ann Thorac Surg*. 2007;83:S757–S763; discussion S785-S790.

14. Brooke BS, Arnaoutakis G, McDonnell NB, Black JH 3rd. Contemporary management of vascular complications associated with Ehlers-Danlos syndrome. *J Vasc Surg*. 2010;51:131-138; discussion 138-139.

15. Oderich GS, Sullivan TM, Bower TC, et al. Vascular abnormalities in patients with neurofibromatosis syndrome type I: clinical spectrum, management, and results. *J Vasc Surg*. 2007;46: 475-484.

16. Doyle AJ, Doyle JJ, Bessling SL, et al. Mutations in the TGF-beta repressor SKI cause Shprintzen-Goldberg syndrome with aortic aneurysm. *Nat Genet*. 2012;44:1249-1254.

17. Schwartz ML, Gauvreau K, del Nido P, Mayer JE, Colan SD. Long-term predictors of aortic root dilation and aortic regurgitation after arterial switch operation. *Circulation*. 2004;110:128-132.

18. Niwa K. Aortic root dilation in tetralogy of Fallot long-term after repair-histology of the aorta in tetralogy of Fallot: evidence of intrinsic aortopathy. *Int J Cardiol*. 2005;103:117-119.

19. Cinà CS, Althani H, Pasenau J, Abouzahr L. Kommerell's diverticulum and right-sided aortic arch: a cohort study and review of the literature. *J Vasc Surg*. 2004;39:131-139.

20. Pasquali SK, Shera D, Wernovsky G, et al. Midterm outcomes and predictors of reintervention after the Ross procedure in infants, children, and young adults. *J Thorac Cardiovasc Surg*. 2007;133:893-899.

21. Regalado E, Medrek S, Tran-Fadulu V, et al. Autosomal dominant inheritance of a predisposition to thoracic aortic aneurysms and dissections and intracranial saccular aneurysms. *Am J Med Genet*. 2011;155A:2125-2130.

22. Beroukhim RS, Kruzick TL, Taylor AL, Gao D, Yetman AT. Progression of aortic dilation in children with a functionally normal bicuspid aortic valve. *Am J Cardiol*. 2006;98:828-830.

23. Fedak PW, de Sa MP, Verma S, et al. Vascular matrix remodeling in pateints with bicuspid aortic valve malformations: implications for aortic dilation. *J Thorac Cardiovas Surg*. 2003;126:797-806.

24. den Reijer PM, Sallee D 3rd, van der Velden P, et al. Hemodynamic predictors of aortic dilatation in bicuspid aortic valve by velocity-encoded cardiovascular magnetic resonance. *J Cardiovasc Magn Reson*. 2010;12:4.

25. Poullis MP, Warwick R, Oo A, Poole RJ. Ascending aortic curvature as an independent risk factor for type A dissection, and ascending aortic aneurysm formation: a mathematical model. *Eur J Cardiothorac Surg*. 2008;33:995-1001.

26. Wooderchak-Donahue WL, O'Fallon B, Furtado LV, et al. A direct comparison of next generation sequencing enrichment methods using an aortopathy gene panel—clinical diagnostics perspective. *BMC Med Genomics*. 2012;5:50.

27. Elefteriades JA. Thoracic aortic aneurysm: reading the enemy's playbook. *Yale J Biol Med*. 2008;81:175-186.

28. Hatzaras IS, Bible JE, Kallias GJ, et al. Role of exertion or emotion as inciting events for acute aortic dissection. *Am J Cardiol*. 2007;100:1470-1472.

29. Kim M, Roman MJ, Cavallini MC, Schwartz JE, Pickering TG, Devereux RB. Effect of hypertension on aortic root size and prevalence of aortic regurgitation. *Hypertension*. 1996;28:47-52.

30. Finkbohner R, Johnston D, Crawford ES, Coselli J, Milewicz DM. Marfan syndrome. Long-term survival and complications after aortic aneurysm repair. *Circulation*. 1995;91:728-733.

31. Yetman AT, McCrindle BW. The prevalence and clinical impact of obesity in adults with Marfan syndrome. *Can J Cardiol.* 2010;26:137-139.

32. Hannuksela M, Lundqvist S, Carlberg B. Thoracic aorta: dilated or not? *Scand Cardiovasc J.* 2006;40:175-178.

33. Davies RR, Gallo A, Coady MA, et al. Novel measurement of relative aortic size predicts rupture of thoracic aortic aneurysms. *Ann Thorac Surg.* 2006;81:169-177.

34. Roman MJ, Devereux RB, Kramer-Fox R, O'Loughlin J. Two dimensional echocardiographic aortic root dimensions in normal children and adults. *Am J Cardiol.* 1989;64:507-512.

35. Elefteriades J, Botta DM. Indications for the treatment of thoracic aortic aneurysms. *Surg Clin N Amer.* 2009;89:845-867.

36. Gersony DR, McClaughlin MA, Jin Z, Gersony WM. The effect of beta-blocker therapy on clinical outcome in patients with Marfan's syndrome: a meta-analysis. *Int J Cardiol.* 2007;114:303-308.

37. Ahimastos AA, Aggarwal A, D'Orsa KM, et al. Effect of perindopril on large artery stiffness and aortic root diameter in patients with Marfan syndrome: a randomized controlled trial. *JAMA.* 2007;298:1539-1547.

38. Yetman AT, Bornemeier RA, McCrindle BW. Usefulness of enalapril versus propranolol or atenolol for prevention of aortic dilation in patients with the Marfan syndrome. *Am J Cardiol.* 2005;95:1125-1127.

39. Everitt M, Pinto N, Hawkins J, Mitchell MB, Kouretas P, Yetman AT. Cardiovascular surgery in children with Marfan and Loeys-Dietz syndromes. *J Thorac Cardiovasc Surg.* 2009;137:1327-1332.

40. Habashi JP, Judge DP, Holm TM, et al. Losartan, an AT1 antagonist, prevents aortic aneurysm in a mouse model of Marfan syndrome. *Science.* 2006;312:117-121.

41. Lacro RV, Dietz HC, Wruck LM, et al. Rationale and design of a randomized clinical trial of beta-blocker therapy (atenolol) versus angiotensin II receptor blocker therapy (losartan) in individuals with Marfan syndrome. *Am Heart J.* 2007;154:624-631.

42. Abdul-Hussien H, Hanemaaijer R, Verheijen JH, van Bockel JH, Geelkerken RH, Lindeman JH. Doxycycline therapy for abdominal aneurysm: improved proteolytic balance through reduced neutrophil content. *J Vasc Surg.* 2009;49:741-749.

43. Yang HH, Kim JM, Chum E, van Breemen C, Chung AW. Effectiveness of combination of losartan potassium and doxycycline versus single-drug treatments in the secondary prevention of thoracic aortic aneurysm in Marfan syndrome. *J Thorac Cardiovasc Surg.* 2010;140:305-312.

44. Tae HJ, Marshall S, Zhang J, Wang M, Briest W, Talan MI. Chronic treatment with a broad-spectrum metalloproteinase inhibitor, doxycycline, prevents the development of spontaneous aortic lesions in a mouse model of vascular Ehlers-Danlos syndrome. *J Pharmacol Exp Ther.* 2012;343:246-251.

45. Ong KT, Perdu J, De Backer J, et al. Effect of celiprolol on prevention of cardiovascular events in vascular Ehlers-Danlos syndrome: a prospective randomised, open, blinded-endpoints trial. *Lancet.* 2010;376:1476-1484.

46. Thomas J, Yetman AT. Management of cardiovascular disease in Turner Syndrome. *Expert Rev Cardiovasc Ther.* 2009;7:1631-1641.

47. Pannu H, Tran-Fadulu V, Papke CL, et al. MYH11 mutations result in a distinct vascular pathology driven by insulin-like growth factor 1 and angiotensin II. *Hum Mol Genet.* 2007;16:2453-2462.

48. Guo DC, Pannu H, Tran-Fadulu V, et al. Mutations in smooth muscle alpha-actin (ACTA2) lead to thoracic aortic aneurysms and dissections. *Nat Genet.* 2007;39:1488-1493.

49. Van de Laar IMBH, vand der Linde D, Oei EH, et al. Phenotypic spectrum of the SMAD3 related aneurysms—osteoarthritis syndrome. *J Med Genet.* 2012;49:47-57.

50. Stulak JM, Dearani JA, Burkhart HM, Sundt TM, Connolly HM, Schaff HV. Does the dilated ascending aorta in an adult with congenital heart disease require intervention? *J Thorac Cardiovasc Surg.* 2010;140:S52-S57.

51. Carlson M, Airhart N, Lopez L, Silberbach M. Moderate aortic enlargement and bicuspid aortic valve are associated with aortic dissection in Turner syndrome: report of the international Turner syndrome aortic dissection registry. *Circulation.* 2012;126:2220-2226.

13 ARRHYTHMIAS IN ADULT CONGENITAL HEART DISEASE

Anish Amin, MD
Steven Kalbfleisch, MD
Naomi J. Kertesz, MD

PATIENT STORY

KG is a 38-year-old woman with the diagnosis of transposition of the great arteries (TGA). She underwent an atrial switch operation at age 2 (Figure 13-1). Her first episode of atrial flutter occurred at age 11 and was refractory to antiarrhythmic drug therapy with multiple cardioversions and ultimately required permanent pacemaker implant to support drug therapy. A prior electrophysiologic (EP) study and radiofrequency ablation (RFA) was unsuccessful. She recently had an episode of atrial flutter while taking sotalol 120 mg bid and metoprolol 12.5 mg daily. Her symptoms abruptly began with exertion and including dizziness and dyspnea associated with ventricular rates greater than 200 bpm (Figure 13-2). She underwent cardioversion and beta-blocker dose titration but unfortunately could not tolerate higher beta-blockade. She was subsequently referred for repeat EP study. Two separate arrhythmias were induced, an atrial tachycardia that had not been seen clinically (Figure 13-3) and atrial flutter (Figures 13-4 and 13-5). Mapping was initially performed on the systemic venous side and the atrial tachycardia location was identified and ablated. In order to map the atrial flutter a transbaffle puncture was performed to access the tricuspid valve and the pulmonary venous side (Figure 13-6). Entrainment mapping was used to identify the circuit (Figure 13-5). The atrial flutter was successfully ablated (Figure 13-7) by placing lesions from the inferior vena cava (IVC) to the baffle on the systemic venous side and then from the baffle to the tricuspid valve on the pulmonary venous side (Figure 13-8). She has since had no recurrence of her atrial flutter.

CASE EXPLANATION

- Over 1 million adult congenital heart disease (CHD) patients are living in the United States.[1]

- About 45% have simple defects (eg, atrial septal defect [ASD], ventricular septal defect [VSD], valve stenosis).

- About 40% have moderately complex heart disease (eg, tetralogy of Fallot [TOF]).

- About 15% have severely complex defects (eg, single ventricle anatomy, Fontan, atrial switch procedure for transposition of the great arteries).

- This case highlights that arrhythmogenic complications increase as patients with CHD get older. These arrhythmias are often the leading cause of hospitalization and morbidity in adults with congenital heart disease.[2]

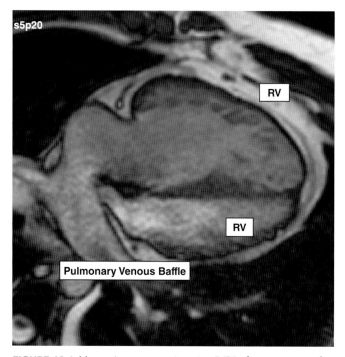

FIGURE 13-1 Magnetic resonance imaging (MRI) of transposition of the great arteries following atrial switch operation. There is no access to the tricuspid valve from the systemic venous side or the IVC.

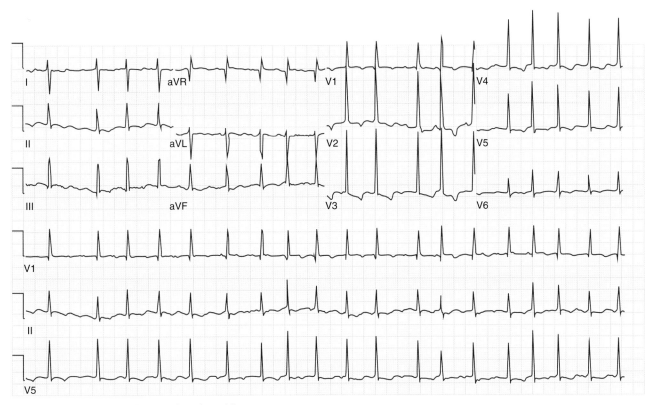

FIGURE 13-2 A 12-lead ECG showing clinical atrial flutter.

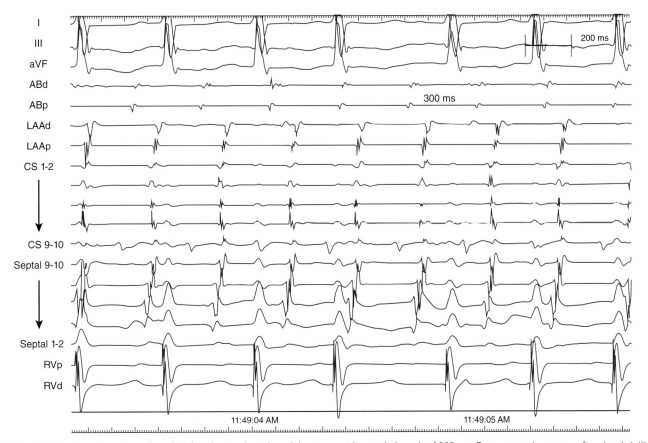

FIGURE 13-3 Atrial tachycardia induced in the electrophysiology laboratory with a cycle length of 300 ms. From top to bottom surface leads I, III, and aVF; ablation distal and proximal, left atrial appendage distal and proximal, 10 pole coronary sinus catheter distal (1, 2) to proximal (9, 10). 10 pole halo catheter proximal (9, 10) to distal (1, 2) and the right ventricular proximal and distal electrograms.

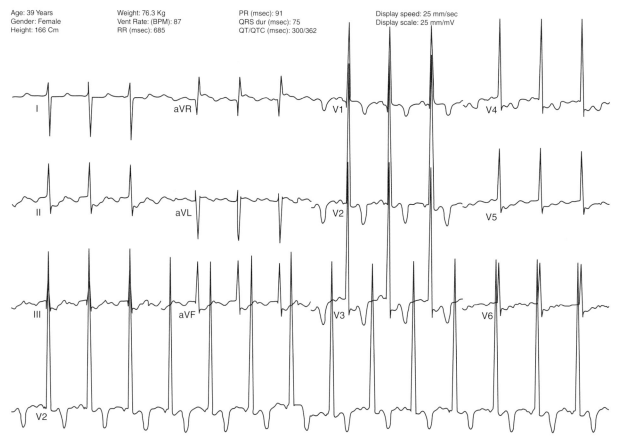

Age: 39 Years
Gender: Female
Height: 166 Cm

Weight: 76.3 Kg
Vent Rate: (BPM): 87
RR (msec): 685

PR (msec): 91
QRS dur (msec): 75
QT/QTC (msec): 300/362

Display speed: 25 mm/sec
Display scale: 25 mm/mV

FIGURE 13-4 Atrioventricular block during catheter manipulation which makes the flutter waves easier to identify.

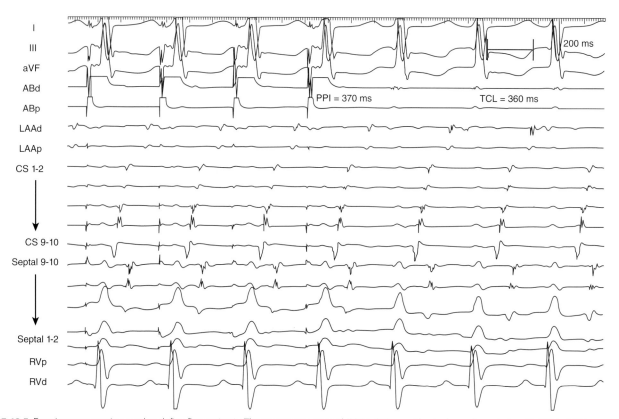

FIGURE 13-5 Entrainment mapping used to define flutter circuit. The post pacing interval (PPI) is 370 ms with a tachycardia cycle length (TCL) of 360 ms. The PPI-TCL of 10 ms suggests that the pacing catheter is within the tachycardia circuit.

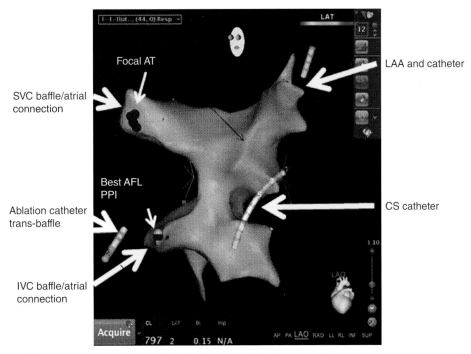

FIGURE 13-6 Carto map of the systemic venous baffle. The site of successful focal atrial tachycardia ablation is in the proximal superior vena cava (SVC) baffle. Note that the ablation catheter is transbaffle on the pulmonary venous side of the atrium.

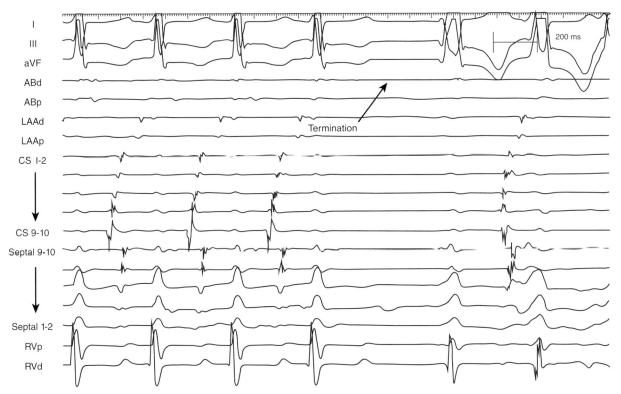

FIGURE 13-7 Atrial flutter terminated with radiofrequency ablation. From top to bottom surface leads I, III, and aVF; ablation distal and proximal, left atrial appendage distal and proximal, 10 pole coronary sinus catheter distal (1, 2) to proximal (9, 10). 10 pole halo catheter proximal (9, 10) to distal (1, 2) and the right ventricular proximal and distal electrograms.

- Cardiovascular anatomy predicts the location of conduction system disease.
- Broadly, arrhythmias should be considered as the following:
  - Supraventricular including bradyarrhythmias
  - Ventricular arrhythmias that pose a risk of sudden death

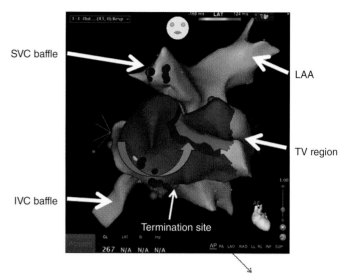

SVC baffle

LAA

TV region

IVC baffle

Termination site

FIGURE 13-8 Both systemic and venous baffles are outlined. In order to completely ablate the flutter isthmus it was necessary to cross the baffle and ablate from the inferior vena cava (IVC) to the tricuspid valve.

Supraventricular Arrhythmias: Bradyarrhythmias and Supraventricular Tachyarrhythmias

EPIDEMIOLOGY

- About 34% of older patients with TOF develop symptomatic supraventricular arrhythmias.[3]
- Older style atriopulmonary Fontans, have up to a 50% incidence of atrial arrhythmias due to atrial dilation and suture lines.[4]
- Bradyarrhythmias occur as a result of sinoatrial node dysfunction, delays in intra-atrial conduction, dysfunction of the atrioventricular (AV) node, or disease of the His-Purkinje fibers.[3,5]

Bradyarrhythmias

- Cardiovascular anatomy and the surgical repair predict the location of conduction system disease.

Tetralogy of Fallot

- Arrhythmias are dependent on the surgical approach with ventricular arrhythmias predominating in older repairs via ventriculotomy and atrial arrhythmias dominant in newer transatrial or transpulmonary approaches.
- About 4% to 8% of patients present with bradycardia.[6]

Transposition of the great arteries

- Complete AV block occurs in 22% of patients, largely in the infra-hisian fibers.[7]
- Following Mustard or Senning repairs bradycardia is mediated by direct iatrogenic injury to the sinus or AV node or interruption of blood flow to the sinus node during surgery.[8]

Univentricular physiology with Fontan palliation

- Arrhythmias are dependent on the surgical approach.[9]
- Atriopulmonary level conduits result in 30% to 40% of patients with sinus node dysfunction and 11% to 18% requiring pacemaker therapy.
- Extracardiac Fontan patients have 7% to 23% incidence of sinus node dysfunction with 3% to 7% requiring pacemakers.
- Lateral tunnel conduits result in 3% to 25% of patients with sinus node dysfunction and 5% to 10% of patients needing pacemaker therapy.

DIAGNOSTIC TESTING

Electrocardiography

- Sinus node anatomy in most patients with adult congenital heart disease is consistent with the normal adult and is located in the high right atrium lateral to the superior cavoatrial junction.[10]
- P-wave axis is 20 to 75 degrees.
- AV nodal and QRS features are based on anatomy and highly variable depending on the type of congenital anomaly.[11]

Tetralogy of Fallot

- Rightward axis with right bundle branch block is almost universal.
- Left anterior fascicular block is seen in 10% of patients.

Transposition of the great arteries

- Mobitz type II or III AV block with a stable narrow complex junctional QRS.
- Third-degree AV block is common in patients with simultaneous VSD repair.

Univentricular physiology with Fontan palliation

- Highly variable electrocardiography (ECG) but universal prolongation in the PR interval.

Electrophysiology Studies

Transposition of the great arteries

- About 80% to 90% of patients have a prolonged and corrected sinus node recovery time.[8]
- About 80% to 90% of patients have a prolonged sinoatrial conduction time (SACT).
- Infrahisian block: Anterolateral position of the AV node and inherent long course of the His-bundle and Purkinje fibers across the anterior aspect of the pulmonary valve puts the His fibers at risk.[12]
- Rare abnormalities in atrial refractoriness.

Univentricular physiology with Fontan palliation

- The Fontan operation for single ventricle, results in extensive suture lines and abnormal hemodynamics that predispose patients to atrial tachycardias and sinus node dysfunction.[13]
- About 50% to 60% of patients have a prolonged and corrected sinus node recovery time.
- About 50% to 60% of patients have a prolonged SACT.
- Common abnormalities in atrial refractoriness in as much as 25% of patients.

Tetralogy of Fallot

- Unlike patients having undergone Mustard or Fontan procedures patients with tetralogy of Fallot are unlikely to demonstrate baseline abnormalities in sinus node or AV node function.[14]
- Electrophysiologic studies conducted to risk stratify patients for sudden death demonstrate inducible monomorphic ventricular tachycardia (VT) in 35% of patients conferring a relative risk of recurrent VT or sudden death of 4.7.
- In 5% of cases polymorphic VT is induced.

Exercise Testing

- Chronotropic incompetence is an independent predictor of mortality in patients with complex congenital heart disease.
- About 70% to 90% of patients with complex congenital heart disease manifest chronotropic incompetence.[15]

Ambulatory Holter Monitoring

- Assess heart rate range and the presence or absence of junctional rhythms or pauses.

MANAGEMENT

Pacemaker Therapy

- Indicated for patients with advanced AV block including second- or third-degree AV block with symptoms related to bradycardia, ventricular dysfunction, or low cardiac output.[16]
- Postoperative second- or third-degree block which does not resolve after 7 days.[16]
- Reasonable for patients with complex congenital heart disease and heart rates lower than 40 bpm at rest or pauses of greater than 3 seconds.[16]
- Reasonable for patients with complex congenital heart disease and impaired hemodynamics secondary to AV dyssynchrony or bradycardia.[16]
- It is not indicated for transient AV block or Mobitz type I block.[16]

ATRIOVENTRICULAR REENTRY AND TWIN AV NODES

- The embryologic abnormalities that cause congenital heart defects may also have a direct impact on the conduction system.
- The AV node and the His bundle may only be displaced or there may be accessory or duplicated AV connections with the possibility of reentrant arrhythmias.

ATRIOVENTRICULAR REENTRY

- Common in some types of congenital heart disease.
- Ebstein's anomaly of the Tricuspid valve, (Figure 13-9) is associated with Wolff-Parkinson-White syndrome in 20% of cases. Nearly half of these patients will have multiple accessory pathways.
- Patients with L-TGA, that is corrected transposition, also have a high incidence of accessory pathways many of whom also have Ebstein's anomaly of their left-sided tricuspid valve.
- Given the atrial dilation in these patients the risk of atrial fibrillation with rapid conduction is becoming increasingly problematic in adolescence and adulthood (Figure 13-10).
- Catheter ablation is considered the standard of care for management of accessory pathways.
- It should be recognized that the short-term success rate and long-term recurrence are higher in patients with Ebstein's anomaly. These ablations are complicated by distorted landmarks, difficulty in identifying the true AV groove, and the high incidence of multiple pathways.[17]

TWIN AV NODES

- This is rarer anomaly typically seen in single ventricle of the heterotaxy variety.
- There are 2 AV nodes with 2 discrete His bundles with evidence of a connecting fiber.[18]
- Treatment is focused on ablation of one of the limbs of the duplicate system.

TACHYARRHYTHMIAS

- Both atrial and ventricular tachyarrhythmias have been described in adults with CHD.

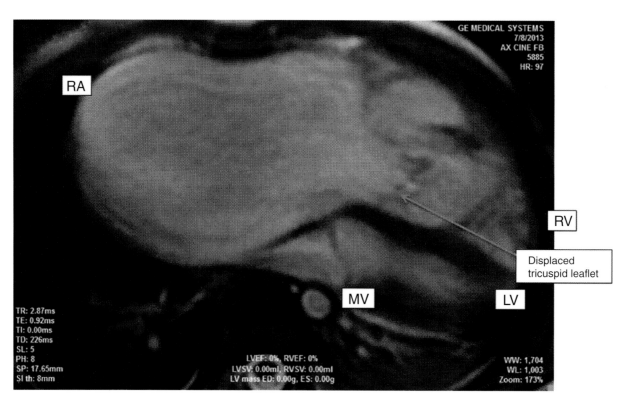

FIGURE 13-9 MRI of Ebstein's anomaly of the tricuspid valve. Note the diminutive right ventricle, the displaced tricuspid valve, and the large right atrium.

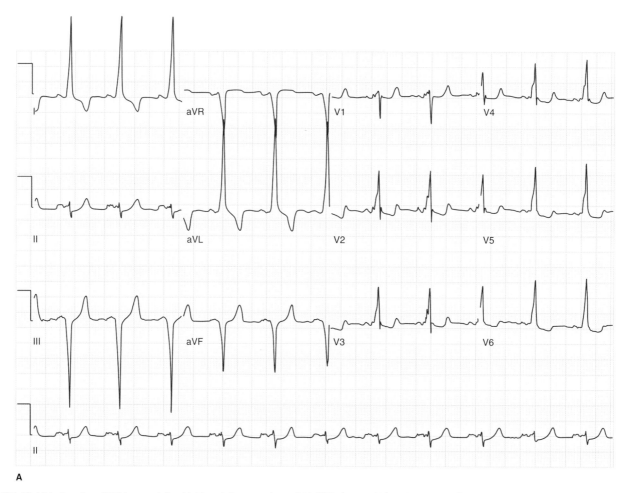

FIGURE 13-10A Baseline ECG in an adult with Ebstein's anomaly and Wolff-Parkinson-White (WPW) syndrome.

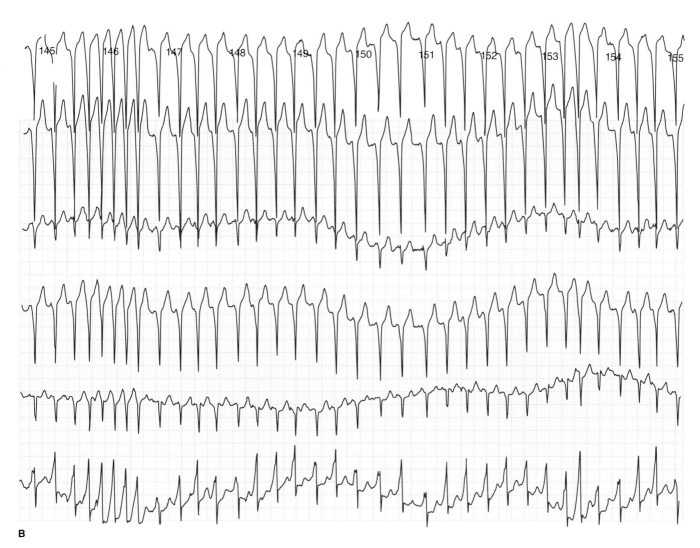

FIGURE 13-10B Atrial fibrillation in a 20-year-old woman with Ebstein's anomaly and WPW.

- The most common mechanism for symptomatic atrial tachycardia in the adult CHD population is macroreentry within atrial muscle. The terms "intra-atrial reentrant tachycardia" (IART) and "incisional tachycardia" have become customary labels for this arrhythmia in order to distinguish it from the typical variety of atrial flutter that occurs in structurally normal hearts.[18]

- Considerable data are available on the natural history data of ventricular tachyarrhythmias and clinical outcomes among patients with TOF, because of its prevalence in the adult CHD population and elevated incidence of ventricular arrhythmias.

Intra-Atrial Reentrant Tachycardia

- It is the most common mechanism of symptomatic arrhythmia in the adult CHD patient.

- IART and incisional tachycardia are customary labels to distinguish this arrhythmia from typical atrial flutter (Figures 13-11 and 13-12). It is a macroreentrant circuit within atrial muscle caused by atrial dilation, thickening, and scarring.

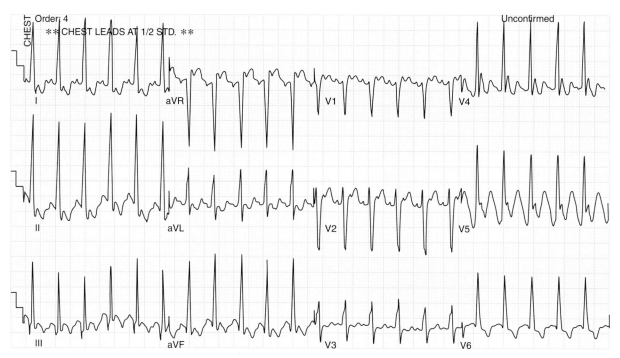

FIGURE 13-11 Atrial flutter in an adult with unrepaired single ventricle.

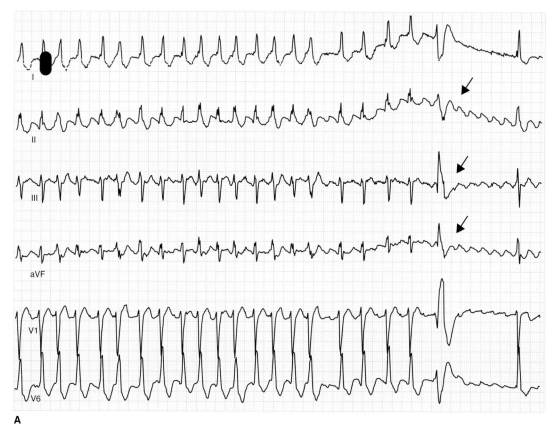

A

FIGURE 13-12 A 19-year-old with Fontan presented with palpitations. Adenosine administration (arrow) makes classic flutter waves easily seen.

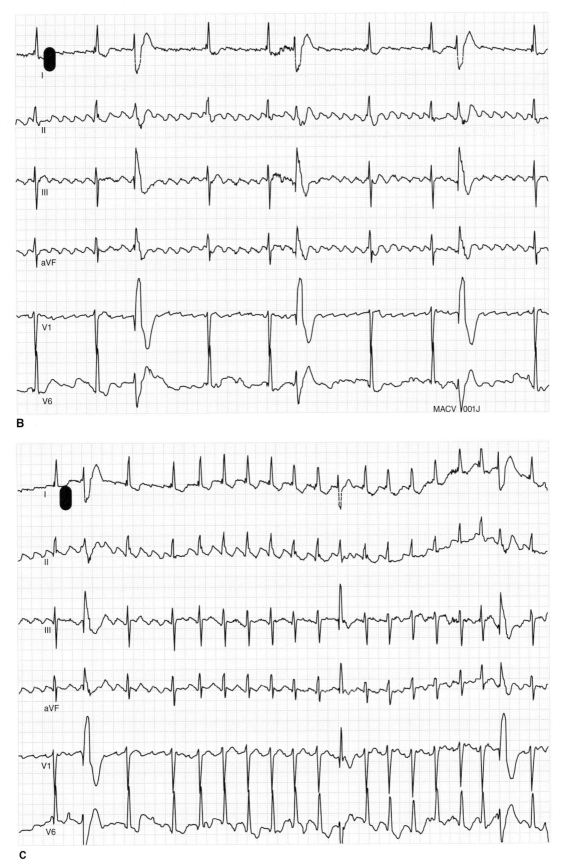

FIGURE 13-12 (*continued*)

- Other risk factors for IART include concomitant sinus node dysfunction with tachy-brady syndrome and older age at the time of surgery.[4]

- IART is seen in 30% of patients following an atrial switch operation (Mustard or Senning) as in Figure 13-3 or 50% of patients following a Fontan palliation (Figure 13-13) though can be seen in any patient who has undergone an atriotomy incision.

- The route of propagation varies depending on the anatomic defect and the surgical repair and is modulated by fibrosis of suture lines or patches.

- The IART rate is generally slower than classic flutter with atrial rates of 150 to 250 bpm. The P-waves are small and separated by a flat baseline and are masked by the QRS and T-waves (Figure 13-14). There may be 1:1 or variable AV conduction.

TREATMENT

- IART can be reliably terminated with electrical cardioversion and sometimes with overdrive pacing.

- Many patients with underlying sinus node dysfunction and may be significantly bradycardic following cardioversion.

- Long-term therapeutic options include antiarrhythmic drugs, pacemakers, catheter ablation, and surgical intervention.

- Pacemakers are useful for treating tachy-brady syndrome, allowing use of antiarrhythmics in patients with underlying sinus node dysfunction, and antitachycardia pacing. One must be careful with antitachycardia pacing as this may cause a shift to a different and faster IART circuit or cause degeneration into atrial fibrillation.

- Catheter ablation using 3D mapping and irrigated or large-tip catheters has a short-term success rate of nearly 90%.[19,20] It is important to remember that in patients with atrial switch procedures that the cavotricuspid annulus is in the pulmonary venous atrium and only accessible prograde via transbaffle puncture.

- Recurrence risk is particularly high, nearly 40%, in Fontan patients due to the large number of IART circuits and the thickness and size of the atrium. However, ablation still may be useful as it may reduce the frequency of episodes or make drug therapy more effective.[17]

- Surgical ablation is an option and consists of a right atrial maze procedure particularly in the Fontan population. Many times this is combined with a revision of the Fontan connection from an older atriopulmonary anastomosis to a cavopulmonary anastomosis or extracardiac Fontan.

Atrial Fibrillation

- Atrial fibrillation arises in response to hemodynamic stress in the left atrium and is most commonly associated with aortic stenosis, mitral valve deformities, and unrepaired single ventricles.

- Patients with isolated right-sided heart lesions are at a higher risk of developing atrial arrhythmias than those with isolated left heart lesions. The 30-year risk of developing atrial arrhythmias in an 18-year old with right-sided heart disease (ASD, Ebstein's anomaly, Fontan, tricuspid valve abnormality) is 18% in comparison to 11% in one with left-sided disease (VSD, aortic or mitral valve disease).[21]

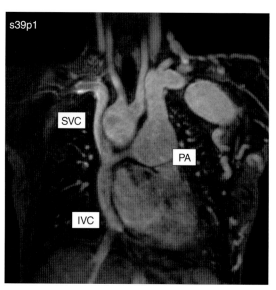

FIGURE 13-13 Lateral tunnel Fontan. Note the superior vena cava (SVC) and inferior vena cava (IVC) directly connected to the pulmonary arteries (PA).

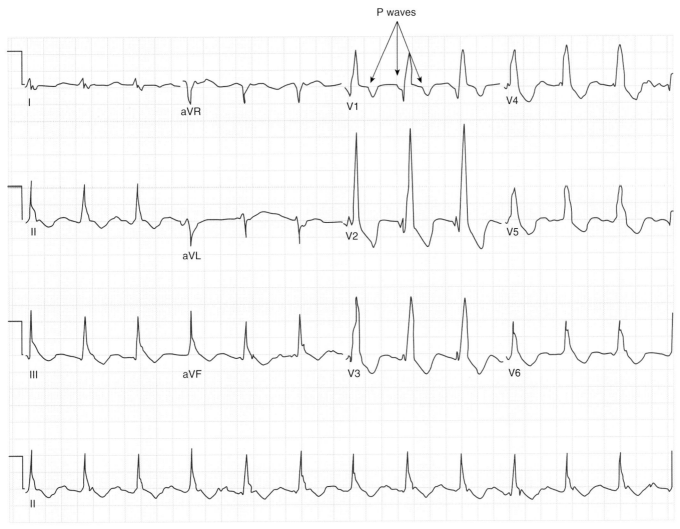

FIGURE 13-14 A 30-year old with history of Mustard operation who presented with complains of tachycardia. The ECG demonstrates intra-atrial reentrant tachycardia (IART) with 2:1 atrioventricular (AV) conduction. Note short PR and P-wave within T-wave.

- Issues regarding hemodynamic instability, heart failure, and stroke are seen in this population just as in those patients with structurally normal hearts. There is no difference in morbidity or mortality between those with right- or left-sided heart lesions.

TREATMENT

- Similar to atrial fibrillation in adults without CHD, there remains an emphasis on anticoagulation and symptom management with cardioversion, antiarrhythmic therapy, and in limited cases ablative therapy.
- Pacemaker insertion may reduce recurrence in those with sinus node dysfunction.
- Ablative therapy is possible with surgical right and left sided Maze. Catheter ablation with pulmonary vein isolation has been reported in the presence of congenital heart disease with the most common defect being an ASD. However pulmonary vein isolation has also been reported in patient's status post Fontan operation.[22]

Ventricular Tachyarrhythmias

- Serious ventricular arrhythmias are rare among CHD patients during their first or second decade of life, but once adulthood is reached, the potential for VT and sudden death becomes more of a concern.[18]

- The bulk of literature and clinical experience regarding VT in CHD has centered on tetralogy of Fallot. The prevalence of VT after tetralogy of Fallot repair has been estimated to be between 3% and 14% in several large clinical series.[18]

- Some patients with slow VT may be hemodynamically stable at presentation, but VT tends to be rapid for the majority, causing syncope or cardiac arrest as the presenting symptom.

- To date, no perfect risk-stratification scheme has emerged, although several clinical variables with modest prognostic value have been identified, including the following:
  1. Older age at time of definitive surgery
  2. History of palliative shunts
  3. High-grade ventricular ectopy
  4. Inducible VT at electrophysiologic study
  5. Abnormal right ventricular (RV) hemodynamics
  6. Wide QRS width (>180 ms)[18]

Sudden Cardiac Death

- Relatively low rate of sudden death in the entire congenital heart disease population.

- High rates of sudden death approaching 20% to 25% of adults with complex congenital heart disease.[23]

- Largely related to an underlying ventricular arrhythmia.

- Data is mostly limited to patients having undergone prior repair of tetralogy of Fallot, Mustard or Senning procedures in patients with transposition of the great arteries.

- Greatest risk in individuals who have undergone ventriculotomy with mechanisms similar to those seen in IART.[24]

- Underlying ventricular dysfunction and prolonged QRS duration may predict those individuals at greatest risk.[25]

- Ablative therapies may be considered in individuals with monomorphic sustained ventricular arrhythmias.

TREATMENT: ICD THERAPY

- There is lack of objective guidelines for VT prediction and treatment in CHD patients, however, implantable cardioverter-defibrillators (ICD) are increasingly utilized in the primary and secondary prevention of sudden death in patients with tetralogy of Fallot.

- These are indicated in individuals with structural heart disease and a history of sustained monomorphic ventricular tachycardia.

- Indicated for individuals who have survived an episode of sudden cardiac death.

CONCLUSION

- Symptomatic arrhythmias occur with increasing frequency for adult congenital heart disease (ACHD) as they move through adolescence and into adulthood.

- These arrhythmias may be intrinsic to the structural malformation of specific congenital defects or acquired related to the surgical scars of early treatments and changes over time related to hypoxemia plus volume/pressure changes.

- Sudden cardiac death (SCD) is the greatest concern in ACHD. The greatest risk of late SCD has been most studied in patients with repaired TOF and TGA.

- The paucity of evidence-based management protocols for arrhythmias in adults with CHD is also a concern, and a need clearly exists for larger collaborative studies involving both pediatric and adult CHD centers to generate more objective treatment guidelines.[18]

REFERENCES

1. Warnes CA, Liberthson R, Danielson GK, et al. Task force 1: the changing profile of congenital heart disease in adult life. *J Am Coll Cardiol.* 2001;37:1170-1175.

2. Khairy P, Dore A, Talajic M, et al. Arrhythmias in adult congenital heart disease. *Expert Rev Cardiovasc Ther.* 2006;4:83-95.

3. Roos-Hesselink J, Perlroth MG, McGhie J, Spitaels S. Atrial arrhythmias in adults after repair of tetralogy of Fallot. Correlations with clinical, exercise, and echocardiographic findings. *Circulation.* 1995;91:2214-2219.

4. Fishberger SB, Wernovsky G, Gentles TL, et al. Factors that influence the development of atrial flutter after the Fontan operation. *J Thorac Cardiovasc Surg.* 1997;113:80-86.

5. Rekawek J, Kansy A, Miszczak-Knecht M, et al. Risk factors for cardiac arrhythmias in children with congenital heart disease after surgical intervention in the early postoperative period. *J Thorac Cardiovasc Surg.* 2007;133:900-904.

6. Nakazawa M, Shinohara T, Sasaki A, et al. Study group for arrhythmias long-term after surgery for congenital heart disease: ALTAS-CHD study. Arrhythmias late after repair of tetralogy of Fallot: a Japanese Multicenter Study. *Circ J.* 2004;68:126-130.

7. Huhta JC, Maloney JD, Ritter DG, Ilstrup DM, Feldt RH. Complete atrioventricular block in patients with atrioventricular discordance. *Circulation.* 1983;67:1374-1377.

8. Gillette PC, Kugler JD, Garson A, Jr, Gutgesell HP, Duff DF, McNamara DG. Mechanisms of cardiac arrhythmias after the Mustard operation for transposition of the great arteries. *Am J Cardiol.* 1980;45:1225-1230.

9. Deal B. Late arrhythmias following Fontan surgery. *World J Pediatr Congenit Heart Surg.* 2012;3:194.

10. Khairy P, Marelli A. Clinical use of electrocardiography in adults with congenital heart disease. *Circulation.* 2007;116:2734-2746.

11. Davachi F, Moller JH. The electrocardiogram and vector cardiogram in single ventricle: anatomic correlations. *Am J Cardiol.* 1969;23:19-31.

12. Anderson RH, Becker AE, Arnold R, Wilkinson JL. The conducting tissues in congenitally corrected transposition. *Circulation.* 1974;50:911-923.

13. Kurer C, Tanner C, Vetter V. Electrophysiologic findings after Fontan repair of functional single ventricle. *J Am Coll Cardiol.* 1991;17:174-181.

14. Khairy P, Landzberg M, Gatloukis M, et al. Value of programmed ventricular stimulation after tetralogy of Fallot repair: a multicenter study. *Circulation.* 2004;109:1994-2000.

15. Diller GP, Dimopoulos K, Okonko D, et al. Heart rate response during exercise predicts survival in adults with congenital heart disease. *J Am Coll Cardiol.* 2006;48:1250-1256.

16. Epstein AE, Dimarco JP, Ellenbogen KA, et al. ACC/AHA/HRS 2008 guidelines for device-based therapy of cardiac rhythm abnormalities: executive summary. 2008;5:934-955.

17. Lam W, Friedman RA. Electrophysiology issues in adult congenital heart disease. *Methodist Debakey Cardiovasc J.* 2011;7:13-17.

18. Walsh E, Cecchin F. Arrhythmias in adult patients with congenital heart disease. *Circulation.* 2007;115:534-545.

19. Triedman JK, Alexander MA, Love BA, et al. Influence of patient factors and ablative technologies on outcomes of radiofrequency ablation of intra-atrial tachycardia in patients with congenital heart disease. *J Am Coll Cardiol.* 2002;39:1827-1835.

20. Jais P, Shah DC, Haissaguerre M, et al. Prospective randomized comparison of irrigated-tip versus conventional-tip catheters for ablation of common flutter. *Circulation.* 2000;101:772-776.

21. Vernier M, Marelli AJ, Pilote L, et al. Atrial arrhythmias in adult patients with right versus left sided congenital heart disease anomalies. *Am J Cardiol.* 2010;106:547-551.

22. Philip F, Muhammad KI, Agarwal S, et al. Pulmonary vein isolation for the treatment of drug-refractory atrial fibrillation in adults with congenital heart disease. *Congenit Heart Dis.* 2012;7:392-399.

23. Verheugt CL, Uiterwaal CS, van der Velde ET, et al. Mortality in adult congenital heart disease. *Eur Heart J.* 2010;31:1220-1229.

24. Horowitz LN, Vetter VL, Harken AH, Josephson ME. Electrophysiologic characteristics of sustained ventricular tachycardia occurring after repair of tetralogy of Fallot. *Am J Cardiol.* 1980;46;446-452.

25. Koyak Z, Harris L, de Groot J, et al. Sudden cardiac death in adult congenital heart disease. *Circulation.* 2012;126:1944-1954.

14 COMMON PERCUTANEOUS STRUCTURAL INTERVENTIONS IN ADULTS WITH CONGENITAL HEART DISEASE

Jamil Aboulhosn, MD, ΓACC, FSCAI

The Adult with Repaired Coarctation of the Aorta

PATIENT STORY

A 48-year-old woman with coarctation of the aorta, ventricular septal defect (VSD), and bicuspid aortic stenosis was followed with progressive aortic root dilation and severe aortic regurgitation. She also had moderate aortic valvular stenosis and underwent aortic valve and root replacement with a 22-mm homograft and reimplantation of the coronary arteries in 2002 at 38 years of age. This operation was complicated by right brachial artery occlusion requiring surgical bypass graft. She also developed third-degree heart block and underwent dual-chamber transvenous pacemaker placement. In the distant past, she had undergone initial repair of her coarctation and VSD closure at age 14 months in 1965 (coarctation resection with end-to-end anastomosis, required reoperation for residual coarctation in 1973 at 9 years of age). She had developed systemic hypertension and was managed with dual therapy using a beta-blocker and angiotensin-converting enzyme (ACE) inhibitor. She continued to have frequent headaches, fatigue with exertion, bilateral lower extremity pain, and fatigue with ambulation.

On physical examination, the patient had evidence of right brachial to left femoral pulse delay, the right femoral pulse was only faintly palpable. A 2/6 mid-systolic murmur was auscultated at the right upper sternal border. A soft systolic murmur was heard over the left scapula, no continuous murmurs or diastolic murmurs were appreciated. An S4 gallop was auscultated over the apex.

A stress echocardiogram in 2009 demonstrated a peak resting instantaneous gradient of 63 mm Hg, mean 32 mm Hg across the coarctation site, increased to PIG of 132 mm Hg with exercise. She had poor exercise capacity, went 6 minutes on a Bruce protocol with right upper extremity (RUE) blood pressure (BP) rising to greater than 200 mm Hg systolic, lower extremity exercise BP could not be measured. The decision was made to proceed with invasive catheterization to further assess anatomy and hemodynamics and to perform palliative intervention if deemed feasible and necessary.

INTERVENTIONAL CARDIAC CATHETERIZATION: CASE EXPLANATION

- The patient was brought to the catheterization laboratory and placed under general anesthesia in expectation of possible transcatheter intervention. The right femoral pulse was faintly palpable, evaluation with ultrasound suggested an obstructed right femoral artery. The left femoral arterial pulse was palpated and a 6-French (F) sheath was placed under fluoroscopic and ultrasound guidance using the modified Seldinger technique.

- Hemodynamic evaluation demonstrated a minimal gradient across the aortic homograft, an elevated left ventricular end-diastolic pressure (LVEDP) of 20 mm Hg, and a peak-to-peak gradient of 40 mm Hg across a focal area of re-coarctation in the proximal descending aorta (Figure 14-1).

- Angiography demonstrated a focal narrowing at the site of prior coarctation repair, the transverse aorta, and descending aorta at the diaphragm measured 17 mm in diameter, the area of stenosis measured 8 mm in minimum diameter. A left femoral angiogram demonstrated complete occlusion of the left femoral artery by the 6-F arterial sheath (Figure 14-2). Intra-arterial nitroglycerin was given and the sheath was downsized to 4 F with manual pressure used to maintain hemostasis. Repeat angiography demonstrated an open but small caliber (<5 mm) common femoral artery. The decision was made to not proceed with percutaneous intervention via the femoral approach given the small-caliber left femoral artery (cannot abide the 12-F sheath needed for large-diameter stent placement).

- The patient was taken off the table and bought back for a hybrid intervention with surgical exposure of the right subclavian artery. A 3-cm horizontal incision was made below the right clavicle and the artery was exposed (Figure 14-3). A micropuncture kit was used to access the artery and "preclosed" the artery with 2 Proglide sutures. A 10-F flexor sheath was positioned in the descending aorta. An EV-3 LD max 26 mm × 12-mm stent was mounted on a 14 mm × 3.5-cm BIB balloon and deployed, residual waist noted despite inflating to 8 atmosphere (atm) (Figure 14-4A). Angiogram

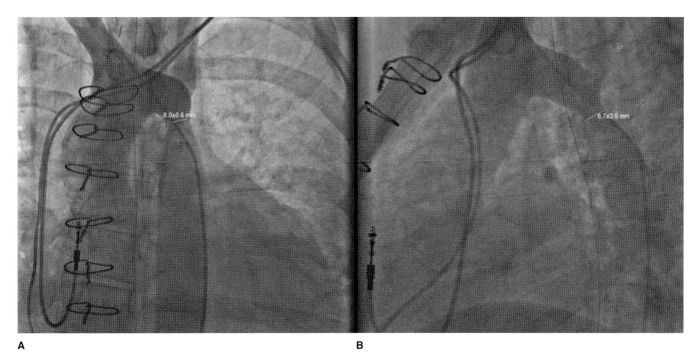

A   **B**

FIGURE 14-1 **A.** Aortogram in the anteroposterior (AP) view demonstrating focal restenosis of a previously surgically repaired coarctation segment; the patient had undergone prior surgical resection of the narrowed segment with end-to-end repair. **B.** Lateral view demonstrating focal restenosis.

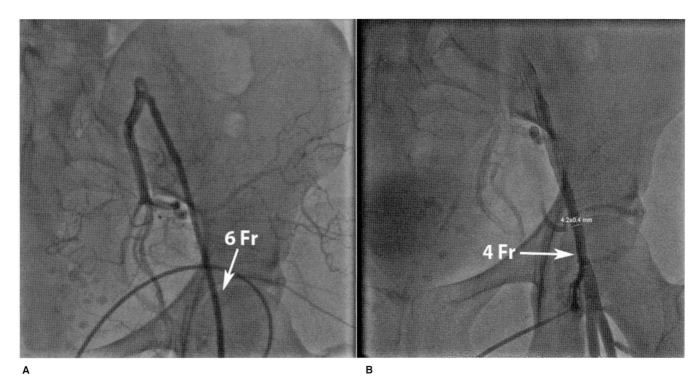

A   **B**

FIGURE 14-2 **A.** Complete occlusion of the left common femoral artery by a 6-F sheath. **B.** One hundred micrograms of intra-arterial nitroglycerine was infused and the 6-F sheath was exchanged for a 4-F sheath with subsequent improvement in distal flow. The common femoral artery measures 4.2 +/- 0.4 mm in minimal diameter and was deemed too narrow to accommodate a large-diameter long sheath necessary for coarctation angioplasty and stenting.

performed post deployment, no evidence of dissection or aneurysm. The stent was postdilated with an Atlas PTA 14 mm × 2-cm balloon to a maximum pressure of 10 atm with minimal residual waist noted (Figure 14-4B).

- Rotational angiography post deployment demonstrated a focal outpouching at the site of stent deployment, consistent with a controlled rupture of the aorta (Figure 14-5). Over 15 minutes, the pseudoaneurysm progressed from 1.5 mm in diameter to 3.5 mm in diameter. The decision was made to proceed with covered stent placement. A Melody valve was used as a "covered stent" by cutting out the valve leaflets (Figure 14-6A) and mounting the covered stent on an 18-mm BIB, placed through an 18-F sheath.

- Angiography demonstrated a patent left subclavian artery, complete coverage of the pseudoaneurysm without residual "leak," and a widely patent aorta at the prior coarctation site (Figure 14-6B). Simultaneous ascending and descending aorta pressure measurement did not demonstrate a residual gradient. The sheath was withdrawn and the Proglide sutures were tightened and cut. The incision was then surgically closed with running sutures (Figure 14-7).

- The patient was discharged within 23 hours of the procedure. A chest computed tomography (CT) angiogram was performed 3 months following the operation and demonstrated excellent stent apposition, no evidence of endovascular leak, and a widely patent aorta (Figure 14-8). Her systemic blood pressure control improved appreciably and the ACE inhibitor was discontinued within 3 months of the procedure.

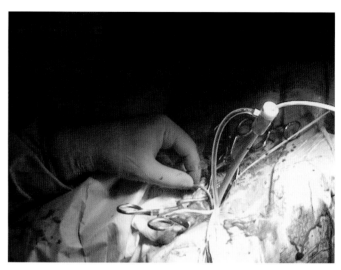

FIGURE 14-3 Surgical approach to the right subclavian artery with exposure of the vessel and subsequent placement of a 10-F sheath.

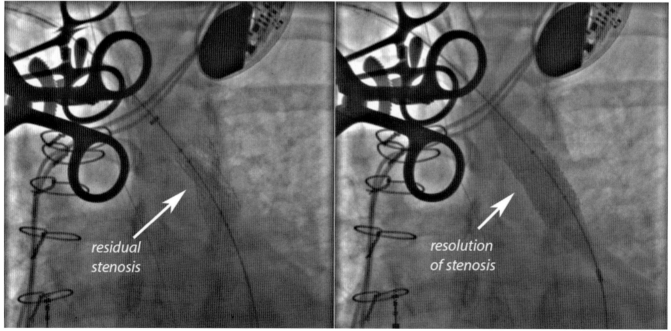

A   **B**

FIGURE 14-4 A. EV-3 LD max 26 × 12-mm large-diameter balloon expandable stent following deployment at a pressure of 8 atm on a 14 mm × 3.5-cm balloon. Note the residual waist at the area of residual coarctation. **B.** Redilation using a 14-mm Atlas balloon, inflated to 10 atm with resolution of residual stenosis.

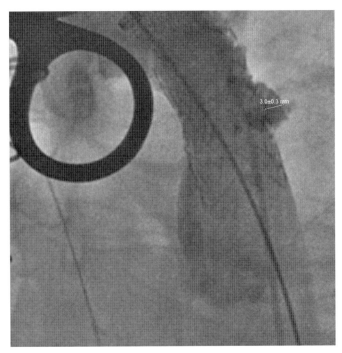

FIGURE 14-5 Right anterior oblique aortogram poststent redilation demonstrates a focal outpouching of the aorta consistent with a contained rupture.

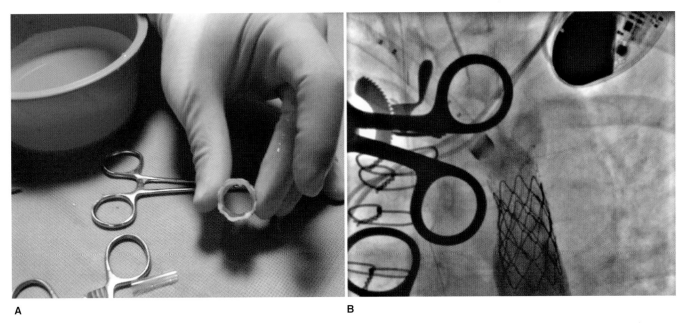

A   **B**

FIGURE 14-6 A. The Melody valve was converted to a covered stent by manually cutting out the valve leaflets. **B.** Aortogram post covered stent placement demonstrating a patent aorta without residual stenosis, no evidence of residual pseudoaneurysm, and a widely patent left subclavian artery.

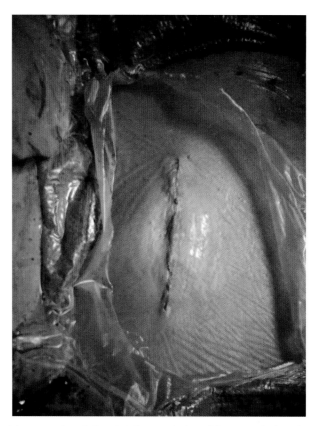

FIGURE 14-7 The right subclavicular incision was sutured closed at the conclusion of the case, the location and length of the incision are reminiscent of that seen with pacemaker placement.

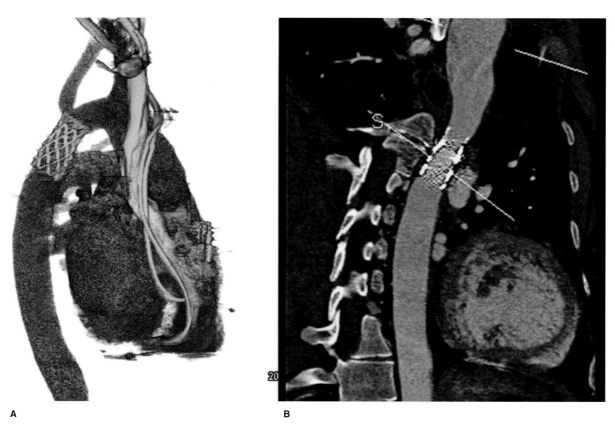

A   B

FIGURE 14-8 **A.** 3D reconstruction, right posterior view of a chest CT angiogram 3 months postprocedure demonstrating excellent stent apposition, no evidence of endovascular leak, a widely patent aorta, and a patent left subclavian artery. **B.** Multiplanar reconstruction demonstrating minimal residual narrowing of the stented segment.

DISCUSSION

- Transcatheter balloon angioplasty of aortic coarctation was first performed in 1982 and has been applied to discrete native coarctation and recurrent narrowing with considerable immediate success and a low rate of procedural complications.[1] While the risk of death is low (<1%), the risk of dissection, aneurysm, or pseudoaneurysm formation is higher with angioplasty alone than with stenting.

- While the immediate results of angioplasty are favorable, the intermediate and long-term results are less impressive, up to 50% of subjects require repeat intervention within a decade.[2] Repeat interventions were for recurrent stenosis or aneurysm formation. The para-coarctation segments of the aorta harbor medial abnormalities that increase the risk of aneurysm and pseudoaneurysm formation (in up to 35% of patients) following angioplasty.[3] Stent placement relieves obstruction and carries a lower risk of aneurysm formation.

- Stent placement has become the treatment of choice for de novo and postsurgical residual coarctation in adults. The immediate, intermediate, and long-term outcomes of stent implantation are excellent. The resting gradient is virtually eliminated in most patients but most patients will continue to have an inducible gradient with exercise given the noncompliant nature of the stented segment.[4]

- Procedural success (<20 mm Hg residual peak-to-peak gradient) occurs in 96% of cases, 4% of patients require repeat interventions and 1.3% may have aortic complications such as dissection or pseudoaneurysm formation.[5] Other complications include stent fracture, access site complications, stent migration, balloon rupture, and arterial embolization. At long-term follow-up, 23% of patients continued to have systemic hypertension, 9% had an upper-to-lower limb blood pressure gradient in excess of 20 mm Hg, and 32% were taking antihypertensive medication.[5]

- Covered stents can be used as a "bailout" in patients with dissection, aneurysm, or pseudoaneurysm formation. Internationally, the Cheatham-Palmaz stent from NuMed has become the stent of choice for most coarctations in adults. Currently, US Food and Drug Administration (FDA) approval of this device is pending in the United States.

The Adult with an Unrepaired Secundum Atrial Septal Defect

PATIENT STORY

A 77-year-old woman with a history of hypertension presented to emergency room (ER) 12 hours after the acute onset of blurry vision and dizziness. A brain magnetic resonance imaging (MRI) demonstrated an acute thromboembolic stroke in the posterior right occipital and parietal cortex. She was treated conservatively with antiplatelet agents. She was in sinus rhythm and telemetry monitoring did not reveal any arrhythmias. Hypercoagulable work-up was negative and bilateral lower extremity ultrasound did not demonstrate any evidence for deep venous thrombosis. She had a gradual reduction in exercise capacity over the past 5 years and became dyspneic with one flight of stairs.

Her physical examination revealed an acyanotic female with resting oxygen saturation of 99%. Cardiac examination revealed a faint right ventricular heave, fixed splitting of the second heart sound, normal jugular venous pressure, a faint systolic murmur was heard at the left upper sternal border, an S4 gallop was auscultated over the apex. The lungs were clear and there was no evidence of extremity edema or ascites.

During the course of her work-up, a transesophageal echocardiogram revealed a secundum atrial septal defect (Figures 14-9 and 14-10). There was no evidence of intracardiac thrombus. Pulmonary venous connections were normal. The atrial septal defect (ASD) measured 1.4 cm with adequate rims and evidence of mostly left-to-right shunt. The right atrium, right ventricle, and left atrium were enlarged. There was moderate tricuspid regurgitation with a velocity of 3 m/s. Pulse wave and tissue Doppler assessment of left ventricular diastolic function suggested abnormal relaxation. The decision was made to proceed with cardiac catheterization and transcatheter ASD closure.

INTERVENTIONAL CARDIAC CATHETERIZATION: CASE EXPLANATION

- The patient was placed under general anesthesia and intubated. Transesophageal echocardiography was used to guide defect closure.

- Hemodynamics were as follows (Figure 14-11):

Predevice Placement

- There was a step-up in oxygenation from the superior vena cava (SVC) to pulmonary artery (PA) of 10%. (66% SVC, 76% right atrium [RA], 65% inferior vena cava [IVC], 76% PA.)

- Right ventricular end-diastolic pressure (RVEDP) = 12 mm Hg. Pulmonary artery pressure (PAP) = 53/23/34 and pulmonary capillary wedge pressure (PCWP) = 16.

- Pulmory blood flow (PBF) = 8 l/min.

- Systemic blood flow (SBF) = 5.3 l/min.

- Qp:Qs = 1.5:1.

- Pulmonary vascular resistance (PVR) = 2.25 Wood units.

- Systemic vascular resistance (SVR) = 10 Wood units.

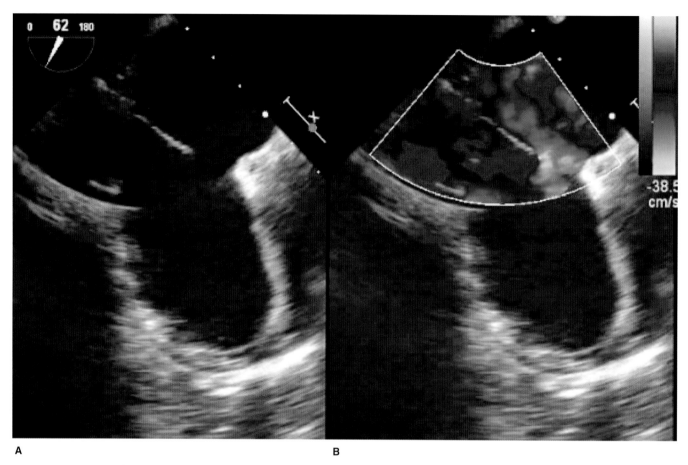

FIGURE 14-9 Transesophageal echocardiogram, demonstrating a moderate-sized (14-mm unstretched diameter) secundum ASD. Color flow Doppler demonstrates low-velocity left-to-right shunting.

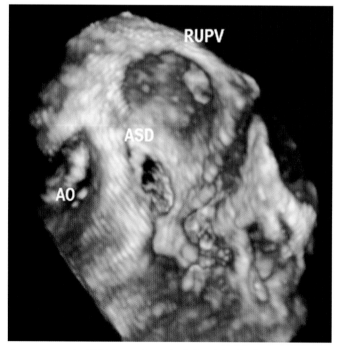

FIGURE 14-10 3D transesophageal echocardiography (TEE) image from the left atrial side demonstrating the special relationship of the atrial septal defect (ASD) to the right upper pulmonary vein (RUPV).

During ASD Balloon Occlusion

- Increase in PCWP to 32 mm Hg mean with V-waves up to 42 mm Hg from a baseline mean of 16 mm Hg (Figures 14-12 and 14-13).

- With balloon deflation, the mean wedge pressure came back down to 16 mm Hg (Figure 14-14).

Postdevice Placement (With Fenestrations)

- RVEDP = 12 mm Hg. PAP = 45/20/31 and PCWP = 15.

- Qp:Qs = 1.4:1.

- PVR = 2.3 Wood units.

- Transesophageal 3D echo with color Doppler demonstrated excellent device position and stability (Figures 14-15 and 14-16).

- The patient was discharged home within 23 hours on full-dose aspirin. At her latest follow-up (3 months), she had improved exertional capacity and there had been a reduction in right atrial and right ventricular size.

- The device fenestrations could not be well visualized by transthoracic echocardiography.

DISCUSSION

- ASDs often go unrecognized for the first few decades of life because of the indolent clinical course and benign findings on physical examination. Initial diagnosis in adulthood is common when symptoms of dyspnea on exertion and palpitations usually occur and are caused by increasing right-sided chamber enlargement, pulmonary hypertension, right ventricular failure, tricuspid regurgitation, and atrial arrhythmias.

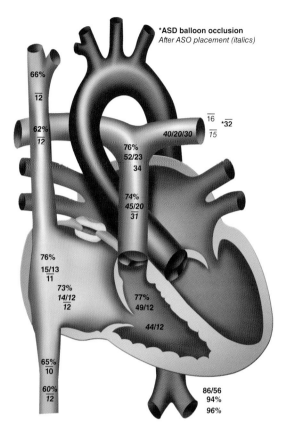

FIGURE 14-11 Hemodynamic measurements and oxygen saturations during the 3 phases of the study: (1) baseline, (2) balloon occlusion of the atrial septal defect (ASD) resulted in a drastic rise in the pulmonary arterial capillary wedge pressure from a mean of 16 to 32 mm Hg, (3) post fenestrated device placement.

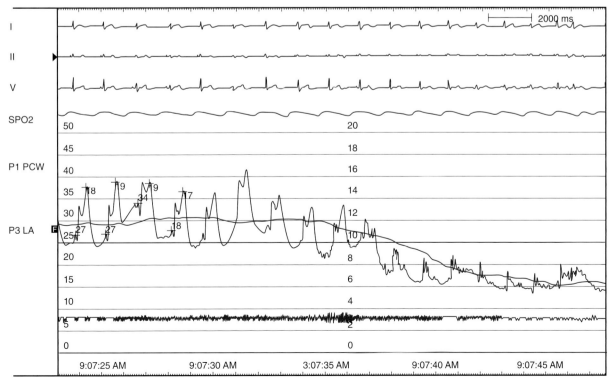

FIGURE 14-12 Pulmonary arterial capillary wedge pressure with balloon occlusion of atrial septal defect (ASD) is elevated to a mean of 32 mm Hg with V-waves up to 42 mm Hg, with balloon deflation the wedge pressure dropped to a mean of 16 mm Hg without accentuated V-waves.

- The degree of left-to-right shunt may increase with age as left ventricular compliance decreases, as was the case in this patient. Paradoxical embolism may occur as it did in this patient.

- Surgical repair had been considered the standard of care until the advent of occluders that could be delivered via transcatheter means.

- Advancements in biocompatible materials, device design and catheterization technology have led to the widespread availability of a variety of closure devices. Transcatheter device closure compares favorably with surgical closure in terms of long-term outcome and is associated with shorter hospital stays and fewer postprocedural complications.[6]

- Appropriate patient selection is imperative.[7-10]

- Transcatheter device closure techniques have supplanted surgery at many institutions as the method of choice for ASD closure in properly selected patients; complications are rare. Short-term complications include device embolization, aortic root or atrial wall perforation, and cardiac tamponade.[11] Mid- and long-term complications include device fracture, thrombus formation, device erosion, atrial dysrhythmias, and infection.

- The use of platelet inhibitors for at least 6 months following device closure is recommended to decrease the risk of device thrombosis.[12]

- The long-term outcomes of device closure using the Amplatzer septal occluder are equivalent to long-term surgical results.[6,13] Older patients with abnormal left ventricular compliance or restrictive physiology may have significant increase in left heart filling pressure with ASD closure.

- Balloon test occlusion of the ASD with simultaneous measurement of pulmonary artery occlusion pressure or direct measurement of left ventricular diastolic or left atrial pressure may be revealing. Manual fenestration of commercially available devices allows for a small "pop-off" for decompression.[14]

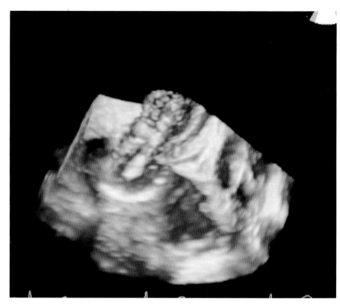

FIGURE 14-13 3D transesophageal echocardiography (TEE) during balloon sizing of the atrial septal defect (ASD).

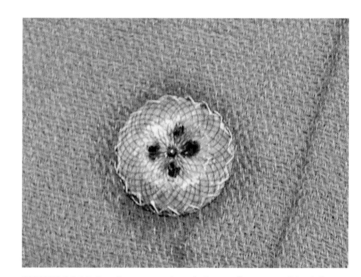

FIGURE 14-14 Amplatzer septal occluder, en-face view of the left atrial disc following manual fenestration with placement of 4 small holes near the center of the device, the cloth mesh was manually cut away to create each hole.

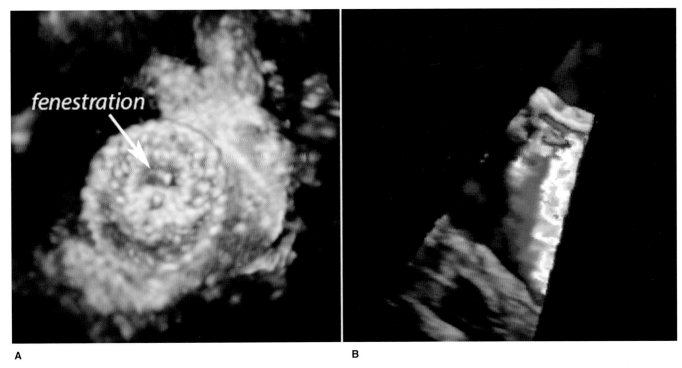

FIGURE 14-15 **A.** 3D TEE demonstrating a fenestration of the left atrial disc. **B.** 3D color Doppler demonstrating left-to-right shunting through a fenestration within the device.

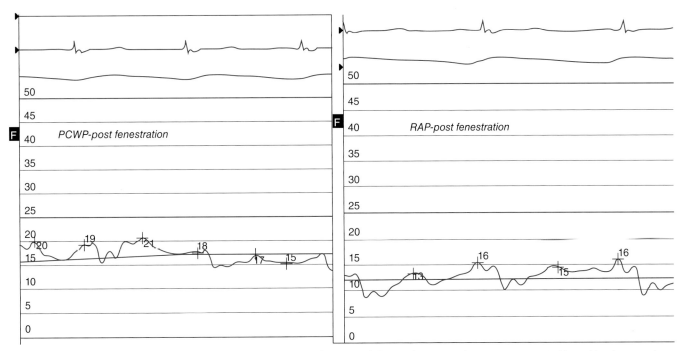

FIGURE 14-16 **A.** Pulmonary arterial capillary wedge pressure post fenestrated device placement, the mean pressure is 16 mm Hg, the wave-form is normal. **B.** Right atrial pressure postdevice deployment is lower than the estimated left atrial pressure, the RA pressure is a mean of 12 mm Hg.

Transcatheter Pulmonary Valve Replacement in an Adult with Repaired Tetralogy of Fallot

PATIENT STORY

A 28-year-old woman with tetralogy of Fallot with pulmonary atresia underwent surgical palliation with bilateral unifocalization at 3 years of age and full intracardiac repair with VSD closure and placement of an 18-mm aortic homograft in the pulmonary position. At 8 years of age she underwent excision of an RV to PA conduit false aneurysm, and replacement of the RV to PA conduit using a Hemashield graft and 23-mm aortic homograft in the pulmonary position. She had been doing well and asymptomatic until 1 year prior to intervention when she began developing dyspnea with moderate exertion and nonsustained palpitations. On physical examination, her vital signs were normal, her resting oxygen saturations were 100% on room air; she was acyanotic.

She had a well-healed midline sternotomy scar and a well-healed right thoracotomy scar. The RV impulse was palpable at the left sternal border. On cardiac examination, she had a regular, rate and rhythm. She had normal S1, S2 with widened splitting of S2. There was a 1/6 mid-systolic murmur at the left upper sternal border (LUSB), 3/4 diastolic murmur at the LUSB and left mid sternal border (LMSB), with no clicks, gallops, or rubs. Jugular venous pulsations were normal.

Her abdomen was soft, nondistended, and nontender with no hepatosplenomegaly. She had no peripheral edema with 2+ carotid, brachial, and radial pulses.

Diagnostic testing included a cardiopulmonary exercise stress test using the Bruce protocol. She went to exercise for 7 minutes and 10 seconds and achieved 7.2 METS and a maximum VO_2 of 25.2 mL/kg/min which is 72% of predicted. Her baseline electrocardiography (ECG) demonstrates sinus rhythm with a right bundle branch block, QRS duration is 160 ms. No ischemic ECG changes or arrhythmias. No desaturation with exercise. Her Holter monitor showed sinus rhythm with ventricular ectopy in singles and couplets as well as some single atrial premature complexes. The event monitor revealed frequent ventricular ectopy including couplets and bigeminy corresponding to symptoms of palpitations.

Cardiac imaging with an echocardiogram showed right ventricular enlargement with mildly reduced RV systolic function and severe pulmonic regurgitation and mild pulmonary stenosis. The peak instantaneous gradient was 18 mm Hg.

A cardiac MRI showed right ventricular dilatation with reduced systolic function and severe pulmonary regurgitation with a regurgitant fraction of 35%. She also had moderate pulmonic stenosis. The right ventricular ejection fraction (RVEF) was moderately reduced, measured at 38%, normalized end-diastolic volume indexed at 115.1 mL/m^2 (48-87), normalized end-systolic volume indexed at 69.3 mL/m^2 (11-27.6), stroke volume 45.8 mL/m^2 (27-57), cardiac index 2.84 L/min/m^2. She had a dilated right ventricular outflow tract (RVOT) measuring 22 × 17 mm and 16 mm at the pulmonic valve level. Ascending aorta was also dilated to 4.3 cm (Figure 14-17).

Based on the presence of severe pulmonary regurgitation, decreased RV systolic function, worsening exercise tolerance, and frequent ventricular ectopy, the decision was made to proceed with cardiac catheterization and transcatheter pulmonary valve replacement.

INTERVENTIONAL CARDIAC CATHETERIZATION: CASE EXPLANATION

- The patient was bought to the cardiac catheterization laboratory and placed under general anesthesia. A 5-F sheath was placed in the right femoral artery (RFA), 7-F sheath in the right femoral vein (RFV), 6-F sheath in the left femoral vein (LFV). RFV preclosed with 2 Proglide Perclose sutures. Unfractionated heparin (UFH) given for activated clotting time (ACT) is greater than 230 seconds.

- 3D MR overlay of RVOT/PA/aorta (Ao) on fluoroscopic image performed with ECG registration. Calcified RVOT patch used to "line up" the 2 images (Figure 14-18). Temporary pacing wires were placed in the RV via LFV.

- 3D rotational pulmonary angiography was performed while respirations suspended and RV paced to 180 bpm. The RFV sheath upsized to 14 F. A 22-mm Mullins-X balloon catheter advanced into the RV to PA. Serial inflations were performed with simultaneous aortography and 3D rotational angiography to rule out coronary artery compression.

- A Melody valve was prepped and mounted on a 22-mm ensemble BIB delivery system and positioned at the pulmonary annulus using 3D MR overlay to guide positioning and deployment with rapid RV pacing to minimize stent motion (Figure 14-19). No pulmonary regurgitation noted post deployment.

- The patient was discharged home within 23 hours of the procedure.

- On follow-up she noted improved functional capacity and significant reduction in palpitations.

DISCUSSION

- The long-term consequences of severe pulmonary regurgitation include irreversible right ventricular dilation, decreased right ventricular systolic function, and increased risk of ventricular and atrial arrhythmias.

- Pulmonary valve replacement is warranted in patients with severe pulmonary regurgitation who are symptomatic or functionally limited and should also be considered in patients with right ventricular dysfunction, progressive dilation, and arrhythmias.

- Adult patients with repaired tetralogy of Fallot may undergo multiple such surgical procedures throughout their lifetime and the risk of ventricular dysfunction and malignant arrhythmias progressively increases with each additional surgical procedure.[15] Over the past decade, nonsurgical transcatheter pulmonary valve replacement has become an acceptable therapeutic alternative to surgical valve replacement.

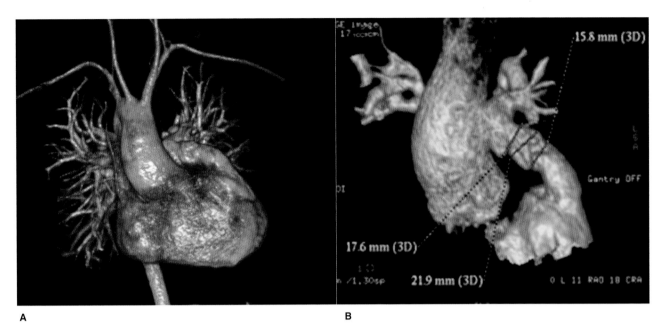

FIGURE 14-17 A. 3D volume-rendered MRA demonstrating a dilated ascending aorta and a narrowed right ventricle to pulmonary artery homograft conduit. B) 3D rendering of the aorta and the RV to PA conduit which narrows to 15.8 mm.

- Bonhoeffer and colleagues spearheaded the development of the Melody valve, a percutaneous stent-based expandable pulmonary valve using a glutaraldehyde-treated bovine jugular venous valve sewn into a covered balloon expandable stent.[16]

- Early and intermediate follow-up results are encouraging and the valve was approved by the FDA in 2010 under a Humanitarian Device Exemption.[17] The Melody valve can be placed in the circumferential right ventricle to pulmonary artery conduit, dysfunctional bioprosthetic valve or native right ventricular outflow tract if there is an adequate landing zone.[18]

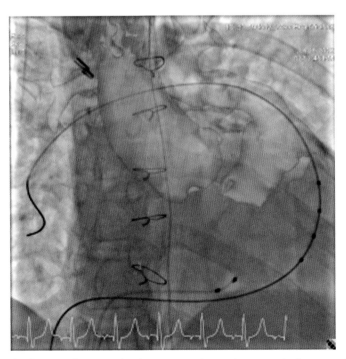

FIGURE 14-18 3D MRA overlay of RVOT, homograft, proximal pulmonary arteries, and aorta on the fluoroscopic image during balloon advancement.

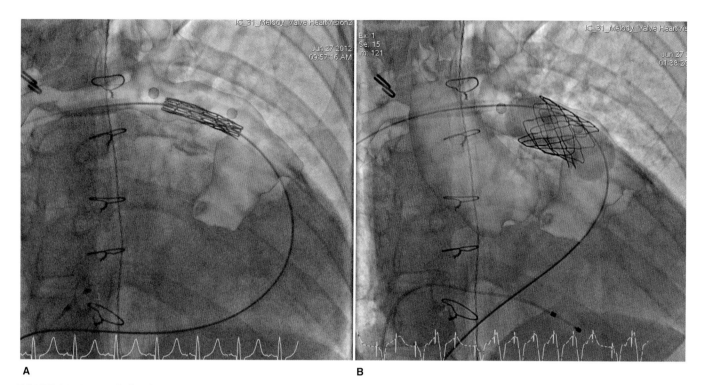

FIGURE 14-19 A. Melody valve positioning using 3D MRA overlay, markers have been placed to identify the proximal, mid, and distal locations on the conduit. **B.** Melody valve deployment with rapid pacing to stabilize the stent valve.

- Patients with native RVOT or trans-annular repair may not be candidates for Melody valve placement because the diameter of the landing zone is > 24 mm, however, the Edwards-Sapien XT 29 mm valve could potentially be used in this setting. There are investigations under way to develop self-expanding RVOT reducers that would enable transcatheter pulmonary valve replacement in such patients.

REFERENCES

1. Singer MI, Rowen M, Dorsey TJ. Transluminal aortic balloon angioplasty for coarctation of the aorta in the newborn. *Am Heart J*. 1982;103:131-132.

2. Cowley CG, Orsmond GS, Feola P, McQuillan L, Shaddy RE. Long-term, randomized comparison of balloon angioplasty and surgery for native coarctation of the aorta in childhood. *Circulation*. 2005;111:3453-3456.

3. Isner JM, Donaldson RF, Fulton D, Bhan I, Payne DD, Cleveland RJ. Cystic medial necrosis in coarctation of the aorta: a potential factor contributing to adverse consequences observed after percutaneous balloon angioplasty of coarctation sites. *Circulation*. 1987;75:689-695.

4. Johnston TA, Grifka RG, Jones TK. Endovascular stents for treatment of coarctation of the aorta: acute results and follow-up experience. *Catheter Cardiovasc Interv*. 2004;62:499-505.

5. Holzer R, Qureshi S, Ghasemi A, et al. Stenting of aortic coarctation: acute, intermediate, and long-term results of a prospective multi-institutional registry—congenital cardiovascular interventional study consortium (ccisc). *Catheter Cardiovasc Interv*. 2010;76:553-563.

6. Kutty S, Hazeem AA, Brown K, et al. Long-term (5- to 20-year) outcomes after transcatheter or surgical treatment of hemodynamically significant isolated secundum atrial septal defect. *Am J Cardiol*. 2012;109:1348-1352.

7. Abdel-Massih T, Dulac Y, Taktak A, et al. Assessment of atrial septal defect size with 3D-transesophageal echocardiography: comparison with balloon method. *Echocardiography*. 2005;22:121-127.

8. Mazic U, Gavora P, Masura J. The role of transesophageal echocardiography in transcatheter closure of secundum atrial septal defects by the amplatzer septal occluder. *Am Heart J*. 2001;142:482-488.

9. AboulHosn J, French WJ, Buljubasic N, Matthews RV, Budoff MJ, Shavelle DM. Electron beam angiography for the evaluation of percutaneous atrial septal defect closure. *Catheter Cardiovasc Interv*. 2005;65:565-568.

10. Aboulhosn J, Shavelle DM, Matthews R, French WJ, Buljubasic N, Budoff MJ. Images in cardiology: electron beam angiography of percutaneous atrial septal defect closure. *Clin Cardiol*. 2004;27:702.

11. Schneider DJ, Levi DS, Serwacki MJ, Moore SD, Moore JW. Overview of interventional pediatric cardiology in 2004. *Minerva Pediatr*. 2004;56:1-28.

12. Franke A, Kuhl HP. The role of antiplatelet agents in the management of patients receiving intracardiac closure devices. *Curr Pharm Des*. 2006;12:1287-1291.

13. Masura J, Gavora P, Podnar T. Long-term outcome of transcatheter secundum-type atrial septal defect closure using amplatzer septal occluders. *J Am Coll Cardiol*. 2005;45:505-507.

14. Kretschmar O, Sglimbea A, Corti R, Knirsch W. Shunt reduction with a fenestrated amplatzer device. *Catheter Cardiovasc Interv*. 2010;76:564 571.

15. Khairy P, Aboulhosn J, Gurvitz MZ, et al. Arrhythmia burden in adults with surgically repaired tetralogy of Fallot: a multi-institutional study. *Circulation*. 2010;122:868-875.

16. Bonhoeffer P, Khambadkone S, Coats L, et al. Percutaneous pulmonary valve implantation in humans: results in 59 consecutive patients. *Circulation*. 2005;112:1189-1197.

17. McElhinney DB, Hellenbrand WE, Zahn EM, et al. Short- and medium-term outcomes after transcatheter pulmonary valve placement in the expanded multicenter US melody valve trial. *Circulation*. 2010;122:507-516.

18. Gillespie MJ, Rome JJ, Levi DS, et al. Melody valve implant within failed bioprosthetic valves in the pulmonary position: a multicenter experience. *Circ Cardiovasc Interv*. 2012;5:862-870.

15 HEART FAILURE IN ACHD PATIENTS

John Lynn Jefferies, MD
Gary D. Webb, MD
Jeffrey A. Towbin, MD

PATIENT STORY

A 25-year-old man presented with a history of bicuspid aortic valve (BAV), moderate aortic valve stenosis, moderate aortic valve insufficiency, dilated aortic root, and left ventricular noncompaction cardiomyopathy.

He was born with BAV and severe aortic valve stenosis and underwent surgical aortic valvotomy at 2 days of age. There was recurrence of the aortic valve stenosis requiring percutaneous balloon valvuloplasty at age 1 year and again at age 2 years. He ultimately required repeat surgical valvotomy at age 4 years which also included supravalvular aortoplasty with a Gore-Tex patch. He was also noted to have short stature and developmental delay. Genetic evaluation was pursued with no definitive diagnosis being established. He has been seen in scheduled follow-up since and had done reasonably well without report of cardiovascular related symptoms until 2 years ago when he began experiencing 2 pillow orthopnea and increasing fatigue with activity. Up until this time, he was living alone and working part time in a factory.

Assessment of his symptoms at that time included an echocardiogram which revealed moderate-to-severe aortic insufficiency with preserved left ventricular ejection fraction (LVEF). However, detailed assessment of the left ventricular apex showed abnormal myocardium consistent with left ventricular noncompaction (LVNC). Diuretic therapy was instituted to manage his orthopnea. He was referred to the care of the Adult Congenital Heart Disease (ACHD) and Cardiomyopathy services for further management. He continued to have heart failure (HF) symptoms and had worsening aortic insufficiency on serial imaging studies with a decline in his LVEF. Treatment with appropriate heart failure therapies was instituted and aspirin was given for his diagnosis of LVNC. Based on his severe aortic insufficiency and worsening LV systolic function, he was referred for elective replacement of his aortic valve.

He underwent successful aortic valve replacement with a 21-mm Carpentier Edwards prosthetic valve. He did well postoperatively and was discharged to home on postoperative day 6 on his preoperative medical regimen with the substitution of Coumadin for aspirin therapy. Outpatient evaluation 1 week after discharge was significant for complete resolution of his heart failure symptoms. An echocardiogram at that time revealed improvement in his LVEF with mild systolic dysfunction (LVEF 48%) and no evidence of significant prosthetic aortic valve stenosis or insufficiency.

CASE EXPLANATION

- Many, if not all, ACHD patients are at risk of HF whether unrepaired, repaired, or palliated.

- Several of these patients may have underlying myocardial dysfunction, valvular heart disease along with exercise intolerance. Some progress to have heart failure.

- Myocardial dysfunction (right, left, or biventricular) is a common final pathway for these patients, which underscore the need for surveillance of systolic and diastolic function as well as resting and provocable HF symptoms.

- Recognition of dysfunction prior to symptoms allows for institution of appropriate medical therapies and more regimented evaluations in an attempt to avoid progression to more advanced stages of HF.

- The above patient underscores the importance of lifelong surveillance for adult congenital patients. Without appropriate ongoing evaluations, myocardial dysfunction may ensue resulting in symptoms of heart failure as well as associated morbidity and mortality.

- Management by providers familiar with heart failure and cardiomyopathy results in opportunity for timely and needed intervention to avoid adverse outcomes.

EPIDEMIOLOGY

- The diagnosis of heart failure continues to be a major cause of morbidity and mortality in children and adults worldwide. There are an estimated 5 million adults in the United States alone living with heart failure with approximately 650,000 new cases diagnosed each year.[1,2] These numbers likely are an underestimate of disease burden as they do not reflect pediatric patients or those adults surviving with palliated or repaired congenital heart disease.

- There are now over 1 million adults with congenital heart defects (CHD) in the USA. Because of these steadily increasing numbers and many have concomitant myocardial dysfunction, the number of patients developing heart failure is also on the rise. The prevalence of HF in ACHD remains poorly defined. More importantly, agreement on appropriate HF treatment strategies does not exist secondary to the heterogeneity of the population and a paucity of published data. Those ACHD subpopulations likely at highest risk of HF include single ventricle physiology, two ventricle circulations with a systemic right ventricle, and repaired tetralogy of Fallot.[3]

- The ACHD is aging secondary to increased awareness and improved care. Patients over the age of 60 with moderate or severe congenital heart defects have high mortality rates and higher utilization of health care resources with symptoms of HF, New York Heart Association (NYHA) class, and systemic ventricular dysfunction being independent predictors of outcome.[4]

- In addition, patients with genetically triggered myocardial disease would also be predisposed to HF in conjunction with congenital heart disease.[5,6]

ETIOLOGY AND PATHOPHYSIOLOGY

- Heart failure is a complex clinical syndrome that is a result of a functional or structural impairment of the ventricular filling or ejection of blood.[7] Historically, heart failure has been defined using the NYHA Functional Classification ranging from stage I (No limitations on physical activity) to stage IV (symptoms of heart failure at rest).[8]

- The diagnosis of heart failure may apply when symptoms of heart failure occur at rest or during exercise, which mainly include dyspnea, and to a lesser extent exertional fatigue, along with objective evidence of systolic and/or diastolic cardiac dysfunction. When the diagnosis is not clear, a favorable response to treatment directed toward heart failure may aid in the diagnosis.

- An alternative classification strategy has been adopted that take into account structural abnormalities as well as risk factors that place individuals at risk for heart failure (stages A-D).
  - Patients who are at risk of HF but without evidence of structural heart disease fall under stage A.
  - Those patients with evidence of structural heart disease but without HF symptoms are categorized as stage B.
  - Those patients with evidence of structural heart disease and either current or prior symptoms of HF categorized as stage C.
  - Patients with refractory HF requiring advanced interventions are categorized as stage D.

- Based on these classifications, patients with ACHD would all be classified in one of these stages with many being stage A or B.

- Heart failure is typically subcategorized by the presence of systolic dysfunction (heart failure with reduced ejection fraction or HFrEF) or absence of systolic dysfunction (heart failure with preserved ejection fraction or HFpEF).

- Our patient progressed from to stage C HF in the face of appropriate medical therapy. He had concomitant valvular disease that prompted a surgical intervention but currently remains in stage C. Many, if not all, ACHD patients are at risk of HF whether unrepaired, repaired, or palliated. Myocardial dysfunction (right, left, or biventricular) is a common final pathway for these patients, which underscores the need for surveillance of systolic and diastolic function as well resting and provocable HF symptoms.

- Recognition of dysfunction prior to symptoms allows for institution of appropriate medical therapies and more regimented evaluations in an attempt to avoid progression to more advanced stages of HF.

- Heart failure in the adult with CHD may occur for a variety of reasons some of which include primary myocardial disease, myocardial dysfunction secondary to structural heart disease, changes in function after cardiopulmonary bypass, and underlying metabolic or syndromic disease.

- Certain lesions, such as Mustard or Senning repair of d-transposition of the great arteries (TGA), congenitally corrected TGA (CC-TGA), and single ventricle circulations (cyanotic patients or patients who have had a Fontan repair), are at risk for systemic ventricular dysfunction. Other congenital heart lesions are at risk for subpulmonary ventricular dysfunction, including repaired tetralogy of Fallot with severe pulmonary regurgitation, Ebstein's anomaly, and patients with pulmonary hypertension.

- Mustard and Senning patients have a 32% to 48% rate of systemic right ventricular systolic dysfunction at 15 to 18 years of follow-up. Clinical heart failure occurs in 10% to 22% of these patients.[9-11]. Notably, the Mustard and Senning procedure were both abandoned in most centers in the 1980s in favor of the arterial switch for patients with D-TGA.

- Arterial switch patients are not particularly prone to congestive heart failure since their systemic ventricle is their left ventricle.

- Patients with CC-TGA usually have a left atrium connected to a right ventricle connected to the aorta, and a right atrium connected to a left ventricle connected to the pulmonary artery. CC-TGA patients often have systemic ventricular dysfunction. To some extent this is a function of age, but it may also be related to the development of substantial systemic tricuspid regurgitation. A group of patients with CC-TGA have associated lesions such as ventricular septal defects (VSDs) and pulmonary stenosis, and many have had corrective surgery which has left the right ventricle in the systemic position.

- Patients with functionally single ventricles are certainly prone to both systolic and diastolic ventricular dysfunction. In an adult series, the prevalence of clinical heart failure in Fontan patients was 40% 16 years after the procedure.[10] The probability of developing heart failure in patients with single ventricles, tetralogy of Fallot, D-TGA S/P Mustard patients, left-to-right shunt patients, valve disease patients, and aortic coarctation patients[3] (Figure 15-1).

- Systemic ventricular dysfunction is less likely to occur but can occur in the settings of uncorrected aortic or mitral valve disease, uncorrected aortic coarctation, or uncontrolled systemic hypertension. Ventricular dysfunction or valvular dysfunction occurs for a variety of reasons. Some ACHD patients may have or develop comorbidities that cause heart failure, such as coronary artery disease or forms of associated cardiomyopathy, such as dilated, hypertrophic, and noncompaction cardiomyopathy.

- Our patient had LVNC which is a primary cardiomyopathy characterized by trabeculations in left ventricle (Figure 15-2). Other comorbidities may precipitate heart failure and/or make it more difficult to manage, such as atrial fibrillation, hyperthyroidism, and infective endocarditis. ACHD patients with heart failure do have elevated neurohormonal markers, but to a lesser degree than heart failure patients with acquired heart disease.

- There are a group of CHD patients who have had coronary artery reimplantation. This includes patients who have had an arterial switch procedure, a valve-sparing aortic root replacement, and a Bentall procedure. These patients may develop stenoses or occlusions of these anastomoses with consequent myocardial damage, myocardial dysfunction, or angina pectoris. Optimal surveillance for asymptomatic patients who have had coronary reimplantation is controversial.

- Patients may also have valvular disease which was seen in our patient. Significant stenosis or regurgitation may lead to myocardial dysfunction as well as symptoms of HF. In the setting of a primary cardiomyopathy or additional structural heart disease, HF symptoms may present at an earlier stage of valvular dysfunction.

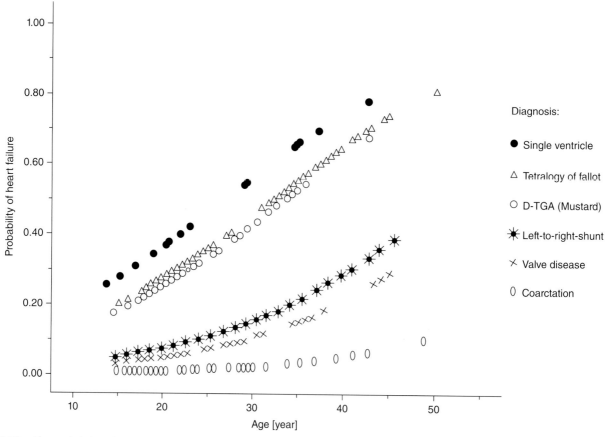

FIGURE 15-1 The probability of heart failure (HF) over age and type of heart defect.

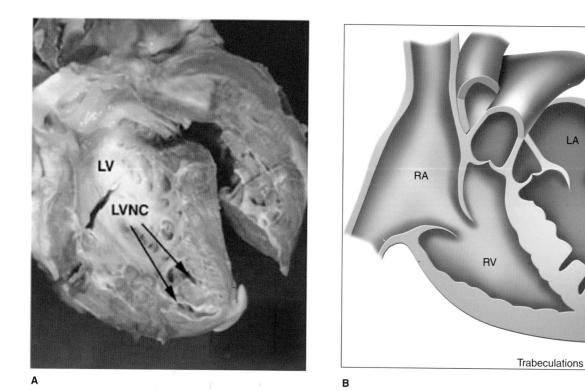

A   **B**

FIGURE 15-2 Pathology specimen of patient with left ventricular noncompaction (LVNC). Note the deep trabeculations throughout the left ventricle (LV). LA, left atrium; RA, right atrium, RV, right ventricle.

DIAGNOSIS

- The diagnosis of heart failure may be made when symptoms of heart failure including dyspnea, and to a lesser extent exertional fatigue occur at rest or during exercise and there is objective evidence of systolic and/or diastolic cardiac dysfunction by echocardiography or cardiac magnetic resonance imaging (CMRI)

- In some cases the diagnosis of heart failure may not be clear; in this case, a favorable response to treatment directed toward heart failure, can aid in the diagnosis.

- We will not discuss the issue of ventricular dysfunction in ACHD patients in the absence of heart failure symptoms, which is beyond the scope of this section.

Clinical History

- Symptoms of pulmonary venous congestion include dyspnea (exertional or at rest), orthopnea, cough, or hemoptysis. All forms of heart failure may be associated with exertional fatigue, reflecting a low-output state.

- Symptoms of systemic venous congestion include dependent edema, symptomatic hepatic congestion, and ascites.

Physical Examination

- Physical examination findings of pulmonary venous congestion include tachypnea, crackles at the lung bases or more extensively, wheezing, pleural effusions, and a third heart sound. Physical findings of systemic venous congestion include elevation of the jugular venous pressure, hepatomegaly, ascites, and dependent edema, notably including presacral edema.

DIAGNOSTIC STUDIES

ECG and Holter Monitor

- Electrocardiographic (ECG) monitoring may be useful in the detection of conduction system disease as well as significant arrhythmias. Findings may include varying degrees of heart block including bundle branch, atrial or ventricular ectopy, brady- or tachyarrhythmias, ST segment abnormalities, Q-waves indicating prior infarction, and T-wave abnormalities.

- Findings of these tests may influence ongoing management such as need for a pacemaker and/or defibrillator[5] (Figures 15-3A through 15-3G).

Radiography

- Radiographic findings offer additional information regarding cardiac size as well as pulmonary congestion. Findings may include cardiomegaly and pulmonary edema. Patients may be postoperative with ongoing chamber enlargement such as mitral valve replacement (Figures 15-4A and 15-4B) or have massive cardiomegaly such as that seen in Ebstein's anomaly (Figures 15-4C and 15-4D).

- Patients with ACHD may also have findings of device placement such as a permanent pacemaker in a young adult with TGA and intact ventricular septum following the Mustard procedure (Figures 15-4E and 15-4F). Cardiomegaly may be secondary to right ventricular enlargement such as in patients who have undergone repair of tetralogy of Fallot with pulmonary regurgitation (Figures 15-4G and 15-4H).

Echocardiography

- Echocardiography is typically used to evaluate patients with heart failure. Findings may include chamber enlargement, myocardial dysfunction (systolic, diastolic, or combination) in one or both ventricles depending on anatomy, valvular insufficiency, elevation of calculated pulmonary artery pressures, dilation of the inferior vena cava (IVC).[12]

- In patients with congenital heart disease, additional findings may be found related to the patients' primary diagnosis and previous catheter or surgical interventions (Figure 15-5).

Cardiac Catheterization

- Cardiac catheterization may be used to further evaluate hemodynamics, define anatomy, and offer potential treatment strategies such as angioplasty, stent placement, or valve replacement. In select cases, endomyocardial biopsy may also be a consideration during cardiac catheterization.[13]

- Hemodynamic findings may include elevated right atrial pressures as well as increased ventricular filling pressures. Angiography may reveal depressed systolic function in the right and/or left ventricles. Coronary angiography may also be considered based on the age and symptoms which may reveal stenosis, dilation, or congenital anomalies.

- Catheter-based assessment in adult congenital patients may require alternative approaches necessitating additional resources and expertise[14] (Figure 15-6).

Magnetic Resonance Imaging

- Cardiac magnetic resonance (CMR) imaging is an advanced imaging strategy increasingly employed in adults with heart failure as it overcomes some inherent limitations of echocardiography. Findings may include dilation of chambers, depressed myocardial function, and late gadolinium enhancement (LGE), which is a surrogate marker of fibrosis[15] (Figure 15-7A and 15-7B). CMR provides more reliable information regarding right ventricular systolic function and vascular anatomy which may be of significant importance in patients with congenital heart disease or vasculopathy.[13]

- An understanding of congenital heart disease is essential for developing appropriate sequencing strategies as well as interpreting results such as in patients with single ventricle physiology[16] (Figure 15-8). In addition, CMR is a very useful modality in patients with tetralogy of Fallot to assess for right ventricular size and function and can be used in conjunction with echocardiography to optimize patient management (Figures 15-9A through 15-9C).

Biomarkers

- A variety of biomarkers are available that have diagnostic and prognostic implications in patients with heart failure. Brain natriuretic peptide (BNP) and N-terminal are well-established markers for heart failure in the non-ACHD population.[17]

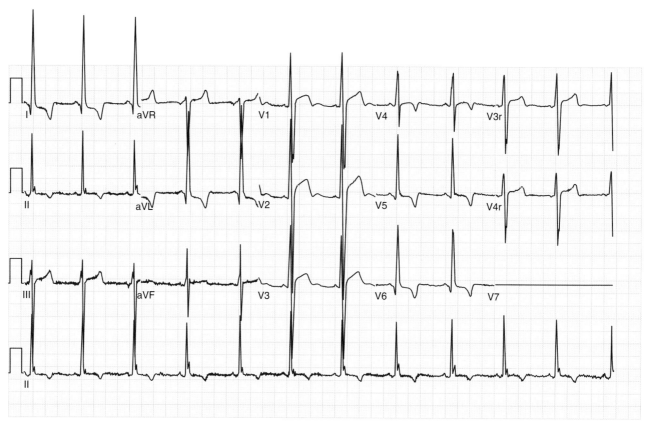

FIGURE 15-3A Electrocardiogram of a patient with left ventricular noncompaction (LVNC) revealing left ventricular hypertrophy, ST segment abnormalities, and T-wave inversion.

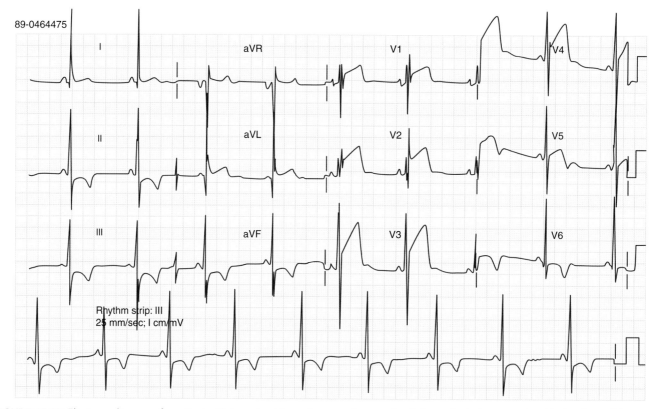

FIGURE 15-3B Electrocardiogram of a patient with hypertrophic cardiomyopathy revealing left ventricular hypertrophy with significant ST segment elevation.

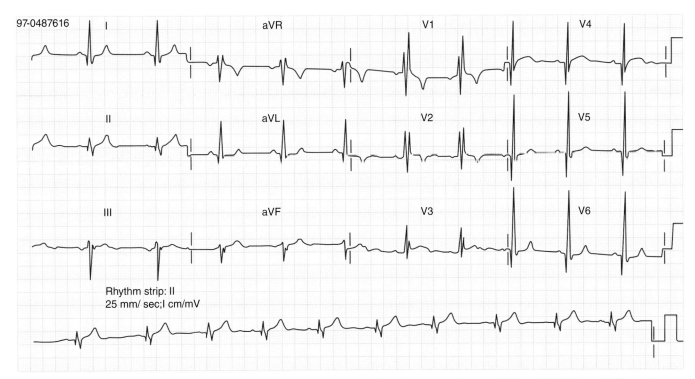

FIGURE 15-3C Electrocardiogram of patient with hypertrophic cardiomyopathy and a ventricular septal defect (VSD) following VSD repair revealing right bundle branch block.

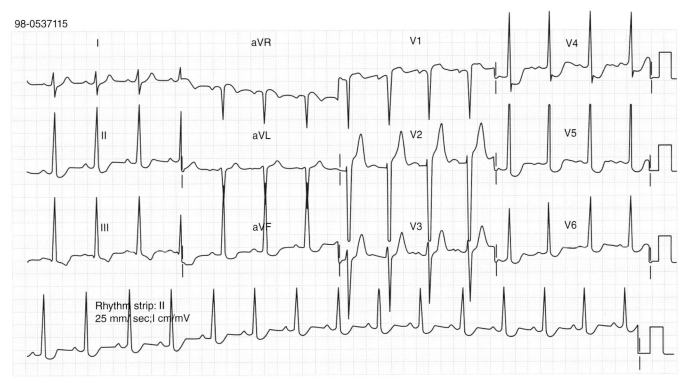

FIGURE 15-3D Electrocardiogram of a patient status aortic valve prosthesis who presented with acute prosthetic valve insufficiency revealing significant ST segment depression in the anterolateral leads.

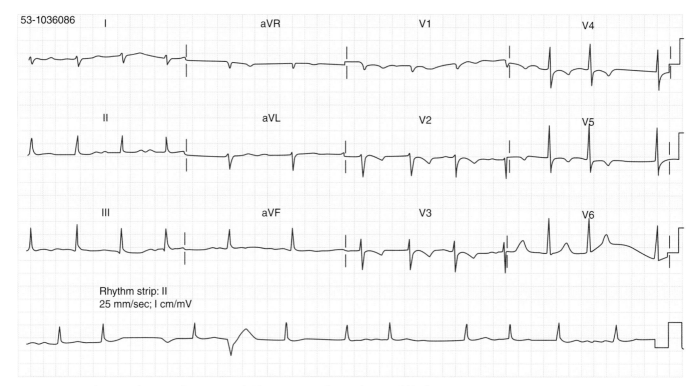

FIGURE 15-3E Electrocardiogram of a patient with Ebstein's anomaly revealing atrial fibrillation.

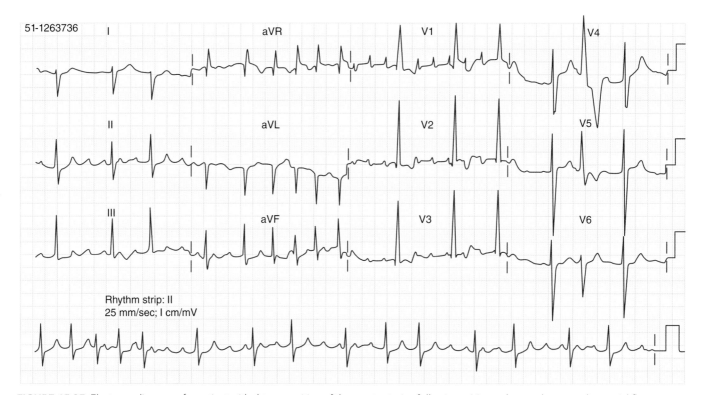

FIGURE 15-3F Electrocardiogram of a patient with d-transposition of the great arteries following a Mustard procedure revealing atrial flutter.

79-1086824

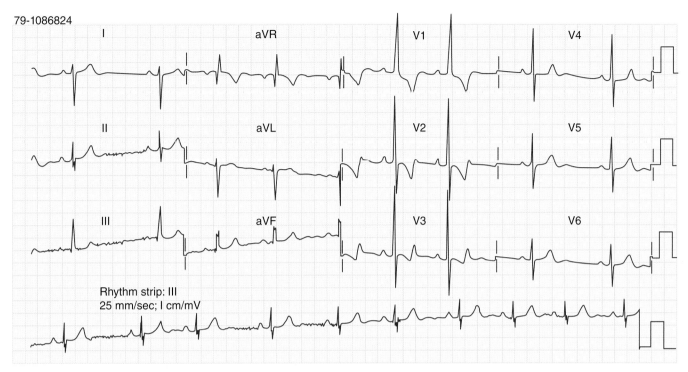

FIGURE 15-3G Electrocardiogram of a patient with unrepaired ventricular septal defect and Eisenmenger syndrome.

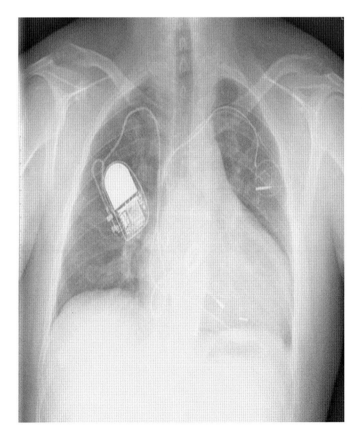

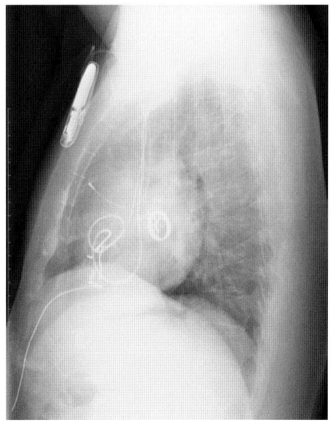

FIGURE 15-4A AND 15-4B Chest radiograph (anteroposterior [AP] and lateral) of a patient who underwent mitral valve replacement and tricuspid valve annuloplasty revealing moderate cardiomegaly with left atrial and left ventricular enlargement.

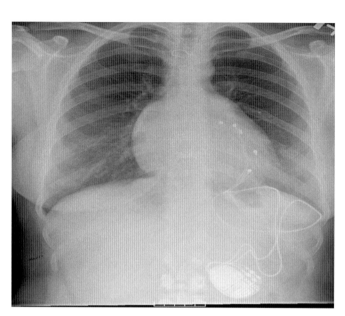
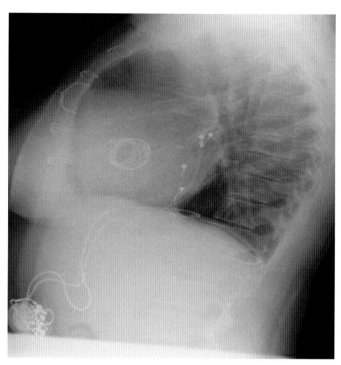

FIGURE 15-4C AND 15-4D Chest radiograph (AP and lateral) of a patient with Ebstein's anomaly revealing severe cardiomegaly.

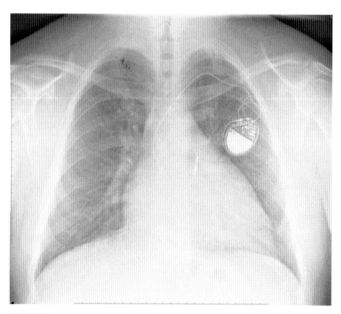
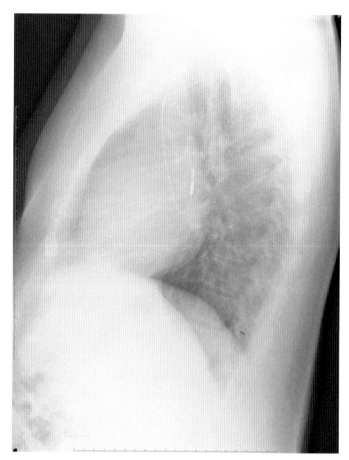

FIGURE 15-4E AND 15-4F Chest radiograph (AP and lateral) of a patient with transposition of the great arteries (TGA) and intact ventricular septum who underwent the Mustard procedure early in life and had a pacemaker placed. The pacemaker wire was introduced into the left atrium through the innominate vein, superior vena cava, and the atrial baffles.

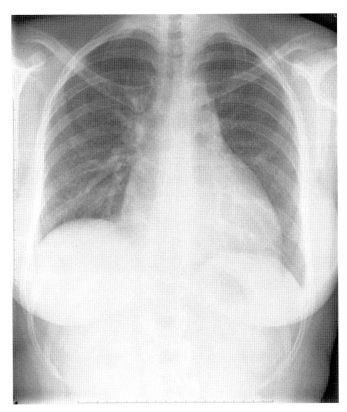

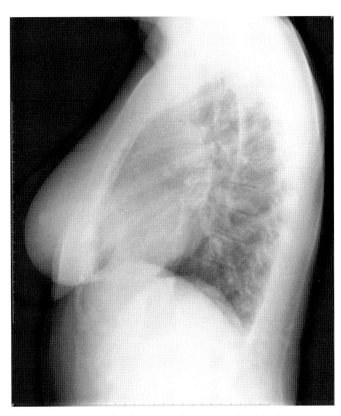

FIGURE 15-4G AND 15-4H Chest radiograph (AP and lateral) of an adult patient with tetralogy of Fallot who underwent a right Blalock-Taussig (BT) shunt early in life with subsequent complete repair which reveals moderate cardiomegaly and bulging of the pulmonary artery segment of the left heart border.

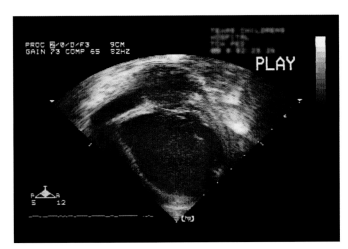

FIGURE 15-5 Apical 4-chamber view of a patient with dilated cardio-myopathy (DCM). Note the dilated left ventricular (LV) diameter and evidence of spontaneous echocardiographic contrast.

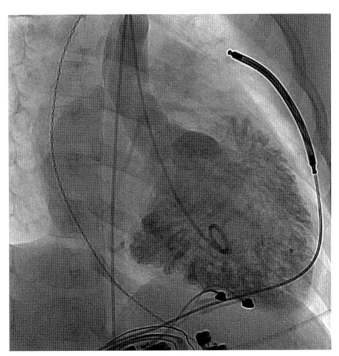

FIGURE 15-6 Left ventricular angiogram in right anterior oblique (RAO) projection revealing deep trabeculations throughout the left ventricle.

• These hormones are synthesized and released into the circulation by ventricular myocytes in response to pressure overload, volume expansion, and increase in myocardial wall stress. Whether these biomarkers might be of clinical importance in the congenital heart disease population has been speculated but some evidence exists to suggest their utility.[18]

• Eindhoven et al performed a literature review of 49 publications regarding heart failure, CHD and BNP levels and demonstrated BNP levels to be elevated in patients after correction for tetralogy of Fallot, and in patients with a systemic RV, while BNP levels correlated with RV dimension and severity of pulmonary regurgitation in patients with tetralogy of Fallot and RV function in systemic RV patients.[19] Patients with a univentricular heart had elevated BNP levels before completion of the Fontan circulation or when symptomatic, suggesting an association between BNP levels and NYHA class.

• Zaidi et al analyzed echocardiographic indices of strain and strain rate and sought to determine whether correlation existed between strain and strain rate and serum biomarkers (interleukin 6, interleukin 8, matrix metalloproteinase 9, procollagen I C-terminal peptide (PCIP), cross-linked carboxyterminal telopeptide of type 1 collagen (ICTP), pro-B-type natriuretic peptide, nitrotyrosine, tissue growth factor beta (TGF-β), tumor necrosis factor alpha (TNF-α), vascular endothelial growth factor, and creatinine (Cr) in adult patients with single ventricles and heart failure.[20] They demonstrated that pro-BNP, Cr, and ICTP had positive correlation with worsening NYHA functional class and suggested that worsening Cr and elevated pro-BNP levels could be considered a maker for poor cardiac output.

• Feng et al previously demonstrated that asymmetrical dimethylarginine (ADMA), an endogenous inhibitor of nitric oxide synthesis, has increased blood levels in experimental heart failure.[21]

• Kielstein et al was the first to show an association between high ADMA levels and heart failure in humans and more recent studies demonstrated that ADMA correlates with disease severity and independently predicts adverse clinical events in heart failure, as well as correlating with parameters of impaired exercise capacity and reduced ventilatory capacity.[22]

• Tutarel et al evaluated ADMA as a biomarker in the assessment of NYHA class for estimation of maximum exercise capacity in adults with congenital heart disease and compared it to NT-pro-BNP in 94 adults with congenital heart disease.[23] In this study, which included patients with D-TGA after Mustard and CC-TGA, tetralogy of Fallot, coarctation of the aorta, atrial or ventricular septal defect, atrioventricular septal defect, congenital aortic or pulmonary valve stenosis, and single ventricle physiology, showed that ADMA increased in correlation with NYHA class while, in contrast, NT-pro-BNP could not differentiate between the NYHA classes.

• The etiology of HF symptoms can be typically be ascertained as described above. However, alternative causes should be considered when caring for ACHD patients.

• Primary genetic causes of myocardial dysfunction may be in the differential requiring consideration of genetic evaluation. In addition, other end-organ dysfunction must be considered when caring for patients with ACHD. Kidney dysfunction may contribute to myocardial dysfunction as well as systemic disease.[24]

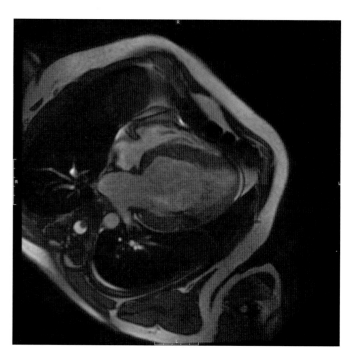

FIGURE 15-7A Magnetic resonance imaging (MRI) of a patient with left ventricular noncompaction (LVNC).

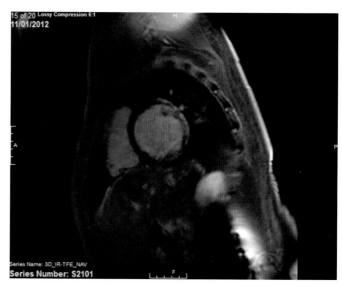

FIGURE 15-7B MRI with extensive late gadolinium enhancement (LGE) in the same patient of Figure 15-7A with LVNC.

Appropriate management of the cardiorenal syndrome may have important effects on ventricular systolic and diastolic function.[25]

- Cirrhotic disease may also lead to secondary myocardial dysfunction and HF symptoms.[26]

MANAGEMENT

Medical Management

- Keys to the successful treatment of congestive heart failure in ACHD patients include the ability to treat both the cause and the precipitating factors that have contributed to the development of heart failure.

- Clinical trials in adult heart failure patients with acquired or genetically triggered heart disease have demonstrated the efficacy of angiotensin-converting enzyme (ACE) inhibitors, aldosterone antagonists, angiotensin receptor blockers (ARBs), and in some cases, digoxin. Loop diuretics are frequently beneficial to aid in symptom control but do not favorably impact outcome. Beta-blockers have also been demonstrated to improved survival and reduce sudden death in chronic heart failure patients due to acquired heart disease.[7]

- The applicability of these adult heart failure guidelines to ACHD patients with heart failure may be limited but is often used in the absence of better options. It may be reasonable to believe that a failing systemic left ventricle may be appropriately treated using the adult heart failure guidelines, but that these guidelines may not apply to patients with a failing systemic right ventricle or single ventricle.[27]

- As noted, the appropriate surveillance of BNP and other biomarkers is not well defined in this patient population. It goes without saying that the prevention of heart failure is superior to simply treating it once it develops. Accordingly, the prevention or treatment of high blood pressure, diabetes, obesity, obstructive sleep apnea, dyslipidemia, and other conditions should be encouraged.[7]

- The role of cardiac resynchronization therapy is also poorly defined and controversial in these patients. One is left to use guidelines derived from patients with acquired heart disease and apply them as wisely as possible. Implantable cardioverter-defibrillators (ICDs) have a definite role in both primary and secondary prevention of sudden death in ACHD patients with risk factors including clinical heart failure and substantial ventricular dysfunction. ACHD patients may have a higher rate of inappropriate shocks than patients with acquired heart disease.[28]

Surgical Management

- ACHD patients with refractory heart failure may be candidates for heart transplantation, heart-lung transplantation, mechanical circulatory assist devices, and total artificial heart (TAH) therapy if other therapies do not suffice.[29] However, there are only limited reported data.

- The use of left ventricular assist devices (LVADs) in ACHD has been reported using a variety of devices including the HeartMate XVE, HeartMate II, Jarvik 2000, and HeartWare devices as a bridge to transplant as well as destination therapy.[30]

- However, current practice of ACHD management does not typically employ use of LVAD therapy as a bridge to transplant which may contribute to lower listing status while awaiting a transplant

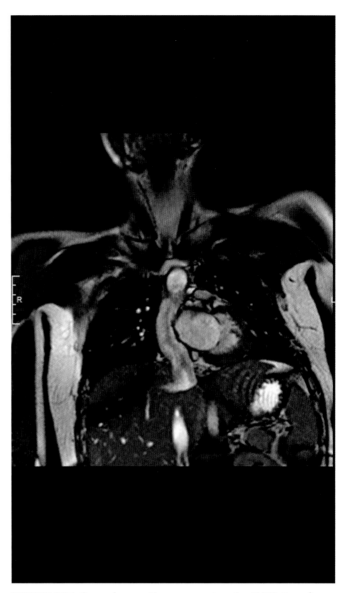

FIGURE 15-8 Coronal magnetic resonance imaging (MRI) view of a patient with a lateral tunnel Fontan.

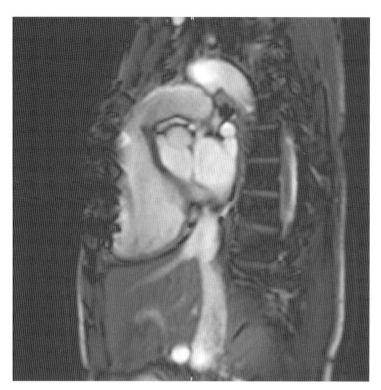

FIGURE 15-9A Magnetic resonance imaging (MRI) of a patient with tetralogy of Fallot following placement of a 22-mm RV to PA conduit earlier in life revealing right ventricular dilation and hypertrophy with depressed systolic function with both stenosis and insufficiency of the conduit.

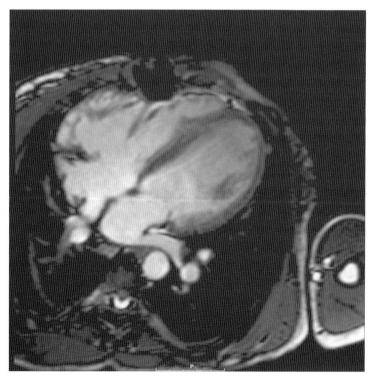

FIGURE 15-9B MRI of the same patient in Figure 15-9A (4-chamber view) revealing dilation of the right ventricle.

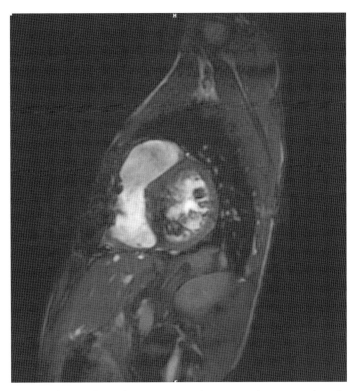

FIGURE 15-9C MRI of a patient with tetralogy of Fallot who underwent transannular repair and most recently underwent placement of a perimount valve in the pulmonary position revealing a severely dilated right ventricle with severe systolic dysfunction and dilation of the main pulmonary artery segment.

and impact organ allocation.[31] Recently, the use of mechanical circulatory support technology is increasing and transplant outcomes appear to be similar to that of the non-ACHD population.[32] Given the complexities of many palliated ACHD patients, VAD technology may not be a viable strategy. Use of TAH support has recently been used in a 17-year-old adolescent boy with congenitally corrected transposition of the great arteries as a bridge to transplant. This may offer an additional option to ACHD patients in the future.[33]

- In addition, surgical interventions should be considered for appropriate cases in an effort to improve myocardial dysfunction if a primary cause, such as valvular disease as seen in our case, can be identified.

FOLLOW-UP

- Longitudinal evaluations are warranted for careful assessment of symptoms and functional class, initiation and uptitration of appropriate medical therapies, and surveillance of the cardiovascular system and end-organ function.

- The clinical requirements for appropriate care of ACHD patients with heart failure are complex and everchanging. This often necessitates a multidisciplinary approach including cardiologists and cardiac surgeons as well as other subspecialists.

Outpatient Evaluations

- Regular surveillance is critical in the longitudinal care of HF patients. Careful attention to changes in functional capacity and medication compliance impact outcome and offer opportunities for intervention. This often requires a multidisciplinary approach given the multiple needs of the ACHD population.

Arrhythmia Surveillance

- Ongoing surveillance for arrhythmias is recommended given the potential for fatal brady- and/or tachyarrhythmias in this population. Findings on surveillance may offer insight into need for long-term pacing or sudden cardiac death protection in the form of an ICD.[34]

Cardiopulmonary Testing

- Cardiopulmonary exercise testing (CPET) has a variety of uses in the long-term care of ACHD patients. Results may inform clinicians on clinical management, capacity regarding daily activity, and sports participation.[35]

- CPET may offer prognostic information and help identify those patients at risk for sudden cardiac death (SCD).[36]

Cardiac Catheterization

- The need for cardiac catheterization may offer opportunities to better characterize hemodynamics and drive medical therapy, especially in those patients with evidence of pulmonary hypertension.

- Cardiac catheterization also offers an opportunity for intervention. The risk of catheterization in ACHD patients, although not negligible, appears to be safer than in children with congenital heart disease when performed at children's hospitals.[37]

End-Organ Surveillance

- Attention to end-organ function is important given the potential for dysfunction secondary to HF. In addition, function may be further compromised in those patients with single ventricle physiology. Referral to appropriate subspecialty care should be considered if end-organ dysfunction is present.

Noninvasive Imaging

- Longitudinal imaging is indicated in ACHD patients with HF to assess for worsening myocardial function, chamber dilation, valvar dysfunction, and myocardial thickening in addition to assessment of palliation or repair of previous congenital lesions including conduits and prosthetic valves.

- This may include echocardiography or cardiac MRI based on clinical need and acoustic windows. For those patients with devices precluding MRI and poor echocardiographic windows, computerized tomography may be considered but radiation exposure must be monitored. Nuclear imaging may be used to assess those patients with concern of coronary artery disease.

Metabolic and Neurologic Testing

- Assessment of metabolic function may be important in ACHD patients. Mitochondrial disease may be present and responsible for structural and myocardial disease. In addition, complex CHD patients often have abnormal skeletal muscle mass and function which may impact exercise capacity.[38]

Genetic Testing

- Genetic etiologies of structural heart disease are increasingly recognized in patients with ACHD.[39] The identification of a pathologic mutation may be of importance in ongoing end-organ surveillance as well as screening of at-risk first-degree family members.

- As above, consideration of primary cardiomyopathy testing may also be considered as congenital heart disease and primary cardiomyopathy disease may coexist.

Psychosocial Surveillance

- Complete care of HF patients must also consider the possibility of psychological diagnoses which may necessitate treatment.[40] There are well-recognized social and insurance issues with ACHD populations which may only be compounded in the setting of HF.[41]

CONCLUSION

- Heart failure is a significant concern in the ACHD population. Given the increasing number of ACHD survivors, the impact of heart failure in this population will only continue to become more important. A thoughtful approach to heart failure in ACHD is required given the multiple etiologies that may be responsible for myocardial dysfunction.

- A team of providers with expertise in ACHD, heart failure and cardiomyopathy, electrophysiology, cardiac catheterization, and cardiovascular surgery is required to deliver optimal care to this growing population.

- Additional study of distinct ACHD populations and therapeutic strategies is needed to effectively manage heart failure in this unique group of patients.

Patient and Provider Resources

- Adult Congenital Heart Association (ACHA): www.achaheart.org
- American Heart Association: www.heart.org

REFERENCES

1. Go AS, Mozaffarian D, Roger VL, et al. Heart disease and stroke statistics—2013 update: a report from the American Heart Association. *Circulation*. 2013;127:e6-e245.

2. Roger VL, Weston SA, Redfield MM, et al. Trends in heart failure incidence and survival in a community-based population. *JAMA*. 2004;292:344-350.

3. Norozi K, Wessel A, Alpers V, et al. Incidence and risk distribution of heart failure in adolescents and adults with congenital heart disease after cardiac surgery. *Am J Cardiol*. 2006;97:1238-1243.

4. Tutarel O, Kempny A, Alonso-Gonzalez R, et al. Congenital heart disease beyond the age of 60: emergence of a new population with high resource utilization, high morbidity, and high mortality. *Eur Heart J*. 2014;35:725-732.

5. Jefferies JL, Towbin JA. Dilated cardiomyopathy. *Lancet*. 2010;375:752-762.

6. Towbin JA. Left ventricular noncompaction: a new form of heart failure. *Heart Fail Clin*. 2010;6:453-469, viii.

7. Yancy CW, Jessup M, Bozkurt B, et al. 2013 ACCF/AHA guideline for the management of heart failure: a report of the American College of Cardiology Foundation/American Heart Association Task Force on practice guidelines. *Circulation*. 2013;128:1810-1852.

8. Hunt SA, Abraham WT, Chin MH, et al. ACC/AHA 2005 guideline update for the diagnosis and management of chronic heart failure in the adult: a report of the American College of Cardiology/American Heart Association Task Force on practice guidelines (writing committee to update the 2001 guidelines for the evaluation and management of heart failure): developed in collaboration with the American College of Chest Physicians and the International Society for Heart and Lung Transplantation: endorsed by the Heart Rhythm Society. *Circulation.* 2005;112:e154-e235.

9. Puley G, Siu S, Connelly M, et al. Arrhythmia and survival in patients >18 years of age after the Mustard procedure for complete transposition of the great arteries. *Am J Cardiol.* 1999;83:1080-1084.

10. Piran S, Veldtman G, Siu S, Webb GD, Liu PP. Heart failure and ventricular dysfunction in patients with single or systemic right ventricles. *Circulation.* 2002;105:1189-1194.

11. Kirjavainen M, Happonen JM, Louhimo I. Late results of Senning operation. *J Thorac Cardiovasc Surg.* 1999;117:488-495.

12. American College of Cardiology Foundation Appropriate Use Criteria Task Force, American Society of Ethnocardiography, American Heart Association, et al. ACCF/ASE/AHA/ASNC/HFSA/HRS/SCAI/SCCM/SCCT/SCMR 2011 appropriate use criteria for echocardiography. A report of the American College of Cardiology Foundation Appropriate Use Criteria Task Force, American Society of Echocardiography, American Heart Association, American Society of Nuclear Cardiology, Heart Failure Society of America, Heart Rhythm Society, Society for Cardiovascular Angiography and Interventions, Society of Critical Care Medicine, Society of Cardiovascular Computed Tomography, and Society for Cardiovascular Magnetic Resonance Endorsed by the American College of Chest Physicians. *J Am Coll Cardiol.* 2011;57:1126-1166.

13. Patel MR, Bailey SR, Bonow RO, et al. ACCF/SCAI/AATS/AHA/ASE/ASNC/HFSA/HRS/SCCM/SCCT/SCMR/STS 2012 appropriate use criteria for diagnostic catheterization: a report of the American College of Cardiology Foundation Appropriate Use Criteria Task Force, Society for Cardiovascular Angiography and Interventions, American Association for Thoracic Surgery, American Heart Association, American Society of Echocardiography, American Society of Nuclear Cardiology, Heart Failure Society of America, Heart Rhythm Society, Society of Critical Care Medicine, Society of Cardiovascular Computed Tomography, Society for Cardiovascular Magnetic Resonance, and Society of Thoracic Surgeons. *J Am Coll Cardiol.* 2012;59:1995-2027.

14. Latson L, Jr., Levsky JM, Haramati LB. Adult congenital heart disease: a practical approach. *J Thorac Imaging.* 2013;28:332-346.

15. Chatterjee K. Is detection of hibernating myocardium necessary in deciding revascularization in systolic heart failure? *Am J Cardiol.* 2010;106:236-242.

16. Marcotte F, Poirier N, Pressacco J, et al. Evaluation of adult congenital heart disease by cardiac magnetic resonance imaging. *Congenit Heart Dis.* 2009;4:216-230.

17. Chowdhury P, Kehl D, Choudhary R, Maisel A. The use of biomarkers in the patient with heart failure. *Curr Cardiol Rep.* 2013;15:372.

18. Alonso-Gonzalez R, Dimopoulos K. Biomarkers in congenital heart disease: do natriuretic peptides hold the key? *Expert Rev Cardiovas Ther.* 2013;11:773-784.

19. Eindhoven JA, van den Bosch AE, Jansen PR, Boersma E, Roos-Hesselink JW. The usefulness of brain natriuretic peptide in complex congenital heart disease: a systematic review. *J Am Coll Cardiol.* 2012;60:2140-2149.

20. Zaidi AN, White L, Holt R, et al. Correlation of serum biomarkers in adults with single ventricles with strain and strain rate using 2D speckle tracking. *Congenit Heart Dis.* 2013;8:255-265.

21. Feng Q, Lu X, Fortin AJ, et al. Elevation of an endogenous inhibitor of nitric oxide synthesis in experimental congestive heart failure. *Cardiovas Res.* 1998;37:667-675.

22. Kielstein JT, Bode-Boger SM, Klein G, Graf S, Haller H, Fliser D. Endogenous nitric oxide synthase inhibitors and renal perfusion in patients with heart failure. *Eur J Clin Invest.* 2003;33:370-375.

23. Tutarel O, Denecke A, Bode-Boger SM, et al. Asymmetrical dimethylarginine—more sensitive than NT-proBNP to diagnose heart failure in adults with congenital heart disease. *PloS One.* 2012;7:e33795.

24. Ronco C, Haapio M, House AA, Anavekar N, Bellomo R. Cardiorenal syndrome. *J Am Coll Cardiol.* 2008;52:1527-1539.

25. Jefferies JL, Goldstein SL. Cardiorenal [corrected] syndrome: an emerging problem in pediatric critical care. *Pediatr Nephrol.* 2013;28:855-862.

26. Zardi EM, Abbate A, Zardi DM, et al. Cirrhotic cardiomyopathy. *J Am Coll Cardiol.* 201;56:539-549.

27. Shaddy RE, Boucek MM, Hsu DT, et al. Carvedilol for children and adolescents with heart failure: a randomized controlled trial. *JAMA.* 2007;298:1171-1179.

28. Yap SC, Roos-Hesselink JW, Hoendermis ES, et al. Outcome of implantable cardioverter defibrillators in adults with congenital heart disease: a multi-centre study. *Eur Heart J.* 2007;28:1854-1861.

29. Jefferies JL, Morales DL. Mechanical circulatory support in children: bridge to transplant versus recovery. *Curr Heart Fail Rep.* 2012;9:236-243.

30. Shah NR, Lam WW, Rodriguez FH, 3rd, et al. Clinical outcomes after ventricular assist device implantation in adults with complex congenital heart disease. *J Heart Lung Transplant.* 2013;32:615-620.

31. Gelow JM, Song HK, Weiss JB, Mudd JO, Broberg CS. Organ allocation in adults with congenital heart disease listed for heart transplant: impact of ventricular assist devices. *J Heart Lung Transplant.* 2013;32:1059-1064.

32. Maxwell BG, Wong JK, Sheikh AY, Lee PH, Lobato RL. Heart transplantation with or without prior mechanical circulatory support in adults with congenital heart disease. *Eur J Cardiothorac Surg.* 2014;45:842-846.

33. Morales DL, Khan MS, Gottlieb EA, Krishnamurthy R, Dreyer WJ, Adachi I. Implantation of total artificial heart in congenital heart disease. *Semin Thorac Cardiovasc Surg.* 2012;24:142-143.

34. Perry JC. Sudden cardiac death and malignant arrhythmias: the scope of the problem in adult congenital heart patients. *Pediatr Cardiol.* 2012;33:484-490.

35. Kempny A, Dimopoulos K, Uebing A, et al. Reference values for exercise limitations among adults with congenital heart disease. Relation to activities of daily life—single centre experience and review of published data. *Eur Heart J.* 2012;33:1386-1396.

36. Diller GP, Dimopoulos K, Okonko D, et al. Heart rate response during exercise predicts survival in adults with congenital heart disease. *J Am Coll Cardiol.* 2006;48:1250-1256.

37. Learn CP, Holzer RJ, Daniels CJ, et al. Adverse events rates and risk factors in adults undergoing cardiac catheterization at pediatric hospitals—results from the C3PO. *Catheter Cardiovasc Interv.* 2013;81:997-1005.

38. Cordina R, O'Meagher S, Gould H, et al. Skeletal muscle abnormalities and exercise capacity in adults with a Fontan circulation. *Heart.* 2013;99:1530-1534.

39. Fahed AC, Gelb BD, Seidman JG, Seidman CE. Genetics of congenital heart disease: the glass half empty. *Circ Res.* 2013;112:707-720.

40. Norozi K, Zoege M, Buchhorn R, Wessel A, Geyer S. The influence of congenital heart disease on psychological conditions in adolescents and adults after corrective surgery. *Congenit Heart Dis.* 2006;1:282-288.

41. Enomoto J, Nakazawa J, Mizuno Y, Shirai T, Ogawa J, Niwa K. Psychosocial factors influencing mental health in adults with congenital heart disease. *Circ J.* 2013;77:749-755.

Note: Page numbers followed by *f* or *t* indicate figures or tables, respectively.